THE SPIRIT OF HOMOEOPATHY

by

RAJAN SANKARAN

**With a foreword by
Dr. Jost Künzli von Fimmelsberg, M.D.**

HOMOEOPATHIC MEDICAL PUBLISHERS
20, Station Road, Santa Cruz (W), Mumbai - 400 054

Printed in India

First Edition   : **1991**

Second Edition   : **1992**

reprint April 1997

reprint January 1998

Third Edition   : **1999**

reprint August 2000

reprint December 2001

reprint November 2002

ISBN-81-900810-0-4

Cover page design

Mr. T. Chatterjee

Printed in India at

Vakil & Sons Pvt. Ltd.,

Industry Manor, Appasaheb Marathe Marg,

Prabhadevi, Mumbai 400 025.

Published by

HOMOEOPATHIC MEDICAL PUBLISHERS

20, Station Road, Santa Cruz (W), Mumbai - 400 054, INDIA

spirit@vsnl.com, www.spiritofhomoeopathy.com

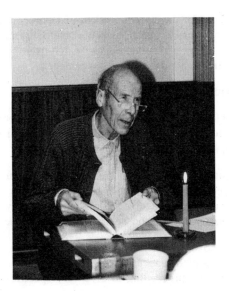

Jost Künzli von Fimmelsberg

FOREWORD

Dr. Sankaran presents us a very original work. But some points will evoke discussion. What I like most in the book are his cases, how he arrives at the solution, his intellectual work, his detective-like way, and his phenomenal knowledge of his repertories. All this together is the true classical way, as Hahnemann gave it to us. There is no place for routine, for laziness, for fixed ideas. Needed are an open mind, sharp intellectual thinking, very acute sense of observation, – and a good memory. As long as Homoeopathy is practised in this way, a golden future is her assured.

St. Gallen, March 24th, 1991

Jost Künzli von Fimmelsberg

PREFACE

This book is meant for the serious student of Homoeopathy and for those who sincerely want to find answers to questions about health, disease and cure. It does not promise solutions, but it does present an honest search over the past several years and contains some observations and ideas from my practice.

The book is divided into four sections.

The first section looks at what disease is. It examines the origine and the dynamics of disease. We shall look at Nature's law of cure and, from this, the evolution of homoeopathic thought and its application in practice.

In the second section I shall focus upon a much talked about, yet still nebulous area in Homoeopathy, namely the understanding of the mental state of the patient. We shall trace my journey to the understanding of delusions and ultimately to the understanding of the mental state as a whole. In this section we shall also examine the body-mind connection.

The third section covers the artistic aspect of Homoeopathy, namely, case taking or the process of understanding the patient. In this section I shall once again emphasize the philosophical aspect before proceeding to give very specific and detailed hints and techniques.

In the final section I shall be laying the foundation for a new way of understanding remedies, and shall present some remedies as examples.

Interwoven into these sections are thoughts on various practical questions such as the importance of pathology, remedy relationship, homoeopathic prognosis and a homoeopathic method of psychotherapy.

Each chapter is illustrated with several clinical cases and also some models for better understanding. I have included as the first chapter the fundamental principles of Homoeopathy ans also kept the language simple so that even the beginner may follow.

The second chapter, namely "The story of this book", is a bird's eye-view of the whole book.

I believe that the aim of the teacher is only to stimulate the teacher within each of us. If this book stimulates you to observe and think, it would have more than fulfilled its purpose.

1st March, 1991, Mumbai

Rajan Sankaran

PREFACE TO THE SECOND EDITION

The last one year has been a time of growth personally and also in my understanding of Homoeopathy. However, I have decided to let this book stay as it is since it represents my first steps in Homoeopathy. I have taken the opportunity to go over the whole book, make some subtle changes, correct the errors, provide a remedy index and also give a better finish to it. I am satisfied that the book is a true reflection of my thoughts on Homoeopathy.

1st August, 1992, Mumbai

Rajan Sankaran

ACKNOWLEDGEMENTS

First and foremost, I must acknowledge with gratitude the guidance and encouragement given to me by my teachers whose wisdom and example continue to inspire me to this day.

I also wish to record my deep sense of gratitude to all my friends and colleagues who have helped me in my preparations for the seminars and in writing this book.

Dr. Jayesh Shah has been my collaborator, who has given me tremendous professional and personal support right from the day we started practice.

Mr. S.M. Gunavante has always encouraged me from the day I started teaching, like a foster parent. He has contributed much to this book.

The trust reposed on me by my friends in England, Dr. Hansjörg Hee of Switzerland and Dr. Kees Dam of Holland has been of great value.

Dr. Nandita Shah has been a good friend. She has also helped me much in tracing and arranging the notes written by me over the last three years, and getting them ready for this book.

Dr. Divya Chhabra and Dr. Prasad Shetye have to put into words my new ideas as they were being formed.

Dr. Sadhana Thakkar gave me considerable support both in writing this book and in managing my clinic.

Dr. Petra Fuchs helped to create an atmosphere in which several new ideas could come up, and then she helped me to shape and organize them.

Ms. Lucinda Dyer performed the skillful job of converting my lecture notes into a form suitable for a book, improving the language at the same time. The last lot of manuscripts was corrected by Ms. Karen Sage.

Dr. Jost Künzli, whom I hold in the highest esteem, has done me the honor of writing the foreword. Dr. Künzli passed away on 5th April 1992.

Last but not least, I take this opportunity to thank my mother who has supported me in all endeavours.

CONTENTS

Tragedy... has been... said by Aristote to be a power, by raising pity, and fear, or terror, to purge the mind of those and such like passions; that is, to temper and reduce them to just measure, with a kind of delight, stirred up by reading or seeing those passions well imitated. Nor is Nature wanting in her own effects to make good his assertion, for so in physic, things of melancholic hue and quality are used against melancholy, sour against sour, salt to remove salt humours.

John Milton (1608-74)
In his introduction to *Samson Agonistes*

Part I

Philosophy

1

WHAT IS HOMOEOPATHY

Homoeopathy is a system of medicine founded by the celebrated physician Dr. Samuel Hahnemann (1755-1843) of Germany. It is based on the principle that "like cures like". In practice, this means that a medicine capable of producing certain effects when taken by a healthy human being is capable of curing any illness that displays similar effects.

Like cures likes

For example, if a healthy person takes a dose of Arsenic, he will develop vomiting, diarrhoea of rice-water stools, a rapid pulse and prostration. His skin will become cold and his expression anxious. In smaller doses or when taken for a longer time, he will develop a running nose, heavy head, cough and bronchial catarrh. Even later there will be specific disturbances of skin and nerves. He will have burning all over which is relieved by warmth, frequent thirst for sips of water, fear of death, restlessness and a worsening of symptoms at noon and midnight.

According to the homeopathic law that "like cures like", countless patients displaying such symptoms have been cured by *Arsenicum*, irrespective of the name of the disease (cholera, colds, eczema, asthma, etc.). This principle has also been mentioned by the ancient Indian poet Kavi-Kalidasa:

Shruyate hi pura loke, vishaya visham aushadam.

Translated, this read: "It has been said of old time in the world that poison is the remedy for poison." Hippocrates postulated this principle in the words: "*Similia similibus curentur*" (likes are cured by likes).

The practice of Homoeopathy is based on certain fundamental principles. Firstly, the remedies that are used are tested on human volunteers (provers) to elicit the symptoms they can produce. The symptoms of each remedy as experienced by the provers are recorded in exact detail and they form the homoeopathic Materia Medica. The symptoms of the patient are matched with the symptoms of the various remedies in the Materia Medica to find out the single remedy whose symptoms are most similar to those of the patient (like cures like).

Potentization

Hahnemann's scientific experiments led him to the process of potentization. A step by step dilution and jerking of the drug makes it extremely powerful and at the same time renders it harmless. This is in direct contrast to the toxic drugs of modern medicine, and their "side-effects".

Potencies employed by the homoeopath are from mother tincture to the 100 000th potencies. The 6th potency will have roughly a dilution of one drop of the original drug substance diluted in a lake full of water. Each potency is 100 times more dilute than the previous one. Imagine the 1 000 000th dilution!

No one has been able to satisfactorily explain how medicines can act when diluted to such fantastic limits. Yet, potencies are found to act very powerfully. It seems that in the process of potentization, stored up energy of the drug is liberated.

The healer within

The practice of Homoeopathy convinces the physician to regard the body as more than a sum of its parts. Unlike a machine, it develops, carries on its function and repairs itself independently. In this sense, everyone carries within himself his own doctor. Ancient physicians were familiar with is natural power of the organism to control disease and they invented for it a beautiful expression: "*Vis medicatrix naturae*" (healing power of nature). This healing power is a function of the life force itself. Hahnemann called it the vital force. Disease is a disturbance of this force. Out of ten people who get wet in the rain, only one gets pneumonia. Most bacteria can affect us only when our own healing power or resistance is low. By removing the bacteria (by antibiotics, etc.) we are doing nothing to correct this lack of resistance. Homoeopathic medicine aims at correcting the disturbed vital force and thus enhances the power of the body to heal itself. It does not aim at removing the symptoms of the parts affected, but treats the cause and restores health. According to Homoeopathy, symptoms are a reflection of the disturbed vital force.

Sickness is like a sitar whose correct tuning has been disturbed. Naturally, all the notes from such a sitar will be far from melodious. There is no use in trying to correct the individual notes. It is the disturbance in tuning itself which has to be corrected.

Treating man as a whole

Another fundamental principle of Homoeopathy is that it treats the patient as a whole and as an individual. There is no medicine for any particular disease, but there is a medicine for the patient suffering from the disease. "The individual, not the disease, is the entity", said the celebrated Sir William Osler. The homoeopath takes into consideration all the symptoms that distinguish a person as an individual. Even a salesman of readymade clothes must try to fit the readymade suit according to the measurements of each individual. The homoeopath thus enquires into the details of the patient's past and family history, his appetite, thirst, bowel habits, sleep, etc., and most important of all, he asks about his temperament.

It is being increasingly acknowledged these days that the mind and body are interlinked. We now see the rapid rise of the holistic concept of disease with an emphasis on the psychosomatic aspect. Hahnemann recognized it long ago, and stressed that bodily and mental symptoms are to be taken together to form the portrait of disease. The homoeopathic Materia Medica is rich in mental symptoms and we especially use these in selecting the remedy.

The present problem of the patient is not usually an isolated occurrence. It is part of a sequence. The family history and the events during childhood are taken into account as Homoeopathy treats not only the present symptoms, but the entire sequence, thereby preventing the progress of disease. Children under homoeopathic treatment grow into more healthy adults, as they find relief from the scourge of bad inheritance as well.

It has been said that the child is father of man. Thus, even in an infant, we can perceive the beginnings of future illnesses. The infant may perspire so much about its head during sleep as to soak its pillow. Perhaps the fontanelles are slow in closing. The child may be slow in walking and teething and also develop the habit of eating mud and chalk. She looks fat, but there is no strength. She may develop enlarged tonsils. She catches cold often and each cold further enlarges the tonsils. The menses occur too soon and are profuse. She feels cold all the time and lacks energy. Slowly a cough begins and there is the faintest trace of fever. There is a desire for cold milk and eggs. The cough further worsens and the evening fever becomes well marked – the X-ray shows tuberculosis.

One can see that T.B. did not appear all at once; *it has evolved from childhood.* The signs of ill-health were all there. They indicate the homoeopathic medicine *Calcarea carbonica.* Had this remedy been given in infancy, the girl would not have developed the later troubles. But it is never too late. Even now Homoeopathy will build up her health. In this way many a problem child has been helped to normalcy by Homoeopathy.

A good homoeopath learns how to perceive disease as a continually evolving process which begins in the womb and, unless arrested and cured, ends in the tomb. There are many measures to palliate and ease the patient, but the progress of the disease continues unless it is treated on homoeopathic principles.

In fact most, if not all, curative therapies (including some forms of psychotherapy, meditation, etc.) are (consciously or unconsciously) based on the "simile" principle. The homoeopath applies this principle scientifically and systematically using carefully tested medicines.

Sometimes in the course of homoeopathic treatment, the history of past illness appears briefly in the reverse order, like a film been played backwards. When this happens, we know that not only the present, but also its cause in the past has been treated and the future is secure.

To a homoeopath, the knowledge of anatomy, physiology, medicine, surgery and gynecology is necessary since he has to examine the patient and come to a diagnosis. This will help him to know the natural course of the ailment and how to manage the case well.

But his most important task is to understand the individuality of each patient fully and correctly, so that he may select the right remedy.

The medicines of Homoeopathy

The process of potentization brings out the latent medicinal energy in those substances. By virtue of this process anything from sand (*Silicea*) to moon light (*Luna*) can be used as medicine in Homoeopathy.

The medicines are derived from the following sources:

Animal kingdom
Ex.   *Tarentula* (spider)
      Cantharis (Spanish fly)
      Sepia (Cuttle fish)
      Bufo rana

Plant kingdom
Ex.   *Aconitum napellus* (Monkshood)
      Belladonna atropa (Deadly nightshade)
      Bryonia alba (White bryony)
      Lycopodium (Club moss)

Mineral kingdom
Ex.   *Sulphur*
      Calcarea carbonica
      (Calcium carbonate)
      Nitricum acidum
      Natrum muriaticum
      (common salt)

Disease products (nosodes)
Ex.   *Tuberculinum*
      Pyrogenium
      (a preparation of pus)
      Hydrophobinum
      (saliva of a rabid dog)

Healthy tissues & secretions (sarcodes)
Ex.   Thyroid
      Pituitary

Imponderables
Ex.   Magnet
      X-ray

A fascinating journey

What has been said so far is a bird's eye-view of the system. We shall now examine each aspect in depth and we will get a very good idea of the homoeopathic way of looking at health, disease and cure. We will see how to take the case and understand the individuality of each patient, how we perceive remedies and how we apply them in practice. Let us begin this fascinating journey.

2

THE STORY OF THIS BOOK

As students of the Homoeopathic College, we found the homoeopathic Materia Medica very dry, the Repertory mechanical and the philosophy theoretical and obsolete. Philosophy was our worst subject because we could not relate it in any way to practice. In fact, we found the lectures so boring that we had literally to be dragged into them. This was just the beginning of our troubles. When we started our practice, we found different schools of thought, different ways to look at Homoeopathy. Some practitioners were giving medicines in combination, some were giving specifics, some were making prescriptions based on pathology, while others were basing them on keynotes, and yet others were using the Repertory. Even among the last group while some were using Kent's method others were working with Boger's, and a select few were following Boenninghausen's. Also while some practitioners gave importance to miasms others criticized them. This situation only added to our confusion.

First steps

Once I got out of College, I started working with the Repertory because of prior familiarity with it, and I started repertorizing cases mechanically. I was trying to use the characteristic and peculiar symptoms mainly because there are fewer remedies in these rubrics which made Repertory work easier. I would choose a few characteristic symptoms, look at the relevant rubrics in the Repertory and prescribe the medicine which was common to them. In some cases it worked, but in many it failed. I remember one early case of mine: my grandmother had difficulty in swallowing and I took her symptoms, "Generalities, food, potatoes aggravate" and "Throat, choking, oesophagus, on swallowing", and from these I came to the remedy *Alumina*, which helped her wonderfully. However, in many cases this approach failed, and so I poured all my energies into the search of a method which would prove a success in every case. I knew that the clinic was the best laboratory I could find and the scientific mind the best tool. The one principle I have adhered to throughout is to use only one remedy or therapeutic method at a time, and I have tried to keep everything else constant as far as possible. This has helped me a great deal in validating my observations.

Precedence of mentals and generals

Together with my colleague Dr. Jayesh Shah, I started studying our cases of success and failure. What became quite obvious was that those cases in which we prescribed on mentals and generals were much more successful than those in which we had relied upon particular symptoms or used pathology as the basis for our prescription. We looked at this idea purely from a practical point of view without really understanding the reason for it, and started trying it out cautiously in some of our cases. I still remember an early case of "vitiligo" (given in detail in the chapter: "Central Disturbance"). I could not get any symptoms from this lady except for my observation that she was a very humorous and talkative person. Also, she was warm-blooded and liked to walk in the open air. Repertorizing the symptoms:

— Loquacity with jesting;

— Walking in open air ameliorates, and

— Warmth in general aggravates,

I found the remedy *Kalium iodatum*. However, *Kalium iodatum* was not even mentioned under the rubric "Skin, discoloration, white spots".

So then, there was the question – Will this remedy work? So far we had been selecting a remedy based on mentals and generals but we also made sure that the remedy covered the local (presenting) problem as well. This was one of the first cases where the pathology was just not covered. I decided to take a chance by ignoring the pathology and gave this lady *Kalium iodatum*. The remedy worked beautifully.

I started asking myself some questions. Why did it work? How did it work? How could the remedy cure something which it is not known to be capable of causing or curing? What was the principle involved? At this time, I suddenly realized that when a remedy is potentized beyond 12C, there is not one molecule of the original substance left; what remains is only energy. Since there is no material substance left, it cannot cause any material changes in the body directly. It can cause no physical, physiological or chemical changes in the body; it can only cause dynamic changes. The sentence that came to my mind was: "*Potentized remedies have dynamic effect only.*"

This sentence was the door to a totally new look at Homoeopathy and my first step to a real understanding of disease. What exactly is a dynamic disturbance? This was the question. We had seen in our practice that a remedy that covers the mentals and generals cures the pathology, even if it is not mentioned in the Materia Medica. We found that in patients, it is the mentals and generals that are common to most patients of a particular remedy, whereas the "particular" or local symptoms differ from person to person.

Central disturbance

So, the general disturbance (represented mainly by mentals and generals), the *central disturbance* as we called it, comes first and this is followed by changes in the various organ systems depending upon each individual's pathological tendencies. Pathology grows on the central disturbance like a creeper grows on a stick. What we have to do is to remove the central disturbance.

Components: rubrics connected by a situation

My understanding progressed further when I started asking the question: What is a mental state? I then got the clue, that understanding the mental state of a person is different from listing his mental symptoms. Initially I had tried to understand the mental state of patients and remedies in terms of essences or cores, but found out that the core did not seem to cover the whole remedy. That is the time when I conceived the idea of understanding remedies in terms of components. Take for example the symptom "Mind, death, predicts the time of", in the remedy *Aconitum*. Immediately two things become clear: one is that *Aconitum* has fear of death, and secondly that it has the ability to predict (clairvoyance). These two components together make up the symptom "Predicts the time of death". In this way I started studying each remedy as a characteristic combination of components. This idea helped me greatly in practice, but then came the question: Are these components merely unconnected phenomena or is there something in the background which connects them?

A hint of the existence of such a background connecting the symptoms can be seen in the study of *Fluoricum acidum*. In *Fluoricum acidum*, there are components like "Indifference to loved ones, yet talks pleasantly with strangers", "Increased sexual desire" and also "Lack of morality". If we look at these three aspects, they seem at first sight to be unconnected. How, we could ask, is "Increased sexual desire" connected with "Indifference to loved ones"? One situation can explain all these components, namely, when a man finds that he has married someone totally unsuited to him, and needs to dissolve the marriage. In such a situation he needs to develop an indifference to his family, to become irresponsible and have increased sexual desire along with sociability. I looked into the Repertory and found the rubric: "Mind: Delusion, marriage, must dissolve", and the only remedy given is *Fluoricum acidum*!

Such observations created a new wave of thinking in my mind and I postulated that *components of a state are not unconnected*; the connection is that *all of them are needed in one particular situation*. A corollary to this is that this remedy represents a particular situation and that each patient's state also comes from a particular situation in the past, in which the components of his present state were necessary. From these observations the idea of disease as being a survival mechanism in a particular situation became clear. The concept of situational Materia Medica was born.

Root of disease

As my thinking along this line progressed further, I saw that even children (with no special past situations) have states, and that adults too have states which cannot be explained on the basis of past situations in their lives. I came to the conclusion that these states may have been inherited from earlier generations. When I looked at cases in this new light, I found a very striking *resemblance* between the state of the mother during pregnancy and the state of the infant. I also found similarities between the state of the parents at the time of conception and the state of the child. This is how the idea of roots of disease developed.

9

Roots are tendencies which, when excited, manifest as specific states of disease. These tendencies are impressions from specific situations in the past (or from previous generations) and make a person feel and react as if he were in that situation (delusion).

Delusion: what they really mean

I also realized the importance of the section on delusions, because a delusion is a false perception of reality, and disease too *is a false perception of the present*. The whole mental state of a person is an expression of this false perception (delusion).

Understanding the mental state

With all this understanding, I tried to find more ways of understanding the mental state of a person and evolved some techniques. One was to use dreams since the theme of a dream represents the prominent components of the state of the dreamer. I also studied the way the patient expresses himself and how he relates to the people around him. Such techniques became an integral part of my practice. With new perceptions in my practice, many ideas were generated. These include ideas about remedy relationships, the situational Materia Medica of several remedies and ideas about pathology and homoeopathic prognosis. Much more importantly, however, I could look at the question of what it really means to be healthy. This could be related not only to Homoeopathy but to Philosophy in general.

Higher purpose of life

Health, I realized, was man's freedom to be in the moment and fulfil the purpose of life. I could now appreciate Hahnemann's vision that man, like all creatures, is an instrument of the Spirit and is assigned a specific purpose by it (Aphorism 9 of the Organon).

Disease comes in the way of the organism's ability to fulfil this purpose, since it does not allow man to react to the present. It makes him react according to a situation from the past.

Cure is the restoration of health. It is achieved when man becomes aware of his false perception of reality. This is made possible through exposing him to his delusion. This is the basis of the Law of similars on which Homoeopathy is founded.

In this way practice became more simple; Materia Medica came alive and repertorial rubrics took on a new meaning. Homoeopathic philosophy, which earlier we had to be dragged into, became one with the spirit of life itself.

Sharing insights

Each chapter in this book deals with a specific question. Each idea seems so obvious to me now, but to get to it was a struggle. In practice an idea or question would flash in the mind. Then came sleepless nights when the mind grappled with the problem. Some solution would appear and this had to be tested the very next day in case after case. Practice, a strict and impartial judge, mercilessly shatters some of your most carefully constructed theories. The ideas that stood the test of practice were subjected to further scrutiny; further observations were made and then I could go to the next step, just like a mountain climber who makes sure of his foothold before going higher. Step after difficult step I came closer to the understanding of Homoeopathy.

I wanted to share all these insights with students who might face the same difficulties as I did. It was with this aim that I gave a series of seminars in Europe and India between 1986 and 1990. I had made some notes for these seminars which, together with some more recent insights, I have now put together and given shape to in the form of this book. It is possible that what I say may not be new, but to have knowledge of and, on the other hand, to actually experience and strongly feel something as correct and true are two very different things.

Generally, most classical homoeopaths would agree with the ideas in this book. However, some of the ideas are new in Homoeopathy or at least are not stated so clearly and pointedly elsewhere. These include the ideas of *roots of disease, components of mind, importance and use of delusions and dreams, compensated and uncompensated feelings, Homoeo-psychotherapy and situational Materia Medica.* My view of remedy-states and understanding them through the situations from which they originate promises to be the basis of a new Materia Medica, of which I have made a beginning through this book.

If you read through all the chapters, I think that you will get a fairly accurate view of my thoughts and approach. As each chapter was written independently, there is bound to be some repetition and a lack of sequence. I must also add that even though my perception of Homoeopathy has become much clearer, I still have the feeling of having seen only the tip of the iceberg. I therefore make no pretence that this book is either complete or final. At best, I can say I have made an honest attempt to tell you the story so far. My aim in doing so is to stimulate the reader to make his own observations and develop his vision. I am confident that in doing this the wonderful spirit of Homoeopathy will touch you. Truth has the quality of striking deep within.

3

WHAT IS DISEASE

The allopathic viewpoint

In common parlance "disease" would refer to the diagnostic label a patient is given. We say, "She has got diabetes" or, "His disease is rheumatoid arthritis." Modern medicine has classified diseases along these lines and now has specialists for each "disease". A lot of money is poured into finding the cure for these problems and from time to time a drug appears with a lot of promise, only to fade away soon or be exposed for its injurious side effects. All in all, especially in chronic cases, the only effect of this type of research is to find drugs that have some temporary relieving effect on the problem and therefore have to be taken lifelong in increasing doses despite their side effects.

The basic idea behind such treatment is that disease is a local problem and if we tackle that part, we can solve it. Diabetes is a deficiency of the islet cells of the pancreas, rheumatoid arthritis is due to malfunctioning of the immune system, epilepsy arises from an excitable focus in the brain and so forth. With such a viewpoint, it is natural that they try to find a drug to stimulate the islet cells, suppress the immune response, or sedate the brain. The very failure of such methods to bring about cure or even a significant reduction of the problem over time should have cautioned them that there are other more important and basic factors involved.

The young homoeopath, eager to keep pace with modern medical "discoveries", may be tempted to try to find the "homoeopathic cure" for such conditions as diabetes and rheumatoid arthritis. He then falls into the trap of trying to find a specific drug or a group of drugs to tackle the problem. He, too, now, narrows his vision to the "part affected" and thus invites failure.

Despite knowledge of homoeopathic philosophy and its fundamental principles, the homoeopath is at times unable to avoid giving importance to the diagnostic label the patient presents with. It is too awesome, often the only thing the patient is interested in is getting rid of, and, with his knowledge of medical science – the etiology, pathology and prognosis of the condition known to him – the homoeopath often finds it impossible to remove the diagnosis from his mind while selecting the remedy. He tries to find a remedy which is known to be useful in the treatment of such a pathological entity.

Characteristic symptoms differentiate between the remedies

Even so, the homoeopath still has to make a choice between several remedies, since each pathological entity has several remedies known to cure it. This information did not come from provings of the remedies (since provings were stopped at the level of functional symptoms), but later from clinical observations. The remedy was used initially in the clinic, not on the name of the disease, but on the symptoms, and when that particular disease was cured or substantially benefited, this remedy was listed as one of the remedies for that disease.

The selection between the various remedies listed for that condition is based on the differences between the symptoms of each patient. Such differences are obvious to anyone who has seen even two patients with the same diagnosis label. Two patients with diabetes will have totally different histories, onset of trouble, symptoms, signs, complications, course, response to therapy, etc. Indeed, except for a few common diabetes signs like increased thirst and urination and increased blood sugar, they will have almost nothing in common.

It is obvious that it is not these common symptoms they are going to help us to select the remedy (since most remedies listed under this condition will have them), but it is the individual differences which will decide. These differences include the time of aggravation of complaints and other modalities, the peculiarities of the location, the side and direction of troubles, the exact sensation experienced , and accompaniments to the trouble. The homoeopath tries to differentiate the remedies listed under the disease condition according to these factors.

Mentals and generals as characteristics

However, slowly but surely, he will see that the most marked difference between two individuals suffering from the same condition lies in their mental state and in their general symptoms like preferences in temperature and food, and pattern of appetite, sweat and sleep. These are far removed from the actual seat of the pathology, but are much more useful in differentiating the remedies since they are most characteristic of the patient. For example, of two patients suffering from rheumatoid arthritis, the common symptoms would be pains in the joints with some deformities, a positive R.A. test and an increased blood sedimentation rate. In order to find a remedy that fits the case, the homoeopath would have to ask about the location, sensation, modalities and accompaniments of the pain. He might find that the first patient has pain more on the right side, increasing between 4 and 8 p.m., and is a warmblooded, dictatorial person with a desire for sweets and warm food. The other patient may have some burning pain in the joints ameliorated by warmth, intolerance of cold, and be a miserably mistrustful anxious person with frequent thirst for sips of water.

The remedies *Lycopodium* and *Arsenicum* can be thus easily differentiate on the basis of the peculiar local as well as the mental and general symptoms of the patient. Both remedies are known for their usefulness in the treatment of rheumatoid arthritis.

So far, this is still on "safe" ground. The homoeopath is prescribing a remedy known in the treatment of the "disease" condition and which also has the peculiarities of the patient. He gradually learns through experience that if the remedy he has chosen does not cover the mental and general symptoms of the patient along with the local peculiarities, it usually fails. Therefore he gives importance to these symptoms in selecting the remedy, but makes sure that the remedy he has chosen is in the list of remedies for that disease condition.

Then, along comes a case where the mental and general symptoms fit beautifully into one remedy which is not listed for the disease condition the patient has presented with. If he takes the chance and gives the remedy, he will see some surprising results.

I had a patient, a woman of around forty, who among other things was found to have a fibroid tumor in the uterus. She was a lean, thin woman and one who was extremely anxious and fastidious. The remedy that suggested itself from the emotional and constitutional nature of the patient was *Arsenicum album*. However, when I looked up in the book, nowhere was *Arsenicum album* listed as a medicine for uterine fibroid. In spite of this I gave it to her and within a few months we confirmed by ultrasonography that the fibroid had disappeared.

Treating patient not pathology

If we keep our minds open, such experiences become the rule, not the exception. I have treated patients with remedies not even remotely associated with the problem they came with! Off hand I remember a case of arthritis successfully treated with *Helleborus* (a remedy which is never thought of in such a condition); a case of vitiligo with the remedy *Capsicum*; the pain of a calcaneal spur with *Aconitum* and a case of angina pectoris due to blocked vessels with *Bryonia*. None of these remedies would be ordinarily considered in the respective conditions, but the mental and general state of the patient fitted the remedy and I was open-minded enough to give it.

Nowadays, I often do not bother to check if the remedy I have selected on the mentals, generals and the local peculiarities is listed under the condition. Through experience, I am quite confident that if I have selected the medicine on the above criteria, this medicine will benefit the patient and the pathology will automatically regress. On the other hand, if the remedy is selected only on pathology, without covering the mentals and generals, it will most likely fail.

What do these observations show? They clearly demonstrate that each patient has a specific mental state with an accompanying specific general state, and if we treat this with the remedy, the pathology automatically regresses.

Disease: centre to periphery

This state comes first and in fact is the real disease of the individual patient. Disease is thus not something local, not an affection of the parts, but it is the state of being of the whole person at the time: the way he feels, thinks, behaves, what he likes and dislikes, and what he tolerates and cannot tolerate on the whole.

15

This is the state which needs to be treated, not the local parts. The local parts will function normally once the state is reversed. If we try it the other way, i.e. treat the local parts, the result is bound to be temporary and harmful.

The whole concept of disease thus changes from being something local to being something general, from being a diagnostic label to being an individual's state of being. From this understanding our whole approach to treatment changes. No longer are we going to look for a specific cure for all the patients of the same diagnosis. From now on we are going to try to understand what is individual to each patient. We are going to understand what the mental and general state of a person is, and how to discover it in each case.

The mental state

No wonder the master wrote:

> "This holds true to such an extent, that the state of disposition often chiefly determines the choice of the homoeopathic remedy."
>
> (Aphorism 211)

In the homoeopathic Materia Medica, the mental symptoms of the various remedies have been beautifully brought out, which make this choice easy. The state of the patient has to be compared with the mental and general state of the various remedies in the Materia Medica in order to choose one which is exactly suitable.

> "There is no powerful medicinal substance in the world which does not very notably alter the state of the disposition and mind in the healthy individual who tests it, and every medicine does so in a different manner."
>
> (Aphorism 212)

When I started studying the mental state of the patients I could only see it as a conglomeration of mental symptoms. For example, the mental state of the lady with a fibroid was for me a group of mental symptoms which included fastidiousness and anxiety. I could not really trace any connection between these symptoms, but since they were both prominent, I decided they both belonged to her mental state. The full significance of what a mental state is, was to come to me later, and it opened my eyes to the real meaning of disease.

My attention was drawn by a peculiar case of an 8 year old boy who was working in our college canteen, cleaning the tables. The boy was dumb. Despite this he was full of life, very active, always busy, very communicative through gestures, ever smiling, and entertaining others through his actions, dancing and generosity. One of my student felt sympathetic and approached a colleague of mine to see if the dumbness could be treated homoeopathically. The boy's history was quite tragic. It came out through several expressive gestures. His mother had died when he was three and his father was a drunkard who had sold off all but one of the family's milk cows. Through this cow the boy had managed to survive. When he was about five years old he fell from a moderate height and lost his voice. One year prior to the time my student talked to the boy, his father had sold off the last cow and put the boy in a train to Bombay while he was sleeping. Due to his being dumb, the boy found some sympathizers who gave him menial jobs and ultimately he ended up at the college canteen.

A peculiar feature that came out in the history was that the boy frequently had a vision that God came and spoke to him, took him around the universe and brought him back. The boy was very religious and never missed his daily prayer, which he performed with a lot of dancing and silent singing.

My colleague suspected that the dumbness was hysterical. He gave the boy a few powders of placebo and within a week the boy fell off a small tree and regained his voice!

Around this time, some doctors attached to the college took an interest in him and started teaching him to read and write.

State comes from situation

This case set me thinking. The remedy I would have prescribed for the boy is *Veratrum album* because it has the following symptoms:

- Religious affections;
- Delusion, God, communication with, he is in;
- Delusion, dumb, he is;
- Activity, restless;
- Singing;
- Dancing;
- Smiling, Laughing;
- Busy, Industrious;
- Loquacity;
- Cheerful.

Again this looks like a group of unconnected symptoms. But a little deeper look gave me the insight I was searching for.

I could see the boy gain sympathy and attention which he badly needed. The very symptoms recorded above were the ones that helped him survive the severe crisis he faced. The dumbness attracted sympathy, the feeling of being in communication with God gave him courage and strength; and the activity and his cheerful nature made him useful and also endeared him to everybody. However, these qualities were outliving their usefulness because the situation was now not so grim. He was in safer hands, among people who cared. They wished to help him further and his being dumb only came in the way. So the dumbness disappeared with mere placebo.

I do not mean that the boy was doing all this on purpose. The whole thing was probably subconscious. But the fact remains that his whole state, with all its symptoms, was a suitable survival mechanism in his situation. When the necessity for his state diminished, it automatically regressed.

This case created a revolution in my thinking and in my concept of disease. I realized that *the disease state is a posture adopted by the organism for survival in a particular situation.* As long as that situation exists, and as long as the posture is appropriate and in proportion to the situation, it cannot be helped by any treatment.

When I started studying my cases I found that the mental symptoms of any case fit into a pattern. Each pattern is a posture that suits a particular situation.

For example, let us take the case of the boy aged three who had the following prominent symptoms in the mind:
  – Desire for music;
  – Desire for dancing;
  – Desire for colours;
  – Desire for painting;
  – Very active;
  – Very industrious;
  – Cunning;
  – Deceitful;
  – Mischievous.

In the body we find similar features:
  – Restlessness, especially of limbs;
  – Choreic dance-like movement;
  – Increased energy.

Homoeopaths have been using *Tarentula* as the remedy for patients with such symptoms. I asked myself the question: How are these symptoms connected? It struck me that a lot of them have to do with attractive behaviour. A person who needs to attract attention could develop the love of music and dancing, colours and painting. When does a person need to attract attention? Naturally, when he does not get it. This can happen in a situation of unreciprocated affection or love. Such a situation also demands features like mischievousness, deceit, activity, and increased energy in order to win the attention and affection of the other person. Thus I could see that this whole state of mind is a posture adapted to the situation of a person with unrequited love. As long as the situation exists, no treatment is necessary or helpful. But in this child there was nothing in the situation that needed this posture.

Disease as a posture

So, the posture may be proportionate and appropriate to the situation, as for example, when a man is being chased by a lion, the posture of running fast, being afraid, etc., is appropriate since his survival depends upon it. However, if a man is in the same state without a lion chasing him, or he adopts the same posture even if a little dog chases him, or he is in such a panic that he cannot think (a reaction far in excess of what is needed in the situation) then this state is to be removed by treatment.

So far we have seen that disease is a state of mind and body and that this state is a posture that is suited in a particular situation and needs to be removed when:
- Such a situation doesn't exist (no lion).
- The situation now is different (only dog).
- The reaction is out of proportion to the situation (excessive panic).

Disease is thus seen as an affection of the whole person, as a posture adopted as a survival mechanism to suit a particular situation which does not exist at the moment. This posture makes us react to the present in an unsuitable way due to our false perception of it. Such an unsuitable and disproportionate reaction to the situation naturally causes a constant stress on the organism, and the stress aggravates the pathology which the person has or brings the tendency to a particular pathology into activity. By treating this reaction we reduce the stress of the whole organism and therefore its aggravating influence on the pathology – thus the pathology automatically regresses.

This leads us to the question of why we react in an inappropriate and disproportionate manner. To answer this we must take each of these two separately:
- Unsuitable postures.
- Out of proportion reactions.

We shall examine these two aspects in the next two chapters.

4

UNSUITABLE POSTURES

We understand disease as a state of mind and body: a particular state of mind associated with a particular state of the body. Disease is not anything external; it is not something from without. It is the posture that is adopted by the organism in order to survive in a *perceived* situation. *The state that the organism adopts is disease.* So, it is not something to be removed, but it is something that has to be changed. The posture is an adjustment to a particular situation, and it has to come back to its original form.

As long as the situation exists, and as long as this posture is in proportion to the situation, it cannot be, and should not be removed. For example, if you are lifting a heavy bag and you have to walk with that heavy weight, in order that you back does not break, you have to bend in the direction opposite to the bag. So, your body adopts a posture to survive in this situation. This posture is healthy, it is going to do you good, in this situation it is needed, and as long as the bag is heavy, the posture has to be maintained.

Hence, we see that posture is an adjustment. As long as this adjustment is in proportion to the existing situation, as long as it is suitable to this situation, and as long as the situation or exciting factor remains, this adjustment cannot and should not be corrected.

In our practice we see that most of the time this adjustment, this reaction to the existing situation, is unsuitable. Unsuitable postures can be encountered in people. Look at the miser, the woman who trusts no one and carefully counts her money to the last penny. She keeps it in a safe, yet feels unsafe, and can almost see thieves at night prowling around the house. Restless and anxious, this lean woman with cold hands, nervously sipping water, lives in a state of constant anxiety. A little pain in the chest and she's sure that death is at her doorstep. She runs helter skelter to several doctors and still feels insecure. Even when visiting the most beautiful place she counts her money as if to protect it from thieves, oblivious of the beauty around her. When she is given love, she reacts with mistrust. She has little space for people and even less space for experiences.

The origin of unsuitable postures

Where did such an unsuitable state originate? It seems logical that at some time in the past this woman must have been in a situation where she was surrounded by thieves and so this posture became necessary for her survival. It is likely that she has been badly cheated by deceitful people and so she can trust no one. Such a situation has left its mark on her and she reacts unsuitably to the present because of this impression from the past.

21

When a person gets used to something for a long time, it creates an impression, a memory. This makes that person react unsuitably or out of proportion from the slightest provocation. Let us take the example of a man who has been living in a terror-stricken area where there is a great deal of violence and killing. He remains very scared; there is a state of fear in him. If he has to go out of the house in the evening for some vital reason, he is so scared that he trembles. He keeps looking backwards and forwards; he feels that somebody will do something to him, as if somebody is ready to attack him. If anyone lightly touches him, he starts violently.

This is the state that is required in that situation of great terror. But when he lives in this situation for a long time, then that whole situation creates in him an impression, or what I call a *root*. So that even if he is in a safe place, inside him there is still a root of fear; and if he hears of even slight rioting anywhere he gets extremely panicky. Since he has gone through a lot of terror, a slightly similar situation creates an out of proportion reaction in him.

Roots can be transmitted

When I started looking at my cases in this light, I did find some cases where I could trace the origin of the present state of the patient in the past. However, in most cases I could not find any such situation throughout the whole life of the patient. Moreover, I could see that states exist even in children and new born babies. So it became necessary to find out from where these states originated. This is when I started noticing that children very often have a state that is identical to the one the mother had during pregnancy. In other children I noticed a striking resemblance, even to minute details, between their state and the state of one of the parents. Here is a case example:

The patient, a boy of 10 years, was referred to me by my colleague for treatment of a very severe and chronic skin problem. He had boils on the extremities which were very painful and itching. For the past month he could not even sit or stand. He was carried into my consulting room, crying, his boils full of pus.

The history of boils began when the boy was four months old. Since then he had been treated by several different doctors and subject to several different therapies, including Homoeopathy, but not to avail.

Describing the itching, the mother said it was so bad that the boy wanted to tear away his skin. With his hands clenched, he would shriek from the severity of the itching almost like an insane person. He would say: "Kill me, I can't take it, I don't want to live." Whenever the itching became too much he would say: "Give me a knife, I want to stab my arms."

As a child, the boy had been very dependent on a particular Goddess. He used to compose and sing songs in her praise. With the itching, the boy had become angry with the Goddess and would say: "I have done so much for her and this is what she has done to me!" Once having said this, he tore up the picture he had of the Goddess.

22

He was very sensitive both in mind and skin. He could not tolerate even a drop of water; he did not like bathing and was thirstless. The itching with its accompanying violence was not continuous, but spasmodic. There was cruel behaviour. He would say: "I will become mad."

Physically there was aversion to vegetables, craving for chocolate, and aversion to the heat of the sun.

In this case we can see the following symptoms on the mental and general level:
–   Violence;
–   Abusive;
–   Striking;
–   Cruelty;
–   Tear, impulse to;
–   Cut, mutilate, desire to;
–   Impulse to stab the flesh;
–   Sensitive, sacred music, to;
–   Desires chocolate;
–   Aversion to vegetables;
–   Aversion to water.

The main feelings connected with this state are:
–   Forsaken (by Goddess) (Rubric: "Delusion, deserted");
–   Tormented feeling (by Goddess) (Rubric: "Delusion, tormented");
–   Feels he has suffered wrong (Rubric: "Delusion, wrong fancies, he has suffered").

From these feelings come the violent reactions. He has skin eruption and reacts as if he were in a situation where he is tormented and forsaken by the person he is serving and on whom he is dependent (the Goddess).

The remedy for such a state is *Lyssinum* (*Hydrophobinum*). This was a peculiar state, with no situation in the past of the boy to explain its presence. In fact, the boy developed the problem as early as four months. So, I examined the history of the mother during her pregnancy and got the following story.

The mother had severe toothache throughout the pregnancy. This was her second pregnancy. Her first child was stillborn. Since the beginning of the second pregnancy the mother had felt that something terrible would happen. She would pray all the time. The baby was ten days overdue. This made her panicky and extremely tense. She would stand before the picture of the same Goddess and with her hands clenched, she would cry: "Why are you doing this to me?" She had a fear of dogs and a desire for chocolate. The prominent symptoms of the mother's state during pregnancy are as follows:

23

- Toothache during pregnancy;
- Fear during pregnancy;
- Fear of evil;
- Praying;
- Fear of misfortune;
- Fear as if something will happen;
- Tormented feeling;
- Desire for chocolate.

The feeling is the same "troubled by someone she is dependent on, a sense of injustice, forsaken feeling". The remedy for her state is *Lyssinum*.

It was for me a remarkable experience to see the same state in the mother during pregnancy, even to such small details. The boy did very well on *Lyssinum*. Incidently, one of the probable reasons this remedy was never prescribed for the boy by the colleague who referred him or by the other homoeopaths who had seen him, is that *Lyssinum* is not known at all for skin disease. In the Materia Medica there is no mention of boils or other skin complaints. This case is another glaring example of the need to understand what disease is, that it is the state of being of an individual and not merely the local problem.

I started noticing this phenomenon in several cases. One of my first observation was: *If the mother had a very intense state during the pregnancy, the child almost always has the same state.*

Once this idea of transmission of disease states from one generation to another occurred to me, I started examining other avenues, besides the state during pregnancy, from which these disease state tendencies or *roots* could be transmitted. I started noticing that the states of the parents at the time of conception, if they were intense, were transmitted as roots to the child.

The formation of roots

Roots are formed in the following ways:
- By the existence of an intense state for a long time in a person.
- The intense state of the mother during pregnancy is transmitted as a root to the infant.
- The predominant disease states of the father and the mother at the time of conception will also become roots in the infant.
- The roots of the father and mother at the time of conception will also become roots in the child.

The order in which I have mentioned these four sources is also the order in which the roots are excitable, meaning the first one is the most easily excited into an active disease state.

There is a joke:

When a thief and a pickpocket married, they were blessed with a bony baby. But, after birth, the baby kept its fist clenched and refused to open it. Later when they had brought it home, it opened the fist, and out fell the midwife's ring!

Why do two children of the same parents manifest different diseases, even though they may have the same roots?

The disease state we shall ultimately suffer from depends upon the following factors:
– Which root is excitable;
– The exciting factors.

The exciting factors play a very important role in determining the disease we suffer from. If there are two roots of equal excitability, then a specific exciting factor will tend to aggravate one more than the other.

The situational differences in both parents at the time of conception of their different children could account for the differences in the roots of the children. This explain why two children of the same parents have different roots, or roots of different strength. At this point it becomes necessary to distinguish between the strength and excitability of a root. The *strength of a root* (or depth) depends upon how long the state has persisted, including in the previous generations. If the state of disease has persisted for a long time (over several generations), a strong (deep) root will be formed. The *excitability of a root* (meaning how easily it can be excited by external factors to produce the active disease state) depends upon how recently the disease state has been active. The more recently the disease state has been active, the more excitable the root. I have found, for example, that the state of the mother during pregnancy forms the most excitable root in the infant. For example, a lady was *Calcarea* before pregnancy, but during pregnancy she was intensely frightened and developed a very strong *Stramonium* state; she probably did not have any *Stramonium* root at all. In the child the most excitable root would not be *Calcarea*, but it would be the root of *Stramonium*. This feature was known to ancient people as they insisted on the mother to remain happy and calm during pregnancy, because the child would also develop such features. The idea of roots also shows us why particular remedies are more often indicated in particular nations. For example, I understand that in England *Stramonium* (with "Terror" and "Praying") is very frequently indicated. One of the possible reasons for this could be the World War, which created a state of panic and terror in the whole country, and the root of this state was passed on to a generation of people who were born at this time.

We quite often find different remedies indicated in twins. This is due to the fact that although they have inherited the same roots, the way they were brought up and the way they were treated excited different roots and created different states in them.

So, upbringing does not make roots, but the way a person is brought up will excite a particular root. For example, if one sibling is treated better than the other and both have "jealousy roots", the root of the one who is treated badly will get excited.

Silent and dominating states

I noticed in some patients that they would have one state quite prominently. During treatment this state would go down and another would manifest. On treatment of this second state a third one would come out clearly. When this was treated, the first state would come up again; it would be less intense and the patient would be in better health, his symptoms going in the direction of cure. One initial case where I observed this clearly was of a woman who came with multiple complaints: backache, hypertension, etc. On taking her history, I could see the state of the remedy *Kalium bichromicum*. On giving her *Kalium bichromicum*, she improved, but brought out new symptoms, which now indicated another remedy, namely *Kalium carbonicum*, which relieved her further, but now the picture of the third remedy, *Sulphur*, emerged. *Sulphur* produced a beneficial effect, but soon I could see the *Kalium bichromicum* picture once again. In this way she went in cycles and with each cycle her health would be one step better.

It is rather like coming down a spiral staircase. So that with each cycle we come to the same point, but one level lower. Similar cycles of remedy states are well known in homoeopathic literature. The most famous is the *Sulphur-Calcarea carbonica-Lycopodiun* cycle. Another trio consists of *Causticum-Colocynth-Staphysagria*. It need not always be three states, but any number. The idea is of the existence of several states in one person, one predominant at a particular time.

This can be tabulated as follows:

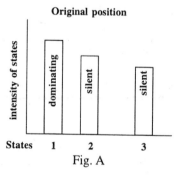

Fig. A

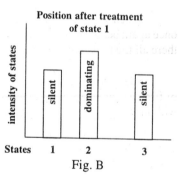

Fig. B

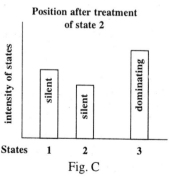

Fig. C

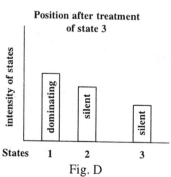

Fig. D

In figure A, I have termed states 2 and 3, when state 1 is prominent, *silent states*, and state 1: *dominating state*. In figure B, state 2 becomes the dominating state.

One could compare this with the parliament of a nation. The party with a majority will rule and impose its policies on the nation. The other parties exist but are powerless. When the strength of the majority party is reduced to less than the strength of the second largest party, this second party takes charge and dominates. When its strength is reduced a third party comes up. Finally the original party would assume power again, the other two being weaker.

But each time this cycle results, the parties are getting less in strength and their ability to make important changes also consequently lessens.

The difference between a silent state and a root

This can be explained as follows. If you have anxiety about health as your main mental state, this is the dominating state at present. Suddenly, you hear a noise and you feel that a thief has entered your house. Now in this situation the state of anxiety about health becomes silent, and a new state becomes dominant. So, the anxiety about health is there, yet it is not seen, Now, as you are ringing up the police to get the thief, you suddenly detect some smoke and think that there is fire somewhere in the house. Here again, the fear of thief becomes silent and fear of fire becomes dominant.

When you call up the fire brigade and the fire is extinguished then the fear of thief once again becomes dominant. The anxiety about the thief and anxiety about health were there all the time, but they were silent. That is why they can be called *silent states*.

Silent states are not roots because if they were roots and not states, then when "fear of fire" has gone away, no state should be left; unless there is an exciting factor. But, if without exciting factor, there is still a state left, it cannot be a root.

Let us take another example. A person has within him the talent to become a doctor, a lawyer and a farmer. He has these three talents within him. He has roots to become any of the three, but at that time in this area a doctor was most required; there was an exciting factor for him to become a doctor. So, he becomes a doctor and he practices medicine for some time. Then there is a war in the country and everyone is enlisted into the army. So this doctor now becomes a soldier. Therefore, "soldier" now becomes his dominating state, and "doctor" becomes a silent state.

We see that in this case "doctor" becomes a silent state, because after the war is over he again becomes a doctor; that the state was within him all the time, although silent.

Therefore the difference between a root and a silent state is that in the case of a silent state, as the dominating state goes down, the disease state is again seen, without any exciting factor. A root requires a specific exciting factor to bring about a disease state.

27

If we represent a root as follows: and a disease as:

ROOT   **DISEASE**

Fig. E

then we can have a chart for each individual as follows:

Model of disease state and roots in a person

Now we are in a position to understand this chart of diseases and roots. We can have:

    – Diseases with roots: A, C
    – Diseases without roots: B
    – Roots without diseases: D, E

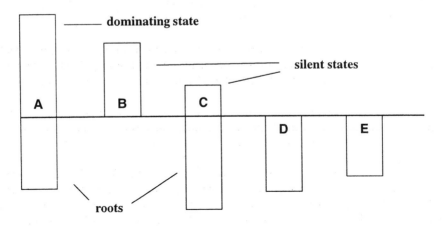

Fig. F

5

OUT OF PROPORTION REACTIONS

In the previous two chapters, we have examined disease and understood that it is the posture adopted by the organism to suit a particular situation. If this posture is either unsuitable or out of proportion to the present situation, then it needs to be treated. We examined in detail the reasons for the development of unsuitable postures and we saw that *they come from memories of past situations*; such memories we call roots.

In this chapter we shall try to understand the reason for out of proportion reactions. Out of proportion reactions can be encountered several times a day; one might even say that a reaction that is in proportion to the stress is the exception rather than the rule. Take any stress, for example a fire in the house or even smoke coming from a room. How many of us will react proportionately to this? Our panic, confusion and anxiety will be far in excess of what is required, and this usually does more harm than good. Such an overreaction creates much more stress in the organism than is needed, and this excess of stress can make a vital difference in some cases as we will see later.

To take the familiar example of a man being chased by a lion, we can see that as long as the lion continues to chase him, he will panic which prevents him from thinking, which creates more panic and this vicious cycle goes on to the point where his state soon blows itself out of proportion. This creates in him so much stress that he may die from this rather than from the lion itself!

This blowing out of proportion can be reduced by a strong force of will. The man who is panicking because of the smoke, can curtail his out of proportion reaction if he voluntarily stops himself and starts thinking. If he stops himself and says: "I must stop overreacting", his stress can be reduced to some extent.

This whole phenomenon can be stated as follows. Under an exciting cause (stress factor) a state tends to blow itself out of proportion, but such a reaction can sometimes be retarded by a strong force of will.

The working of this phenomenon is slightly different in diseases with a root and without a root, and we shall study these two individually.

Disease without a root

Some diseases are without a root. They occur due to a very strong, intense exciting factor. The big epidemics, for example, occur due to intensely pathogenic organisms

29

which, no matter what state the individual is in, overwhelm his defences and set up their own state. Normally in such epidemics, the state of most individuals suffering from disease will be the same.

One such epidemic of cholera occurred during Hahnemann's lifetime and he was able to identify that this epidemic required specific medicines. These medicines could successfully treat countless patients suffering from the disease.

We can see the same epidemic-like phenomenon in several acute conditions such as burns, dehydration, loss of blood, massive injury, severe emotional shock, etc. Again here, the severity of the stress factor ensures a uniformity of reaction. Most people will develop similar states from these factors and will respond to similar remedies. These remedies can very often make a vital difference between life and death.

The question arises, how does the homoeopathic remedy make the difference in such a situation? We have already mentioned that if the disease state is in proportion to the stress factor, then it cannot be treated. This much is obvious. So, if a remedy helps to reduce the reaction, then it must mean that the reaction is in excess of the stress factor, and by reducing the reaction to the level which is proportionate, the homoeopathic medicine makes the vital difference, and prevents death which would have been caused by the excess reaction.

If the stress factor is too intense and the body cannot cope, then death will surely result. However, in many cases the stress factor is not so intense, but the out of proportion reaction causes a tremendous strain which the body cannot bear. Such an excessive reaction is due to the phenomenon described earlier, namely, under the influence of the stress factor, the state tends to blow itself out of proportion.

Diseases with a root

So far we have examined the working of the phenomenon of excessive reaction in diseases without a root, where it can be easily and simply understood. The same phenomenon however applies, albeit in a more complicated way, to diseases with a root. The difference is that when there is a root, even factors that are innocuous for healthy people (those without the root) become exciting factors. The more excitable the root, the more likelihood of smaller and smaller factors exciting the disease state. Therefore, when we look at the phenomenon of excessive reaction in these people, we find they are under the constant influence of an exciting factor (exciting for them), and therefore their state keeps going out of proportion as well as being unsuitable to the present situation (due to their root). Thus, in most chronic cases we shall see not only unsuitable reactions, that is reactions which are suitable to some other situation, but also that the reaction to that situation is out of proportion.

To repeat once again our example of a man being chased by a dog reacting as being chased by a lion. We shall find that he is not only reacting as if a lion was chasing him, but also that his reaction is out of proportion even if the lion were chasing him.

Conclusion

Over the three last chapters we have seen that disease is a posture adopted by the organism for survival in a particular situation. We usually find that this situation does not exist and/or the reaction is excessive. This can be a strain on the whole organism and will aggravate the person's pathology, pathological tendencies. In the next chapter we shall examine the meaning of disease in our life and how it affects our thoughts, feelings and actions. We shall also see that the homoeopathic concept is very similar to concepts from other disciplines.

6

HEALTH AND DISEASE: PSYCHOLOGICAL AND PHILOSOPHICAL CONSIDERATIONS

Disease consists of two parts: generalized disturbance of the whole organism and localized problems. It can be seen that generalized disturbance (which includes physical, general and psychological changes) precedes localization of the problem. This generalized disturbance is probably what Hans Selye (the authority on stress) described as the *General Adaptation Syndrome*. The whole of this generalized disturbance or change can be understood as a posture of adaptation for survival in a particular situation. It is obvious that if the situation does exist or is intense enough, such an adaptation would ensure survival and therefore cannot be treated. Conversely, if such a situation does not exist, or is not proportionately intense, this general adaptation would be a maladaptation and needs to be corrected.

Disease as a posture

In sum, disease is a posture, a state of being, which is suitable and appropriate in a particular situation, a situation that does not exist at present. Disease originates from severe situations which demand this posture or state of being for survival. This state leaves an impression which we call a root which gets activated later on.

Disease sets up several conditions for feeling OK. When we imagine a lion is chasing us we will not feel OK unless we are running. In the same way, if your disease originated in the situation where you needed to achieve in order to be loved or to survive, you will not feel OK unless you achieve. These conditions restrict your being in the present and your reacting to the situation appropriately. The miser's constant need is to check his purse. He will do this even when visiting the Taj Mahal, rather than admiring its beauty.

Disease thus sets up a lot of conditions for feeling OK. It has the quality: "I am OK only if..." Such conditions for feeling OK (compulsive actions) usually arise from our feelings or fears, especially from our fixed ideas regarding the situations in front of us (obsessions). The miser's fear comes from the fixed idea that he is being cheated by the people around him. Obsessions or fixed feelings are needed in the particular situation in which we imagine ourselves to be. We view most situations from our basic delusion and this is our disease, which is a remnant of a past situation and has left an impression on us (root).

Conditions for feeling OK

Due to these conditions (compulsions) and obsessions (fixed feelings) our ability to react to the situation becomes restricted. This restriction is a measure of our disease. When such a restriction takes place we no longer remain open to what is in front of us. We are not-OK in most situations, and are OK only when our conditions for feeling OK are satisfied. The achiever feels insecure in all situations which do not have anything to do with his achievement. One can say that he needs the situation much more than the situation needs him. An achiever needs the situation of achievement much more than the achievement itself, and therefore he opts for no other situation. A diseased man is like one who feels that his car's gears do not function except for the first, and so he has to choose the path of climbing a hill because this is the only situation in which he can feel OK. On every other road he feels he would lag behind the others. Not-OK feelings and conditions of feeling OK are the most prominent effects of disease.

As against this, *health has unconditional OK-ness*; one feels OK without any conditions. Health allows man to be in the moment and react appropriately and proportionately to the situation he faces. If the situation calls for achievement he will achieve. If it calls for passivity he will be passive. He does not need to achieve or be passive in order to feel OK with himself. He is like a man who knows that in his car all the gears are working. He does not stick only to mountain paths but can travel freely. *Health signifies freedom, spontaneity and being in the present*; the spirit within is able to fulfil the requirements of the situation. A sick man can fulfil only those special situations in which his conditions for OK-ness are fulfilled. Health also signifies space in which a person has freedom to be and to express unconditionally. He can take others as they are without wanting them to be in this or that way. Thus health can be expressed in those famous words of Thomas Harris: "I am OK, you are OK."

The philosopher Sosan (Third Zen Patriarch) says:

> "The Great Way is not difficult for those who have no preferences; when love and hate are both absent, everything becomes clear and undisguised. Make the smallest distinction, however, heaven and earth are set infinitely apart. If you wish to see the truth then hold no opinion for or against. The struggle of what one likes and what one dislikes is the disease of the mind."

In health, therefore, man has no preferences, no compulsions, and he accepts things as they are.

Healthy man as instrument of the Spirit

Hahnemann wrote in the Aphorism 9 of the Organon:

> "In the healthy condition of man the spiritual force (autocracy), the dynamis that animates this material being (organism), rules with un-bounded sway, and retains all the parts of the organism in an admirable,

harmonious, vital operation, as regards both sensations and functions, so that our indwelling reason-gifted Spirit can freely employ this living, healthy instrument for the higher purposes of our existence." (Some translations use the word "mind" instead of "Spirit" – but the original German word is "Geist" – here meaning spirit.)

Reflecting the same sentiment Rabindranath Tagore wrote:

> *Thou hast made me endless,*
> *Such is thy pleasure.*
> *This little flute of reed*
> *Thou hath carried over the hills and dales*
> *And breathed into it*
> *Melodies eternally new.*
> *This frail vessel*
> *Thou emptiest again and again*
> *And fillest again and again*
> *Ever with fresh life.*

All these quotations reflect the same idea. The human organism is only an instrument of the Spirit. Health has the quality of being fully usable. This instrument can be used to its fullest extent; it is not blocked. Disease implies a block in its use. A healthy flute is one which is quite clear, all its holes are open and it can be used to make any melody to suit the situation. Disease of the flute would be when some of its holes are blocked and so it can play only one or two notes. It cannot be used in all situations but only in those where these notes are operative – it can be used as a whistle. The flute that is sick has a compulsion to be used only as a whistle.

The measure of disease is: how much does a man need a situation to feel OK and how much does the situation need him to act in that particular way. In the lives of healthy men we find that the situation needed them much more than they needed the situation. The amount of OK feeling determine health in a man. Without conditions, he can react in an appropriate manner in all situations and does not need any particular situation to exist in order to feel OK.

Block as a delusion

Why is the flute blocked anyway? Why is it OK only as a whistle? Is it really blocked? *In reality there is no block.* The flute, having been blocked at some time in the past, imagines that it is still blocked. This delusion creates conditions for it to feel OK and it does not allow the flutist to use the other notes (which it imagines are blocked). Therefore, the block is nothing but a condition for feeling OK. He feels not-OK unless certain conditions are fulfilled. These conditions come from his delusion about himself and his situation. For example, he may feel, "If I can achieve, only then will I be cared for and loved." Delusion prevents us from seeing things as they are. The reader is asked to do this exercise: look around where you are sitting and count all objects which are green in colour. We are trying to test your observation. Now answer the following question: How many blue objects did you see? When you look at a particular thing in a particular way, everything else will get shut out from your observation.

Disease is a restriction of vision, it is a narrow way of looking at things. Only awareness of this delusion can remove it, just as light removes darkness. Delusion disappears only with awareness. Much of what meditation, philosophy and psychoanalysis have to do with is creating awareness of a person's false perception of the present. Homoeopathy is also based on this. Awareness of your delusion is created by the remedy by putting you in touch with the original situation from which this delusion came. Thus, it is based on the same truth: *Disease is delusion, awareness is cure.*

All this talk may sound esoteric and theoretical unless the reader looks at himself in the light of what he has understood so far. If you honestly look at yourself, you will see how you feel uncomfortable in many situations and how you cling to certain roles in which you feel OK. These situations in which you feel OK fulfil your conditions for feeling OK. You are compelled to act in a particular way even though some other type of action is appropriate. In most situations you have the option of deciding how to react, but always you almost choose to react in just one or two ways, no matter what the situation is. This fixed type of reaction, compulsion, comes from the fixed way you view yourself and the situation in front of you (obsession). *Both the obsession and the compulsion come from the perception you have of yourself in the situation; this is your basic delusion.*

Somewhere in the past or in earlier generation you will find that somebody had gone through a situation which necessitated this kind of behaviour. You may find more often than not that you were conceived when one of your parents was exactly passing through such a state of being, or such a situation might have originated sometime in your childhood, especially from the circumstances in your own family. If an orphan received no love from anybody and felt that nobody cared for him, there was therefore no sense in expressing his feelings for anybody. This reaction was appropriate in his childhood as it ensured his survival, but when he becomes an adult it persists and he still cannot communicate with anybody. He has the compulsive need not to talk even in situations where he is listened to. When he receives love he cannot accept it, he feels frequently (obsession) that he is uncared for, and therefore is forced to be reserved (compulsion). This comes from a fixed feeling about himself, that no one loves him. The remnant of the past situations will make him judge all situations in the same way even though he may be exposed to several situations where he is cared for, wanted, respected and loved. Still he will persist in this same type of reaction. He will also choose to be in places where he does not receive love, which will confirm his feeling of being unwanted. When he is loved, he may move away.

Look at yourself

The idea of this example is for you to look at yourself, and to see what your obsessions and compulsions are, in what way you feel restricted and in which situations you are more comfortable and why. From this you will get an idea of your own fixed ideas and fears, and your own actions and compulsions, and you are able to glimpse your viewpoint of the whole situation and find that this is a delusion. Such an awareness can make a change.

Health as adaptation

When we examine the qualities of a healthy human we find general and psychological qualities as well as his local anatomy and physiological structure. In his general and psychological state we may be able to point out a certain range of qualities as normal or healthy. For example, normal temperature, sweating pattern, appetite, heart and respiratory rate, blood pressure, posture, sleep pattern, menstrual pattern, sexual pattern, etc. In the mind such a quantification is more difficult as regards to emotional and intellectual qualities, yet we are able to judge that there is a certain range of anger, fear, memory, intelligence, reasoning, affection, etc., which can be said to be normal. In the local parts too there are ranges of normalcy like the amount of acidity in the stomach or renal and liver functions, etc. The structure of the body also has a normalcy: height, weight, structure of the hands and feet, the face, etc. Any change in the structural alignment can be considered abnormal or unhealthy.

In the healthy condition of man too, we see a posture of mind and body. This posture is an adaptation response, i.e. it has been erected to suit or to survive a particular situation. Man evolved from the ape and developed special qualities and his own individual posture in order to survive in the new situation. The ape lives on trees and eats fruits. At some point in time, the situation (probably destruction of forests in some parts) necessitated that the ape come down from the tree and start hunting in order to survive. This is the original situation of man for which a change was necessary, a new adaptation was called for. Man had to build a shelter for himself and he had no natural talent for this since he was used to living on the tree tops. To build a house, protect himself against natural dangers and to hunt (that too, without any natural advantages like speed or claws), man required:

- Intelligence and creativity;
- To live in groups and identify with a group;
- To maintain peace within the group, yet fiercely protect it and its territory from other groups;
- To develop tools and weapons to help him hunt and construct.

All this, which he had to do in order to survive, created the changes which we call evolution from ape into human. So he had to:

- Adopt the straight posture so that he could use his instruments;
- Develop dexterity with his hands;
- Have an intelligent and creative mind;
- Have social feelings and peace within the group, and yet be defensive.

The whole general and local adaptation to the original situation resulted in the human form, and in this human form the mental and the general state are in perfect harmony with the functioning and the structure of all parts and systems. They are in tune with each other, made for each other, and have come as an adaptation to the same situation.

In health too, man has conditions to feel OK. For example, one of the conditions is, "I am not-OK if my life is in danger and I am OK if I reach the position of safety." Another could be: "I am not-OK if the group around me is in turmoil and I am OK if everything is going well within my society." Therefore, even the healthy man has conditions to feel OK. But there is a big difference between these conditions and the conditions of a diseased man.

The differences between situational stress and the stress of a diseased state

When the stress is produced by the situation alone, the state is proportionate and suitable to that stress factor. So, when the situation is over and there is another one, the healthy man will be able to change the posture entirely to suit the new one. One major difference between situational stress and stress from disease is that *in situational stress (i.e. when man is healthy), he feels OK about himself and experiences himself to be no different from others. In a disease state he feels himself separated and special in a negative way.* Let us take the following example.

Mahatma Gandhi and his son Harilal

Gandhi writes in his autobiography that he initially imitated the British ways and customs, trying in some way to establish an equality with the British. Despite his efforts, his sense of self-respect was no doubt still quite unsatisfied when his son Harilal was born. Gandhi later went to South Africa and was thrown out of the white man's compartment, from which time his sense of suffering an injustice aggravated and he realized that unless he fought back and disobeyed, nothing would change. His main features were:

– Sensitive to injustice;
– Sensitive ego; to hurt;
– Disobedience.

These were almost justified by his circumstances and therefore quite healthy. In fact, we know the circumstances needed Gandhi much more than Gandhi needed them.

Harilal's is however a totally different story. Born with the root of the state of his father (the *Staphysagria* root) he developed the same feelings (of injustice and hurt ego) but there was no situational cause to justify this state.

Harilal no doubt had a censorious father but, unlike the British, Gandhi was well intentioned. Harilal could have easily seen this and would not have needed to react badly. But, the root within him, brought about the same state even though the situation did not call for it.

Harilal broke away from his father, became a Muslim, took to alcohol, did not even attend to his father's funeral and six months later died in a brothel. He had the same symptoms:

- Sensitive to injustice;
- Sensitive ego; to hurt;
- Disobedience.

Harilal reacted to Gandhi in the same way as Gandhi reacted to the British. But Gandhi was healthy, his state was situational, so he was OK with himself; he had space for others too. Harilal's state was due to his delusion about his situation. He had tried to create a situation to justify it. He must have felt very much not-OK with himself – and consequently had very little space for others.

Ego and delusion

There are many situations which call for an adaptation response for survival. In these actual situations, man feels OK because he feels at one with the whole world, even though he is at a disadvantage. *The man who feels separate is not one with a disadvantage, but is one with the delusion of a disadvantage.*

A lame man has a specific disadvantage compared to the rest of the world, but he never feels separate from the rest of the world. He feels equal to everybody, only he is lame. So, he will adopt a survival mechanism; but whilst adopting this survival mechanism he still feels OK about himself. He is really not in an OK situation, but he feels OK himself. He knows that basically he is OK but for this particular disadvantage. It is not he who is not-OK, but it is his situation. The situation is the problem, and not he. The coping mechanism or the adaptation posture he adopts are still OK. Because he is OK, he has space for other people, he is without conditions for others, and so he can allow them to be.

The tragedy, therefore, is that one who is really at a disadvantage feels more OK than one who is not. The man who has two feet and can walk and run, but feels he is lame, has a big problem. *He does not know that he feels he is lame.* If he knew that, he would not feel lame anymore. *The delusion is hidden, never explicit.* The man feels disadvantaged in some way, but he does not know which way. All his pattern and reactions are coming from the hidden past.

Delusion

The lame man, with a lame man's behaviour, has a son, and the son adopts the pattern of behaviour of a lame man though he is not lame. He feels disadvantaged but he does not know why. He holds on to other people for support; he has conditions for others; he has fears, obsessions and compulsions all of which he cannot understand. He has an established pattern of reaction without the cause. When he feels disadvantaged without knowing why, severe not-OK feelings come to him. He feels (though being unaware of it) like a lame man, without being lame; therefore, something must be wrong with *him* not with the situation. He feels more and more isolated from the rest of the world. In order to feel OK with these feelings he has severe conditions for other people, and the moment he has conditions, his space has gone, he can no longer allow them to be as they are and can only think of others in terms of what they can give and take away from him.

Ego

The delusion attaches itself to the ego. The ego feels at a disadvantage, with loss of identity, individuality, security or prestige, etc., but does not know why. Then the ego tries to set up the situation exactly, so that it can justify its own feelings and conditions without justification; so it attempts to bring in the justification by creating the very situation.

The situation created the state, the state created the pattern of behaviour, the pattern of behaviour affected the ego and the ego created the situation so that this pattern of behaviour can be justified. A vicious cycle is formed. However much the ego tries to create the situation, it is not fully able to do it, and so the feelings always remain unjustified and out of proportion. Also, somewhere inside, the person knows that he has created the situation. *Awareness* of the significance of one's fears, compulsions and obsessions in terms of the situation which justifies such behaviour can result in cure.

To summarize: a situation where a man is disadvantaged creates a posture, a pattern of behaviour and thinking, with certain fears, compulsions and obsessions. This helps the man to survive in that situation. When the situation has passed, the pattern of behaviour, with its obsessions and compulsions, will remain. So, the man has the feeling that unless he acts in that way, his survival is threatened. Out of this delusion, he develops his feelings and compulsions, and this is disease. This applies to both body and mind. We have referred to this concept of disease earlier as "unsuitable reaction".

Disease hooks on to the ego very easily. Why, and what is the effect of this? Ego is that part of man which make him feel individual or separate; it gives him a feeling of identity. It is healthy because it also gives him motivation for doing something on his own and for making progress. A cow is chewing the cud, sitting quietly; whether you call it by one or another name, English cow or Indian cow or king, queen or servant cow, it will chew the cud in the same fashion without any change whatsoever. It just does not bother about its separateness, individuality, name or identity, and so the cow remains the same for millions of years without building houses or nuclear weapons. The quality of its milk cannot change; it does not pasteurize it or set up dairies! This example is to highlight the role of the ego in man's development – it gives him separateness. It also gives him the urge to protect his identity and keep him on par with others, if not ahead, and it is that in him which makes him value his name or identity as more important than his life. Man is prepared to neglect his health, his life even, for the protection of his identity, name or ego. Individual identity is fiercely protected – countries go to war for this and millions have died. *My* religion, *my* country, *my* name, *my* family – these may become more important than life itself.

Once we understand this, we can see that in disease there is a pattern of compulsion and obsession. For survival, a man develops fears and conditions, or compulsions. For example the man who has been surrounded by thieves develops a compulsion to lock his doors at night, and develops fear of being robbed. This pattern persists. If his money gets stolen, he will be poor and so may not be able to eat. The urge for survival creates caution; this is common to all beings, but the much greater stress is from the ego. If I become poor, what will happen to my name and position? What will others think about me? So, the ego question becomes equally or even more important, which creates a much greater stress. He feels more and more disadvantaged, his fear will make him feel more and more separate and this has to do with his ego.

Animals do not have this ego problem and therefore disease affects them only at the level of survival. It will be survival stress alone. If an animal is subjected to long periods of pursuit, it will develop fear, and the pattern may persist. But it will not develop the feeling "I will lose my position because I am pursued and I am therefore at a special disadvantage." It will only feel, "I am being chased; what will happen to me?" Much more is involved in a human because these fears put man at a special disadvantage compared with other people. His ego is easily excited: this is because his ego is always trying to keep up with others – his individuality and identity are important. The feeling is: "I am not as good as other people are; I am not-OK, unless I do this or that, and I have to be OK because my ego is involved."

Therefore, humans have many more disease states than animals; the animal Materia Medica would be smaller, because the situations which animals are exposed to are less varied and stressful; they have only to do with survival.

In an animal, it is how to survive in a situation; but in a human, how to keep the ego up becomes very important. A woman in her in-laws' house is being insulted, but she is secure enough, she is being given food; so, survival is not the issue, ego is. Her importance, her name, her identity are important and this creates problems for her.

Some of our problems are ego problems, others are survival problems. But many involve both. In health, a man's ego makes him feel individual but not special. He has an identity and name but he is not above or below others. He is OK. He feels equal to others and basically OK with himself – this is health. Health is affected by a delusion, which create separateness; he feels not-OK and at a disadvantage and must fulfil conditions to feel on par with others.

We have seen then, that disease is a delusion, but there is a bigger delusion that this and that delusion is ego. Ego is a delusion, even in health. So we may say that ego is a healthy delusion. It is healthy because it keeps man progressing, but in reality the ego is part of the survival mechanism of the human species. In the human there is his own survival and his ego, but ego is a part of the urge for survival of the whole species; it makes the species survive. Ego, mind, sexuality, the survival instinct, are all in-built mechanisms in a human for the survival of the species, and this survival is part of the plan of the universe. In reality our sense of identity is a delusion that makes this "machine" work better. Man is like a car which is given a name by its Builder, and so given a feeling that it is something different and special so that it will work faster and better.

Therefore, we have two identities: one as the human with an individuality or the ego, and secondly our deeper identity as the spirit or consciousness or energy that vibrates with the energy of the whole universe. At this second level, the ego is a delusion and at the first level, disease is a delusion. At the level where ego is a delusion this has not to do

41

with health but with spirituality. To be healthy one need not be spiritual, one can and must have an ego. Ego is not an unhealthy part of us. Just as we transcend disease through awareness, the delusion of the ego can also be transcended by awareness. The difference between these kinds of awareness is that in the first case, namely to see one's disease as a delusion, the mind itself can be used to create the awareness, whereas in the second case, i.e. to see that ego itself is a delusion (spiritual awareness), the mind itself has to be transcended and consciousness has to become aware of itself, aware of this delusion. One has to still the mind and then the delusion of the ego can be seen or experienced.

This is spirituality – it is experimental. Disease is a delusion; if you cure disease, you come to health; in health there is ego. Ego is a delusion, the body is a delusion, the sense of identity is a delusion – transcend these and you will reach the highest level of spirituality. *The mission of the physician is to restore the sick to health, to cure as it is termed.* It is enough to understand that there is a difference between spiritual awareness and awareness of one's disease.

7

NATURE'S LAW OF CURE

Discoveries in science and progress in art, literature, spirituality, philosophy, technology and other fields of human endeavour, all fit into a pattern. Similarly, progress in medicine and medical discoveries occurred when they were most wanted.

The earliest sensible practice in medicine was to alleviate the symptom or pain of the patient. When a finger is burnt, we automatically dip it in cold water. This is a natural reflex. When pain in some part of the body becomes unbearable, we naturally seek relief in some way or other. If there is bleeding, there are in-built mechanisms which try to stop it. If there is much pain, pain-killing substances are produced by the body itself. As human technology progressed, more stress, more accidents and hence more pain resulted. Nature, by itself, could not handle these and therefore prompted human ingenuity to discover extensions of its relieving methods. A part of modern medicine has to do with drugs aimed at giving instant relief. Surgery too is an extension of nature's idea. When there is a cut on the skin, natural processes of closing the wound and healing are set in motion. When there is a foreign particle in the body, the system will try to throw it out. It is as if the body had an in-built surgeon. Human progress demanded more than the capacity of this in-built surgeon, and surgery came into being. The fight against infections too was originally the domain of pure nature, but as human civilization crowded people together, infections increased to an intensity beyond nature's capacity to fight them alone. Antibiotics became a necessity and this led to Dr. Alexander Fleming discovery of penicillin, the first antibiotic.

Despite the progress in pain relievers, surgery and antibiotics, the biggest and most basic problem in human health remained unsolved. What remained unsolved was disease itself, the dynamic unhealthy state of the whole being.

We have seen in the previous chapters that disease is a posture, a state of being of the person which is inappropriate in his present situation. How do we naturally cure ourselves of such states? Take the example of the person who is to appear for an interview. You see him trembling with fear, pacing up and down, panic writ large over his face. What do you tell him? You tell him: "Why are you so scared? Are you going to face a lion?" From this you will often see him tense up a little more for a moment and then he will relax.

Let us examine how this happened. Firstly, we realize that the man was reacting disproportionately to the situation. By asking him: "Are you going to face a lion?", you were in fact telling him: "You are reacting as if you were facing a lion, but that is not the situation now." By confronting him with an imaginary situation to which his present reaction would have been appropriate, you make him perceive that the reality is different. This perception checks his overreaction.

Let me give a personal example. One day I started my car and heard a funny noise from the engine. The car was moving in a jerky fashion. I was quite hesitant to take the car out. There was a fear that it would break down on the way. When I looked at my fear, I found it disproportionate to the situation. I asked myself: "After all, why am I acting as if I were going to drive in the middle of an African jungle?" This made me feel relaxed and I could take the car without much hesitation or fear.

Here, too, the same process worked. By becoming aware of my false perception of reality (delusion, as if the city were a jungle), my inappropriate and exaggerated response was checked and reversed.

Now, we can relate these examples to our favourite illustration, namely the man, dog and lion.

When a man who is being chased by a dog is running as if from a lion, this is his state of mind (disease). How does he naturally cure himself? He does so by saying to himself: "Hey! Why am I running from this dog as if it were a lion?" This will allow him to calm down. Palliative or diversionary measures will not help; telling him to be bold or telling him a joke will do no good. The only way he can be cured is by the homoeopathic way, which is to paint before him an imaginary (non-existent) situation for which his reaction would have been appropriate. In other words, when he says to himself: "Why am I running as if there were a lion?", he realizes that he is creating (without any external reason) in his imagination a situation for which his actions are appropriate, and as soon as he does so, he realizes that he is overreacting, and the process of cure starts.

So far we have given examples concerning the mental process. This may give the impression that the Law of cure applies only to mental states. This is not so. The same process which we can easily identify in mind, also takes place in the whole organism without our being mentally aware of it. When the body overreacts, the same process takes place, just as when there is mental overreactions. For example if the inflammation is out of proportion to the factor which caused it, the organism checks this overreactions by becoming conscious of it.

In fact (as we shall see in later chapters, especially in "Mind and body"), the body and mind are not separate but form a part of the underlying unity which is pure consciousness. It is at this level that true awareness and perception occur and cure takes place by the *Law of similars*. This is nature's way and it has been the curative method from time immemorial. Homoeopathy is based precisely on this natural process of cure. A homoeopathic medicine is one that is capable of producing a state similar to the state in which the person already is. By producing such a state, it creates an impression or image of the original situation for which that state would be an appropriate response. This is just like creating the impression of a lion in the man who trembles before the interview, or creating the image of an African jungle when I am scared of taking out my troublesome car. The homoeopathic remedy works by the same process, i.e. by making the organism aware of its delusion and thus checking its overreactions. Homoeopathy is thus the human application of nature's Law of cure, a law that existed as long before Hahnemann as the Law of gravity did before Newton. Human progress and society created dynamic disturbances too intense and deep for the organism to handle on its own. The discovery and hence application of nature's method of cure of (dynamic) disease was not an accident.

The time was ripe for the discovery of the Law of Homoeopathy (like cures like) and it led Hahnemann to perceive the dynamic concept of disease, which also provides the basis for an understanding of disease and its cure.

Hahnemann's major contribution was the discovery that drugs produce specific states of being which they can cure when given to people with similar states. Here we can make a comparison between Psychotherapy and Homoeopathy. The aim of both is to make the patient well. Both recognize that illness is an emotional state of being and that it is a survival mechanism which is good in a particular situation, but persists after the situation is over. The idea of Freudian analysis seems to be that cure is possible through reliving the experience or situation and thereby understanding the origin of the state. Other methods of psychotherapy are also based on similar principles. These methods possibly represent a way of applying the Law of similars. As far as I can see, one of the big disadvantages of this method is in the treatment of (inherited) emotional states where the original situation that caused the state may not be in the lifetime of the person but in the lifetime of his parents, or even may date back to earlier generations. Thus, the person is born with a state, and even as a child without any situation, he manifests great restlessness, irritability, fear, jealousy, etc. Just as it sounds ridiculous to subject such an infant to Psychotherapy, we often see the same state continuing in adulthood. Here, Homoeopathy scores over Psychotherapy since it handles not only states originating in the lifetime of the person, but also what comes over from previous generations.

The homoeopathic method concerns itself with *what* is rather than *why* is (which is often not easy to trace). The totality of the patient's emotional state is taken as fact and it is not mandatory to know exactly why it exists in order to find the remedy. This eliminates a lot of theorizing and interpretation because different schools of Psychology have different theories about the origin of particular states.

The third and probably greatest practical advantage is that Homoeopathy uses the physical general symptoms of the patient in order to confirm the impression about his or her emotional state. More than any other system so far, we have a tested connection between the emotional and physical states. This not only makes it easier to find the similar remedy but also greatly enlarges the scope of therapy to include ailments with predominantly physical problems. Thus, Homoeopathy acts more quickly, surely and gently than Psychoanalysis and therapy in most cases; and its application is much wider.

Homoeopathy does the job beautifully of making the man look at himself and the set up he has made. It allows him to be more in the present, which is the real measure of health.

45

8

THE EVOLUTION OF HOMOEOPATHY

Hahnemann's famous experiment of Cinchona bark was the beginning of a new method of treatment. It took place in the year 1790. Hahnemann discovered that Cinchona, which was famed for its curative power on malaria, when taken by him in a healthy state, produced in him symptoms similar to malaria. It gave him the clue that drugs can cure in the sick what they can cause in the healthy.

From this idea, Hahnemann started testing several drugs on himself and some volunteers to ascertain what effects they could produce on healthy people, so that he could use these drugs when he found similar effects in sick people. These testings are called provings. Initially, Hahnemann employed crude (material) doses of drugs for proving and treatment.

Local action of drugs

In 1796, Hahnemann published his first treatise called "Essay on a New Principle for Ascertaining the Curative Powers of Drugs". On reading this essay it is evident that Hahnemann's ideas were far from fully mature at that stage. He believed that drugs act merely on organs and cause functional and structural changes locally. He tried to use this new idea in relation to individual organs. Let me quote some examples:

> "Since *Conium* produces pain in the glands, it may be the best remedy for painful induration of glands and cancer."

One quotation in particular is worth citing (page 271, 3rd paragraph; all quotations in this chapter are from Hahnemann's "Lesser Writings"):

> "The water hemlock (*Cicuta virosa*) causes, among other symptoms, violent burning in the throat and stomach, tetanus, tonic cramp, true epilepsy; all diseases for which we require efficient remedies, one of which, it may be hoped, will be found in this powerfully acting root, in the hands of the cautious but bold physician."

Here you can see that Hahnemann considered tetanus, cramps and epilepsy all as diseases. He doesn't as yet seem to be clear about the difference between the terms "disease" and "symptoms of disease".

He also says: "Coffee produces and therefore cures headache." Again, the distinction is not made between curing the symptoms and curing the patient.

47

He also tries to explain the drug effects in pathological terms, for example: "*Bella-donna* produces torpor of the lymphatic system", and "*Conium* produces excitant action on the lymphatic system." Though he mentions the term "totality of symptoms", yet he mainly refers to a single symptom as being caused and cured by a drug.

At page 281, paragraph 2, he says:

> "The pansy violet (*Viola tricolor*' at first increases cutaneous eruptions, and thus shows its power to pruuuce skin diseases, and consequently to cure the same, effectually and permanently."

He uses the word "skin disease" which became an anathema to him in his later works, where he insists that there are no skin diseases but diseases which manifest on the skin. In 1796 we see him still trying to fit the proving symptoms into nosological patterns. For example, he says of *Nux vomica*: "It may be useful in apoplexy or intermittent fever." He first used *Nux vomica* in cases of dysentery with cramps in abdomen. It is obvious that his provings were in crude doses. At that time Hahnemann also used for treatment fairly large doses of drugs. However, we have to admit that even at this early stage, in the various examples he has given, he has mostly referred to the nervous and mental effects of the drugs and only sometimes to the organ affinities. Another thing that is evident from this article is that in the initial provings he was not particular in recording exact symptoms. He was content to ascertain the broad effects of drugs like headaches, cramps, fever, etc. He also talks a lot of pathological effects of drugs, for example: "*Arsenicum* diminishes the tone of muscular fiber, by diminishing the proportion of cohesion and coagulability in the blood." Though he mentions "vital power", he is vague about it. For example he says: "Thus, *Arsenicum* generally seems to kill more by extinguishing the vital power and sensibility than by its corrosive and inflammatory power."

In this way, Hahnemann attempted to study the pathology of drugs in crude doses and tried to guess the pathology in which they may prove beneficial by similarity of action.

Discovery of potentization

In 1798, we see Hahnemann still prescribing drugs in crude doses. In an epidemic of fever he prescribes *Arnica* in a few grains and *Ignatia* from 2-3 grains. Then in 1801, in an article on "Cure and Prevention of Scarlet Fever", Hahnemann gives the first hint of a new process of drug preparation which is now called potentization.

Page 375, paragraph 1:

> "For external use I employed a tincture formed by adding one part of finely pulverized crude Opium to twenty parts of weak alcohol, letting it stand in a cool place for a week, and shaking it occasionally to promote the solution. For internal use, I take a drop of this tincture and mix it intimately with 500 drops of diluted alcohol, and one drop of this mixture likewise with other 500 drops of diluted alcohol, shaking the whole well.

Of this diluted tincture of *Opium* (which contains in every drop one five-millionth part of a grain of opium), one drop given internally was amply sufficient in the case of a child of four years of age, and two drops in that of a child of ten years, to remove the above state."

From this quotation, it is evident that Hahnemann considered the diluted drug as being weaker. It was yet to strike him that he stumbled upon one of the greatest discoveries in science!

The reason for this abrupt change is not very clear. The commonly held view is that Hahnemann wanted to diminish the toxicological effect of the drug and was experimenting to find out dilution upto which a drug could act beneficially.

This state of affairs continued until the year 1810 when the first edition of his book, the "Organon", was published. In this "Organon", there is no mention of the word "dynamic" or even "potency". He does however mention the term "vital force".

In 1809, he wrote a brilliant article which was entitled "Observation on the Three Current Methods of Treatment". In this article, he clearly differentiates between:

- Treatment of the name;
- Treatment of the symptom;
- Treatment of the cause.

He asks us to prescribe for the cause of disease, not on their symptoms nor on their names.

Dynamic concept of disease

The years between 1809 and 1813 were crucial as they witnessed a change/evolution in Hahnemann's thinking. In 1813, he wrote in "The Spirit of the Homoeopathic Medical Doctrine":

"Hence it is obvious that the diseases excited by the dynamic and special influence of morbific injurious agents can be described only as dynamical derangements of the vital character of the organism."

Two of the most important paragraphs contain these statements:

"Now as the condition of the organism and its healthy state depend solely on the state of the life which animates it, in like manner it follows that the altered state, which we term disease, consists in a condition altered originally only in its vital sensibilities and functions, irrespective of all chemical or mechanical principles; in short it must consist in an altered dynamical condition, a changed mode of being, whereby a change in the properties of the material component parts of the body is afterwards affected, which is necessary consequence of the morbidly altered condition of the living whole in every individual case."

"Moreover the influence of morbific agencies, which for the most part excite from without the various maladies to us, is generally so invisible and so immaterial that it is impossible that it can immediately either mechanically disturb or derange the component parts of our body in their arrangement and substance, or infuse any pernicious acrid fluid into our blood vessels whereby the mass of our humours can be chemically altered and destroyed – an inadmissible, improbable, gross invention of mechanical minds. The exciting causes of disease rather act by means of their special properties on the state of our life (on our health), only in dynamic manner, very similar to spiritual manner, and in as much as they first derange the organs of the higher rank and of the vital force, there occurs from this state of derangement, from this dynamic alteration of the living whole, an altered sensation (uneasiness, pains) and an altered activity (abnormal functions) of each individual organ and of all of them collectively, whereby there must also of necessity secondarily occur alteration of the juices in our vessels and secretional abnormal matters, the inevitable consequence of the altered vital character, which now differs from the healthy state."

Two stages in disease

These two paragraphs are most significant in terms of practice. Here Hahnemann splits up disease into two stages:

- Initial disturbance of organs of the higher rank and of the vital force;
- The above results in altered activity of other organs of the body.

These quotations represent a very great change in Hahnemann's thinking. Whereas you remember that in 1796, he had said *Ipecac* exerts an action on the nerves of the stomach and *Viola* produces skin disease, i.e. drugs act locally. He was now saying that drugs cannot act locally, they act through the centre.

How did this change in thinking come about? To me it seems obvious that this change is coincidental with his discovery that drugs act even when diluted beyond a point where they can have any physiological or toxicological properties. Not only do they act, but with each dilution and succussion (vigorous jerking) the effect of the drug gets stronger and stronger. If drugs still act in these dilutions and so powerfully too, then how do they act or where do they act?

At about the time Hahnemann was discovering the Law of similars, there was a resurgence of the vitalistic idea in medical thought. The vitalistic idea traces its origin very far back and had been coming up from time to time. The whole idea is of the presence of a force of life. The presence of this force differentiates the living from the non-living, and it is this force that tries to keep the organism healthy, that unites, controls and coordinates the various functions of various organ systems. This force can neither be seen nor measured but can be judged only from its effects.

The vital force

Disease is not an affection of the organs, but a disturbance in the vital force. As long as the vital force is in control, no part of the body can be affected. This idea of the vital force is opposed to the still popular concept which implicates individual organs as the cause of sickness and so leads to the practice of trying to make changes in them or even sometimes removing them.

It is only recently that medical thought is slowly changing and evolving into a holistic concept of man and his health, which means it is gradually realizing that man falls sick as a whole and that all the organ systems of the body are intricately connected to each other, and the body itself has a tremendous recuperative potential.

Medical philosophy is coming more and more to the conclusion that the mere treatment of symptoms and organs can only help temporarily and that it is the healing power of the body as a whole that has to be enhanced. But it is at a loss to know how this can be done.

In 1796, popular medicine was very much worse than it is today. Bloodletting and such other harmful treatments were very popular. But even at that time some medical philosophers were actively considering the idea of the existence of a vital force. One of them was Reil. Reil had published in Hufeland's Journal in 1796 an article entitled "Dissertation of Life Force". In the same year Hahnemann had published in the same journal his first major treatise, entitled "Essay on a New Principle..."

There is no doubt that Hahnemann must have read this article, and probably even agreed with it. But in 1796, he had still not discovered the significance of potentization. The idea of vital force must have remained in the back of his mind until 1810 when he started questioning how and where a potentized drug works.

Being also a chemist he must have known that beyond a particular dilution there is hardly any material of the drug left. Probably he must have reasoned that drugs, once diluted, have an effect on a different level. The only other level than the material one, could be that of energy. So, these drugs, when diluted and succussed, must be liberating some energy or force. Since one force can interact with another, there must be a force in the body on which these drugs must be acting. This force can be no other than the vital force. As a corollary, since drugs produce artificial diseases, diseases should be understood as a disturbance of this force.

This was the shift in Hahnemann's thinking – from considering disease as a material effect, to regarding it as a disturbance of the vital force. From this time onwards he would not refer to drugs as having local organ effects. From then on, the whole level of Homoeopathy changed.

Dynamic action of drugs

By 1813 he had come to the conclusion that the curative action of a drug does not lie in its local organ effect but rather in its dynamic effect, i.e. its effect on the vital force.

The initial disturbance, he said, is in the organs of the higher rank. What he meant was – the vital force acts primarily through certain controlling organ systems. The drug disturbs the vital force producing functional disturbance of these systems, and it is only through this that a drug produces local effects on various organs. Hahnemann did not exactly define which the organs of the "higher rank" are.

It is reasonable to assume that Hahnemann is referring to those organ systems which have a controlling influence on the rest of the body and whose disturbance produces a general effect on the whole organism. Which could these organ systems be? In other words, which are the organ systems whose disturbance produces a generalized effect?

With our present medical knowledge we can identify four such organ systems:

- *The Mind*: The disturbance of which can produce far reaching effects on the heart, lungs and almost every single part of the body. For example, when we are frightened there is palpitation, breathlessness, sweating, trembling, increased frequency of urination, etc.
- *The Nervous system*: Disorder of which produces various types of sensations, pains, sensitivities, etc., in various organs and parts of the body.
- *The Endocrine system*: We know that disturbances of the endocrine system (increase or decrease of hormones) can produce changes in various parts of the body. For example, the growth hormone can produce changes in bones, etc., the male and female hormones produce changes like puberty, menopause, etc. Cortisone can also produce several changes in the system.
- *The Immunological system*: The disturbance of this function can result in allergic and autoimmune disorders as well as the tendency to recurrent infections in several parts of the body.

P-N-E-I axis

The mind acts on the body through the other three systems (Neuro-Endocrine-Immunology). These four systems are intricately connected to each other, so that specific changes in the Psyche (P) can be associated with specific symptoms in the N-E-I systems, and these systems form together one axis, namely the P-N-E-I axis.

It is this axis that controls and regulates the other systems of the body. A specific disturbance in this axis will cause a specific state of the whole organism. The dynamic disturbance which a homoeopathic drug can cause must act through this axis. The symptoms experienced in this axis will therefore be observed first, rather than the local symptoms.

Each person is born with (or acquires during his lifetime) tendencies to certain specific organ pathologies. For example, a person may be born with a tendency to ischemic heart disease or rheumatoid arthritis or both together. These tendencies are not activated when there is a normal functioning of the P-N-E-I axis. But when there are changes in this axis, that is, when there is an unhealthy mental state associated with disturbed functioning of the nervous, endocrine or immunological systems, naturally these tendencies will be activated into pathological entities.

Central disturbance

The symptoms of the P-N-E-I axis together represent what I like to call the *central disturbance*. This central disturbance will naturally create disturbances in each organ system to a greater or lesser extent. The organ systems in which it will create most trouble do not depend only on the nature of the disturbance; they will also vary according to the organ susceptibility or weaknesses of different people.

Even though the drug *Bryonia* is known to have an affinity for pleura, if the person has a predominant tendency to thyroid problems, he may land up with thyroidis. But the thyroidis will have the characteristics of the *Bryonia* disturbance, such as pain in the thyroid worse from slightest motion. And even though *Bryonia* may not have been previously indicated in cases of thyroidis, it will still cure such a case. It is for this reason that we say that *if a remedy covers the central disturbance, then it will cure the particulars/ pathology even if that pathology is not typical to that remedy.*

We shall now examine which symptoms can be considered to be symptoms of the P-N-E-I or central disturbance in clinical terms.

–   *Symptoms of the mental state*: About the symptoms of the *mental state* of the patient Hahnemann writes in paragraph 211 of the "Organon" that to an accurately observing physician the symptoms of the mental state are the most obvious symptoms of the disease. They often chiefly determine the choice of the remedy.

–   *General symptoms*: They include:

1.   General modalities, for example reaction to heat or cold, noise, movement, etc. These are due to nervous sensitivity and show the peculiar sensitivity of the nervous system.

2.   Changes in appetite and thirst also represent a general disturbance of the body.

3.   Cravings and aversions may also represent a peculiar desire of the whole being.

4.   Sleep and dream are functions of the mind and the nervous system.

5.   Sweating patterns are related to the autonomic nervous system; the odour and stain of the sweat are due to generalized metabolic changes and do not represent pathology of the sweat glands. So, sweat symptoms are general symptoms.

6.   Disturbance of the sexual function and impulses, such as menstrual symptoms and climacteric in the female or increased or diminished libido in both sexes, etc., are a property of the endocrine system, as well as the mind and nervous systems.

7.   Tendencies to catch infections, to colds, warts, allergies, etc., are due to

immunological changes. These symptoms too are included in the general symptoms.

- Highly peculiar and characteristic symptoms which have no organic basis also directly represent the central or the P-N-E-I disturbance.

Certain symptoms in particular parts of the body should not be regarded as local problems; they have to be treated as a manifestation of the central disturbance. For example, the burning sensation of soles (as in *Sulphur*) does not represent any pathology of the feet but is rather a specific change in the nervous system. Similarly, the offensive urine of *Nitricum acidum* does not represent a disease of the kidneys but a manifestation of metabolic changes produced by the central disturbance. This can be understood when we see that *Nitricum acidum* also produces the same urinous odour of the sweat.

Similarly, the sun-headache of *Natrum muriaticum* also represents the nervous sensitivity to sun, the nerves of the head being most susceptible to this influence; so are the sweaty palms of *Silicea* or *Calcarea carbonica* manifestations of the central disturbance. Thus, many important characteristics of remedies do not represent pathology, but rather are a manifestation of the central disturbance.

- Though the above three represent the central disturbance, the peculiarities of the local pathology will be often found to be in tune with the central disturbance. In other words, the remedy that covers the central disturbance will also be found to cover the local peculiarities of pathology.

For example, swelling of the thyroid is a local symptom. It could be due to the person's tendency or susceptibility to develop thyroid problems. But if we say that the pain is aggravated from the slightest motion, we can see that a peculiar nervous element is added which, by no logic, can be explained merely by the person's organ susceptibility or tendency. Therefore, the peculiar nervous element, this modality, must be taken as a local expression of the central disturbance. In this way any modality or sensation that cannot be explained by the local organ pathology must necessarily be understood as representing the central disturbance.

Importance of the central disturbance

Therefore, when we seek to identify the central disturbance, we should first look at the mentals, then the generals and the characteristics. Only after this shall we check if the local peculiarities fit into the remedy. Lastly we may, out of curiosity, see if the type of pathology is also known to be curable or has been cured by that remedy. Even if this is not the case, it is enough if the central disturbance does so.

We often see that the remedy that covers the central disturbance in a case also covers the local symptoms, since both are produced by the same disturbance. But if we find that it is not so in a case, then it is safer to give the remedy which covers the central disturbance. We can assume that in a susceptible prover a drug would have produced the same local symptoms if only the proving had been thorough. This is because the central disturbance comes first and does not depend on the prover's individual organ susceptibility. The only exception to this is in the case of remedies, of which only a few particulars are known while the mentals and generals have not been well brought out. If the local peculiarities are covered by such a remedy, we must give it serious thought. Even a hint that it could produce a similar mental state is enough ground for us to prescribe it. Of course, in this case, we must make sure that the mental and general symptoms of the patient are not clearly covered or do not clearly fit into another remedy.

Most often, if we can clearly map out the mental state of the patient, the remedy emerges quite clearly, only to be doubly confirmed by its similarity also with the general and characteristic particular symptoms.

In the next section we shall thoroughly examine the ways and means to determine the exact mental state of remedies and patients.

Notes

1. Some so-called organ affinities of some remedies are not due to their dynamic effect (provings with potencies) but have come down as a remnant of their toxicological properties.

For example, the local irritant action on the bladder and urethra of crude *Cantharis* led many authors to mention the urinary tract as its sphere of action. This is very misleading. In a potentized dose, there is too little of *Cantharis* to produce such an irritant action. *Cantharis* becomes a remedy when its dynamic properties are found. It cannot have direct local action anywhere; it can only produce an effect on and through the central state. *Potentized remedies have no sphere of action except on the vital force*, as represented by the mind and the three controlling systems. When potentized, a drug loses its toxicological and local effect, but gains in its general/dynamic effect.

Bacteria in large numbers elicit a vital reaction and also produce local organ pathology. But when they are attenuated into vaccines, they lose their organ pathology and retain only the power to stimulate a vital reaction (they lose pathogenicity and retain antigenicity).

2. Despite the distinction between the toxicological and dynamic properties of a drug, many symptoms of our Materia Medica have been drawn from toxicological effects as well as provings in their crude form.

3. From Hahnemann's initial experiences with Homoeopathy, i.e. from 1790 to 1796, we can see that a second type of Homoeopathy is also possible: namely organ Homoeopathy or crude Homoeopathy. Here a remedy can be prescribed on the basis of the fact that in its crude form it has a direct action on the organ that is affected. It seems likely that the remedy may act locally, albeit in a homoeopathic fashion, and alleviate the local organ pathology for some time. But since the local pathology is born out of the central disturbance, this effect of the "local remedy" will be short. What is also possible

is that the local pathology might disappear and the disease may express itself in a more important organ, thus complicating the whole case further.

The question arises whether the whole of toxicology is useless to a homoeopath. Are there any symptoms that can be taken from toxicology as dynamic symptoms of the drug? The answer is simple. We have already defined the dynamic effect of a drug on the P-N-E-I system; therefore, even in toxicology, the functional effects of a drug (even in a crude or toxic dose) on the P-N-E-I system are to be taken as the dynamic symptoms of the drug. We can use only these symptoms for prescribing for patients. These symptoms alone will persist when the remedy is proved in potency. For example, in *Opium*, we are to take the toxicological effect, not its action on the kidney, spleen, etc., but the dullness or sopor it produces on the nervous system, and the joyous state it produces on the mind. These symptoms will yield to potentized *Opium*, together with any pathology or functional disorder that goes with them.

9

CENTRAL DISTURBANCE

Vital to developing the homoeopathic vision is the understanding of what is to be cured in disease. It is to be able to perceive, to feel and to know as the truth that disease is not something local but a disturbance of the whole being. It is to have the unshakable conviction that if we treat the disturbance at the centre, the local problems will be lessened. It is to understand that remedies in potency produce the central disturbance alone.

These points need to be stressed repeatedly, explained and exemplified so that they become a part of our thought process. This and only this conviction can make us staunch and successful homoeopaths and remove from our minds the confusions that arise in practice. This vision will make several things clear, and the rules and principles of Homoeopathy will become absolutely logical derivatives and no longer dogmas. Questions about the importance of mind, the differences in the various approaches to totality, the evaluation of symptoms, the importance of pathology, the site of action of a remedy, selection of potency and the prognosis of the case – all these questions will be solved quite easily once the vision develops. It is for this reason that I am writing this chapter.

We are going to examine the very same idea as in the previous chapters but this time from a new angle, namely through observations in practice. We are to begin with one of Hahnemann's most profound observations which he mentions in Aphorism 211 of the "Organon", namely that the mental state often chiefly determines the choice of the remedy. We are going to examine what a "mental state" means. We are going to talk about peculiar and characteristic symptoms and how they too represent the central disturbance. We will see the oneness of Kent's, Boger's and Boenninghausen's philosophies. We will use case illustrations to bring home all that we have said.

Mental state, not mental symptoms

Aphorism 211 from the "Organon" reads:

"This holds good to such an extent, that the state of the disposition of the patient chiefly determines the selection of the homoeopathic remedy, as being a decidedly characteristic symptom which can least of all remain concealed from the accurately observing physician."

Look at the words. It says "the state of disposition" – "the state" and not the "symptoms". Hahnemann did not write, "This holds true to such an extent that mental

57

symptoms determine the choice of remedy." Try to understand. He did not ask us to record the symptoms. He asked us to *understand* the "STATE" of the patient's mind. Don't write "Contradiction, intolerant of", or "Dictatorial", these are all mere symptoms. Understand the state of mind from which these symptoms come. If you look at the symptoms, you will be led to many remedies. But if you look at the state, there will be only one.

Every remedy has a different state of disposition

Aphorism 212:

> "The Creator of the therapeutic agents has also had particular regard to this main feature of all diseases, the altered state of the disposition and mind, for there is no powerful medicinal substance in the world which does not very notably alter the state of the disposition and mind in the healthy individual who tests it, *and every medicine does so in a different manner.*"

Each remedy has a particular state of mind which is characteristic to it. Each remedy produces a state. Each patient has a state of mind. If you compare symptoms, you will be lost in the jungle. If you understand the state, you will find that there is only one remedy which produces that state.

Aphorism 211 says: "The state of disposition... being characteristic, which can least of all remain concealed from the accurately *observing physician.*"

Look at the words. We say mental symptoms are most difficult to get, and Hahnemann says: "It can least of all remain concealed." From whom? "From the accurately observing physician". The word is "OBSERVING". If you are able to observe, no patient can hide his mental state from you. He never wrote: "It can least of all remain hidden from the accurately *enquiring* physician." The physician is an observer. Mental state has to be found mainly by observation, and not by enquiry. You have to look, you have to see, you have to understand and you have to feel the state. You have to experience the experience of the patient. This is the art of case taking, especially with mental symptoms. It is not just asking questions like: "Are you angry? Are you sad? Are you depressed?"

"The state of disposition of the patient often chiefly determines the *choice* of the homoeopathic remedy." The meaning of this can be beautifully illustrated through a case example.

Case

A woman with leucoderma came to me with the history that she had had a dark complexion earlier. Then she went to America where she spent three to four months. This was eleven years ago. In those three to four months, she did not know how, but the skin colour started fading on both arms and legs and both sides of the face together. Slowly over two to three months all the colour faded and she became absolutely white.

There was not a single brown (her natural skin colour) spot when I saw her. She had been to many skin specialists and after trying several therapies they told her that her melanocytes had been completely destroyed, and that she had no hope of ever getting back to her normal skin colour. They asked her to forget about it, since there was no treatment for this.

She did forget about it, but after nine years she developed a leucorrhea, which was very acrid and caused intense itching. She attempted to have the leucorrhea treated with allopathic medicines but without result. So, she came to me for the treatment of her leucorrhea.

When I asked her whether this was her normal colour, she said: "No, doctor, but forget about it. Nothing can be done, so don't bother about treating skin. You only give me medicine for the leucorrhea."

I explained to her the homoeopathic approach and told her that ours was a holistic treatment, and that she might get her skin spots back. She said: "Well, it's good if I get them back." I told her that it may not be all that good since she would be spotted like a leopard, but she was a sensible lady, and said: "If it's going to make me well, I don't mind looking like a spotted leopard for some time."

Then I began taking her case. I was asking her to tell me about her appetite, thirst, urine, stool, sleep, sweat, etc., but got nothing! No symptoms, damn it! Absolutely nothing. Now, what should I be doing? I did get a few symptoms. One was that she was a very warm-blooded patient, the second was that her leucorrhea was acrid and itching, and the third was that she liked to take long walks.

These were the only three symptoms I had elicited. After 1½ to 2 hours questioning, my pages were blank except for these three symptoms. What should I do? The pages were blank, my mind was blank. There was no remedy!

I was asking her:
— Tell me, are you irritable?

And she said:
— Sometimes.
— Are you anxious?
— No, nothing abnormal.

But then I noticed something. I observed that the interview was going on very beautifully, and I was enjoying it very much. It was very pleasant to be with this lady. She was very talkative but nothing she said could be used as a symptom. But she was very expressive, and in her talk there was a lot of humour and joking. I asked her a question and she gave humorous reply. I was laughing, she was laughing, my assistant was laughing, but there were no symptoms, on paper.

I asked her:

— How is your sleep?

She said:

— Sometimes it get disturbed.

— What time?

— Around two in the morning. I wake up sometimes and I don't go back to sleep for one or two hours.

— What do you do at that time?

— Oh, doctor! What can one do! I sit and talk with God. In fact we have a very pleasant conversation!

So, I said to her:

— Don't you think it is very wrong on your part to disturb God at these odd hours?

Look at the answer which came, quick and spontaneous. She said:

— Doctor, you have got it all wrong. I think when God doesn't sleep, he wakes me up to keep Him company.

The interview was going beautifully. But no symptoms. What should I do?

Perceiving the state of mind

And then, suddenly, I got it. She was expressing the most beautiful symptom of her case and that was "Loquacity with jesting" (Synthetic Repertory). So, I took these two symptoms, "Loquacity with jesting", and then added the symptoms, acrid leucorrhea, hot patient and desire for motion in open air.

From this, you come to the remedy *Kalium iodatum*, and you can be sure of your prescription, absolutely sure. I also found in Phatak's Repertory, that *Kalium iodatum* is listed in the rubric "Symmetrical affections".

"Loquacity with jesting" is one of the facets of the state of mind produced by *Kalium iodatum*. If you refer to the particular symptom "Skin, discolouration, white spots" in Kent's Repertory, you will find that *Kalium iodatum* is missing.

That is the point I want to emphasize. If you start with that rubric, you will certainly miss *Kalium iodatum*. That is why Hahnemann writes: "This holds true to such an extent that the state of disposition of the patient often chiefly determines the choice of the homoeopathic remedy."

The first principle supported by practice

So, the first principle that we derive from this case is:

> *A remedy that covers the mental state and general symptoms of a
> patient has got a greater possibility of curing than the one that covers
> the particulars.*

This is one of the lessons I have learned from practice. In so many cases, I have prescribed on mentals and generals, missing the particular symptoms in the Repertory, and I have been successful. But when I tried the reverse, I have always failed.

In the follow-up of this case, progressive changes in her skin could be seen. Slowly the skin colour was bilaterally symmetrically coming back.

Case

Another good case example comes from Dr. Jayesh Shah. It was a case of swelling of the thyroid gland, which was extremely painful. It had come up acutely, and they had done the blood test and found that it was autoimmune thyroidis (Hashimoto's disease). It is very difficult to treat and is an acute condition. The patient came to him for the first time and she wrote down the symptoms, because it was so painful she could not speak. She wrote: "I am not able to swallow, it pains me very very much in the thyroid."

So, he opened the Repertory: "External throat, goitre painful, swallowing, on". Look at this beautiful symptom. He found there one remedy: *Spongia tosta,* and he said: "Wonderful, what else can I ask, Kent has given me a gift." He gave *Spongia tosta* 200, and felt sure of his prescription.

The next day the patient came back and she wrote: "Previously I could spit the saliva out, but now, I cannot even do that; it so painful. It has doubled in intensity – the pain. Absolutely no relief!"

And then Dr. Jayesh suddenly realized that what she was expressing was "Aggravation from least motion". When you swallow, the thyroid moves up and down. So, when she swallowed, the thyroid moved and when she spat or spoke, the thyroid shook. The slightest motion, least motion, any motion causes not mere pain, but intense pain. *The least motion causes intense pain.* This expression is not to be found in *Spongia.* This is not the generality of *Spongia. Spongia* has: "Goitre, painful on swallowing". But when the patient says: "When I move that part a little bit, it causes such intense pain", that is not the expression of *Spongia.* This modality is met with by *Bryonia alba.* He gave *Bryonia,* and within twenty-four hours there was a dramatic improvement. *Bryonia* is totally missing in the rubric "Goitre" in Kent's Repertory!

The remedy that covers the particular symptoms, without covering the general symptoms does not cure; it does not act.

Remember, this remedy *Bryonia* does not have merely aggravation from motion. If a patient has acute inflammation of his knee and he moves his little finger and the knee pain gets worse, then it is *Bryonia.* Any patient with an inflamed knee will tell you that when he moves it has pain. That is not *Bryonia*. We should know how to select the symptom. It is aggravation from *any motion*. Our teachers have described it like this – the patient with an inflamed knee is lying down on the bed and the curtain is moving and he shouts: "Oh, stop that first!" That is the extent of aggravation from least motion in *Bryonia*. If this modality is found in any part of the body, it is only *Bryonia* in the whole Materia Medica, and no other remedy; and that is why *Spongia* failed.

This symptom was not a particular symptom. It was a general modality of *Bryonia*, expressed in the goitre.

Case

I will give you one more case. This is the case of a 9 year old child. He came with a cough, and it was a paroxysmal cough which he had for four months. I had given him *Drosera, Cuprum metallicum*, and several other remedies but they did not benefit him.

What can a homoeopath do when the indicated remedy fails? He has to look at the case again and prescribe. This is what I had been taught: "When the indicated remedy fails, it was not indicated. Find the correct one and it will work." I was not told: "When the indicated remedy fails give *Tuberculinum* or give *Sulphur*." They did not advocate these escape routes. They told us: "Break your head like a coconut and the case will open up." So, that is what we do.

I called the child to the clinic one day, at around 8.30 p.m., after I had finished my practice and made him sit down. I told him that it was either me or him today and that he was not moving from this spot until I found the remedy. I observed him for forty minutes, and then suddenly I noticed a strange thing. The child was coughing in a very peculiar manner. He would hold the side of his chair, and every time he coughed, the knees would go up and the head go down. I opened the "Cough" chapter in Kent's Repertory, trying to look up for this particular symptom, and read from the first to the last page, since I did not know from where to look for it; probably the whole chapter, because it was not until the very last page that I found the rubric "Cough, violent, spasmodic jerking of head forward and knees upward"! The remedy that is mentioned is *Theridion*.

Now, I was not very sure about *Theridion*, I asked his mother whether he coughed liked that always. She said: "Always. Even when he is lying down in his bed on his side, his body just comes together during the cough, doubles up, and it has been like this since the beginning."

When the mother was telling me all this, her voice was quite loud, and the child said to her: "Keep quiet mother, I am getting the vomiting sensation."

I looked up this second symptom, "Nausea, noise, from" in Kent's Repertory. There are only two remedies listed, *Cocculus* and *Theridion*, both in italics. I now had the courage to give *Theridion* 200 because it covered the generality of the case, the general modality of the case, and that was "Aggravation from noise". Tremendous sensitivity to noise, so much that it causes nausea. *Theridion* cured the child within twenty-four hours. Remarkable! I observed this child for six years and there was no more cough. To the very next child that came to me and coughed like that I gave *Theridion* with a lot of confidence, and failed miserably. The reason, there, was no sensitivity to noise or any other concomitant to indicate it.

Second principle – corollary to the first principle

So we may say:

If a remedy covers the particulars, without covering the generals and mentals, it is bound to fail.

Most of you agree with me that the two principles that I have given are not entirely novel. They have been emphasized by many masters of Homoeopathy.

Now, what is the explanation for these observations? The explanation is the key with which many doors of our philosophy can be opened and reduce the differences between various approaches and schools of thought in Homoeopathy.

One of the principles of Logic is that controversies arise out of ignorance. When there is knowledge, there is no quarrel, because truth is one. So, in persons who quarrel, there must be ignorance. We will try to resolve the conflict between the various schools and one explanation will resolve many of them.

Know what is curable in disease

In the third Aphorism of the "Organon", Hahnemann describes something very fundamental. The third Aphorism is perhaps one of the most important of the Organon. He says:

"If the physician clearly perceives what is to be cured in diseases, that is to say, in every individual case of disease (knowledge of disease, indication), if he clearly perceives what is curative in medicines, that is to say, in each individual medicine (knowledge of medicinal power), and if he knows how to adapt, according to clearly defined principles, what is curative in medicines to what he has discovered to be undoubtedly morbid in the patient, so that the recovery must ensure, to adapt it, as well in respect to the suitability of the medicine most appropriate according to its mode of action to the case before him (choice of the remedy, the medicine indicated), as also in respect to the exact mode of preparation and quantity of it required (proper dose) and the proper period for repeating the dose; if, finally, he knows the obstacles to recovery in each case, is aware how to remove them, so that the restoration may be permanent; then he understands how to treat judiciously and rationally, and he is the true practitioner of the healing art."

Get the meaning of it. "If the physician, clearly perceives, clearly understands what is to be cured *in diseases*." Does this make sense? Diseases have to be cured. Hahnemann writes in his first and second Aphorisms:

"The physician's high and only mission is to restore the sick to health, to cure, as it is termed.

The highest ideal of cure is rapid, gentle and permanent restoration of the health or removal or annihilation of the disease in its whole extent, in the shortest, most reliable and most harmless way, on easily comprehensible principles."

Cure is removal of disease. So, the disease has to be cured. Then why is he writing in the third Aphorism: "What is to be cured in disease?"

I consider the word "in" as being very important. The person who knows what is to be cured "in disease" will succeed. I am stressing this point again and again because it needs to be stressed. If we have a clear concept of what is to be cured *in* disease, we will cure. If we don't, we will not cure.

Step by step, we are going to use logic to try and find the answer to this question.

The first is Aphorism 116:

"Some symptoms are produced by the medicines more frequently – that is to say in many individuals, others more rarely or in few persons, some only in very few healthy bodies."

This refers to provings. When a remedy is proved, it produces some symptoms which are common to all the provers, some symptoms which are the symptoms of the individual provers. This means that a drug, when given to hundred provers will develop some symptoms which are common to all of them, some which are common to thirty or forty, and there will be some symptoms that only individual provers will produce.

Now, which are those common symptoms, that all provers will produce? If you read the "Materia Medica Pura", in the introduction to *Bryonia* and *Rhus toxicodendron*, Hahnemann observes that whoever be the prover, whatever be the symptom, *Bryonia* will be aggravated from motion and *Rhus toxicodendron* will be ameliorated by it. These are pure data of observation.

Mental state versus mental symptoms

This means that general modalities are common to all provers. In Aphorism 212, we have already read that each remedy produces a mental state in all provers which is peculiar to that remedy. Whoever be the prover, *Aconitum* will produce violence in the mind, *Stramonium* will produce terror and *Pulsatilla* will produce a tearful disposition. Hahnemann writes of *Aconitum* that it cannot be given to a calm person. So, the second thing a remedy produces that is common to all provers is a *mental state*.

Let us understand this "mental state" a little more. Why did he not write "mental symptoms"? Does a difference exist between "mental state" and "mental disease"? In Aphorism 211, Hahnemann says that all patients have a mental state on which a remedy is to be prescribed. That means every patient, whatever he may be suffering from, has a particular mental state. In much later Aphorisms, Hahnemann talks of the treatment of mental diseases. He says that mental disease symptoms are one-sided local diseases affecting the mind. Therefore, there would be symptoms and these symptoms will be mental symptoms, but they are not important because they are particular symptoms, local symptoms and one-sided symptoms. They belong to mental disease and to mental state. "Mental state" exists in everybody, in every single person. Whatever he is suffering from, eczema or asthma, he will have a mental state, and from this state you will select your remedy.

I would like to go a little further into this difference. In children you will get very prominent mental symptoms. If we want to get cases with fear of dark and of being alone of *Calcarea carbonica*, we will find it most prominently in children. If fear of dark and being alone represent an effect (pathology) at the level of mind, if they represent a disease of the mind, then we may rate these children as very much sick, because their highest level is affected intensely. Are they really so seriously sick even though they are full of vitality? If the fear of dark and being alone represent the mental disease, then these children must be the sickest people on this earth, and the person who is dying of cancer must be the healthiest, if he has only a few mental symptoms.

I am trying to point out that having mental symptoms does not necessarily mean that the mind is affected. Mind is a state which is produced in all diseases, and in all the provers. In "Lectures on Homoeopathic Philosophy", Kent mentions that you will find a *Calcarea* child who will not have any pathology for many years. If you leave the child untreated, only then will he develop pathology.

That means, those initial symptoms did not represent pathology at the level of mind; they represent a "state" that appeared first and then came the pathology. *The "state" comes first and it will be the last to go. The mental disease comes last in the hierarchy and it should be the first to go.*

The idea that unless the mental symptoms go, the person is not cured, is wrong. It is wrong if we think that he is not progressing in the direction of cure.

A person comes with lack of self-confidence and eczema. He says that his eczema is going, but the lack of confidence is still there. What would the interpretation be?

The lack of confidence preceded the eczema. The *Lycopodium* state came first and the eczema came later, just as in the child who is healthy and full of vitality, the *Calcarea* state is there but the pathology comes later.

So, what happens in a proving? *In a proving, a remedy produces a state of being, a state at the level of mind and a state at the level of generalities first. Then, depending upon individual susceptibility, it will produce symptoms in various organs.*

First comes the central disturbance, the affections of parts later

The centre has to be captured first, this is the law of disease: *there can be no affection of the parts without the affection of the whole.* There can be no disease in the organs without central disturbance.

Our medicines are potentized. This means that there is no material dose remaining in them. There is no physiological effect. *Digitalis* has an effect on the heart in Physiology, not in Homoeopathy. In Homoeopathy, *Digitalis* potentized becomes a dynamic agent that causes a central disturbance at the level of mind and generalities *first*, and then there is tendency to heart trouble then it will be affected; and if his prostate is susceptible, this will be affected; if his liver is a weak point, it will affect his liver and if he has a tendency to insanity, he will become insane. *Digitalis* no longer remains a heart remedy.

Kent writes that it is one of the best remedies for prostate! Somebody writes that it is a good remedy for liver troubles and jaundice. Somebody else writes: "Vertigo from hunger is *Digitalis*." *Digitalis* is not vertigo, not heart, nor liver, lung or spleen. *Digitalis* is a dynamic disturbance, which it produces in all provers.

Potentized remedies have only dynamic general effect, not local

The term "local remedy", when it is used for a potentized drug is a misnomer. There are no local remedies when they are potentized. It is clearly written in "Organon" that remedies have dynamic effect *only*. Potentized remedies have dynamic effect *only*. There is no physiological, no pathological, no organic effect. The only local effect it has is on the tongue – it tastes sweet, or on olfaction – it smells alcohol!

So, what is the local affinity of homoeopathic medicines? What is their sphere of action? This point has to be clearly understood.

Particular symptoms depend on susceptibility of provers – hence incomplete

A well proved remedy, if proved further, will give you many particulars, but not as many more generals. All the particular symptoms for which you are searching can be missing. *Kalium iodatum* was not proved nor given as a remedy to a person who had a tendency to leucoderma. Therefore, you missed it, but the craving for motion in open air, bilaterally symmetrical affections, and the state of mind with loquacity and jesting, were produced in most of the provers.

Therefore, *if a remedy clearly produces mentals and generals, you can assume that remedy would have produced the same particulars (local effects).* But if you see a remedy that produces particulars, can you assume that it will produce the same mentals and generals? Impossible. Because it had the opportunity and it did not produce them.

That is why we say the remedy that covers mentals and generals has got much greater possibility of curing than one that covers particulars without covering mentals and generals.

It is the *central disturbance* that comes first, and then this central disturbance will go and act upon those organs which are more susceptible, and will produce the local trouble to which the patient is more susceptible, but with the modus operandi (type of characteristic action) of the central disturbance.

For example, if a person is susceptible to gastritis and you prove on him *Arsenicum album*, *Arsenicum album* will produce all its general symptoms and in the stomach it will produce burning better by warmth. If the same prover takes *Phosphorus*, he will have gastritis with burning in the stomach better by cold drinks.

Modalities represent the central disturbance

So, does the modality represent the central disturbance or the pathology? *The peculiar modality represents the central disturbance and not the pathology*. The peculiar modality will show you who is the culprit, the cause, *Arsenicum* or *Phosphorus*.

Suppose your house is susceptible to robbery and the robbery has taken place. Does this information give you the name of the culprit? No. The way in which the act of robbery was executed will give you the identity of the fellow at the centre who is causing all this trouble. The name of pathology will only point to the individual's tendency.

What is to be cured *in diseases*? It is the central disturbance that has to be cured in diseases, and not the pathology. That is the secret.

I like to compare disease with the Mafia. The Mafia organization (we may assume) is governed by certain rules and principles. The first rule of the Mafia is: *Only one Don can rule at the centre. Unless the Don controls the centre, he cannot act on the periphery.* The reverse is not applicable. They will not allow a second godfather to operate; there will be only one godfather, and *he has to control the centre*, otherwise he cannot operate his smuggling and other rackets.

This central disturbance is what we have identified in the previous chapter as P-N-E-I disturbance. Once you cure the central disturbance, then its aggravating influence on peripheral pathology will disappear. Once you remove the central disturbance, once you remove the P-N-E-I disturbance, its aggravating influence on the pathology will automatically disappear. If you remove the Mafia boss, all the smuggling and other activities will automatically stop. Try and stop the smuggling locally, and nothing will happen. Try to stop the drug racket and it may stop for the time being, but it will come back again. But if you identify the boss and hit him on the head, then everything will stop.

As long as you handle particulars as particulars, you will not succeed. The moment you catch the central thread of one remedy, the central thread of the patient, his P-N-E-I disturbance, everything will become clear.

The other thing that becomes clear is that since there is only one central or P-N-E-I disturbance, all the four systems must indicate the same remedy state.

67

That means, if a person has a mental state, you cannot prescribe on it alone. You must expect concomitants in the neuro-endocrine-immunologic systems. If you have a nervous symptom, you cannot prescribe on it alone, unless there is no contradiction at the level of mind-endocrine-immunologic systems.

Kent's non-pathognomonic symptoms

Once you understand this, three of the deadliest confusions and controversies in Homoeopathy will disappear. The first is that Kent said that in evaluation of symptoms, write them down in two columns: all those which are common to the pathology, write on one side and all those which are not common to the pathology, write on the other. He called these pathognomonic and non-pathognomonic symptoms. Those symptoms which do not represent pathology are important. Why? Because they represent the central disturbance. That is what he meant.

I say, treat the central disturbance. What is its significance? In a local complaint, all those symptoms which do not represent pathology must belong to the central disturbance.

Generalization of Boger

What did Boger say? Boger said: "All those symptoms which are characteristic (characteristic means uncommon), all those modalities which are characteristic, *generalize them*. They are not local, but general."

In the case cited earlier, that characteristic of *Bryonia* was not a local modality because it was peculiar. We can generalize it and take the general modality, "Least motion aggravates", and give *Bryonia*. This is Boger's approach; he generalized. What does he mean by the term "generalize"? He means that the characteristics of the locals are no longer local symptoms, but they are the symptoms of the central disturbance. We take them as our guides.

Concomitants of Boenninghausen

Boenninghausen uses the term "concomitants". What does he mean? He means that if you find a particular mental state, you cannot prescribe on it unless you have a concomitant from another sphere. What he meant was that there is only *one* disturbance. There cannot be two disturbances, and as there is only one disturbance, the "mental state" will necessarily have concomitants in other spheres. (The same Don has to operate every-where. Everywhere we have to see no one but him.) This is the basis of Boenninghausen's doctrine of concomitance.

The concomitant is to the totality what modality is to the symptom: *it is the differen-tiating factor*. In the symptom "Pain in joints" the modality of aggravation or amelioration from motion will differentiate remedies. Similarly in selecting from two or more remedies with a common symptom in one sphere, the concomitant from another sphere will make the choice clear.

Case

Here is the example of a man aged 23 years. He said; "Doctor, when I drink tea in the morning, the cup falls from my hand." This was his chief complaint. I asked:

— How does it fall? Do you drop things or do you feel weak or awkward?

He replied:

— No, doctor, actually what happens is that when I am holding the cup, my hand jerks and it falls.

— Does this happen every time you drink tea?

— No, no, it happens only in the morning after I get up.

— Does this happen every day in the morning?, and he said:

— No, doctor, it happens only if I could not sleep adequately the previous night. My normal time of going to sleep is 11.30 p.m., but if I am not able to sleep until 1 or 2 a.m., and I have to get up next morning at my normal time to go to work, then on that day, when I wake up, the cup will jerk from my hand, sure hundred percent.

I asked:

— This jerking will last for how long?

— It lasts only for one hour and then it goes.

He had been to famous neurologists in Bombay. One neurologist said that he could not really understand it. He called his condition "myoclonus", myoclonic jerks, and he advised the use of plastic cups!

So, what is the remedy? Let us assume that there were no other important symptoms in his case. This information led me to the remedy. I asked myself the question: "If it is worse from loss of sleep, why does it last precisely one hour, what can explain that?"

What happens when you lose sleep the previous night and get up in the morning at the same regular time, what is your state? Are you still sleepy, and for how long? For about one hour. That one hour is the time when you are sleepy, and after it, you get into a routine and become awake. But that one hour you are groggy, you are not fully awake, and this was the time he jerked. The symptom is not precisely "Loss of sleep aggravates", but he is aggravated when he is *half asleep*. Not fully sleepy, not fully awake. At this time, his nervous system is most sensitive and produces jerks.

I confirmed this symptom by one more question. I asked him: "Has it happened that you had to wake up much earlier than usual, say 4 or 5 a.m., if you have to welcome someone at the airport or the train terminal, and you are sitting there waiting for him, and at this time you are feeling sleepy, but you cannot sleep (that is also half asleep); does it happen at that time also? He replied instantly: "Yes doctor, how did you know? I jerk at that time also. That it the only other time I get these jerks, except in the morning.

It is when I have to remain awake for a long time and I am feeling sleepy but cannot sleep. That time I jerk."

Now, it was clear. He was aggravated when he was half asleep. I did not take "Jerking, when half asleep". I generalized this symptom – Boger's generalization – into the general modality, "Aggravated when half asleep". It is not given in Kent's Repertory. It is given in Phatak's Repertory. Four remedies are listed against this symptom, out of which I selected one, based on some other symptoms, and that was *Nitricum acidum*.

This modality was generalized because it was so peculiar. It was his "jerking" that was worse when half asleep. It was the modality of his central disturbance, his peculiar nervous sensitivity which was worse when half asleep.

So, once you understand that there are no local troubles and that medicines produce a general effect even from the local modalities, you can generalize and use Boger's approach.

Phatak's Repertory is based on Boger's approach. Boger's "Synoptic Key" is also based on this approach, and so is Boenninghausen's "Therapeutic Pocket Book". Boger's "Boenninghausen's Characteristics and Repertory" has to be used with this method: *by generalizing the characteristics which are local.* The local characteristics are not local symptoms, but they belong to the central disturbance: this is the philosophy. It is the central disturbance which has to be cured.

Summarizing

To summarize, we have to focus in every case on the central disturbance. It is the factor behind all local problems. It can be identified from the mental state and general symptoms. The local peculiarities are also indicative of the nature of the central disturbance and hence can be generalized (Boger). The central disturbance being the same all over, we can find its indications concomitantly in more than one sphere (Boenninghausen). The easiest way of identifying it (especially in illnesses with body pathology) is to under-stand the mental state (Kent). In the next section we shall focus on this last method and try to find the means of reaching into the mind of the patients.

10

DYNAMICS IN DISEASE

The following quotations from Hahnemann's "Organon" throw abundant light on the different levels of the human organism at which disease operates, and the relative importance of these levels in guiding us to an understanding of the nature of disease and its treatment.

Aphorism 201 of the sixth edition of the "Organon" reads:

"It is evident that man's vital force, when encumbered with a chronic disease which it is unable to overcome by its own powers, instinctively adopts the plan of developing a local malady on some external part, solely for this object, that by making and keeping in a diseased state this part which is not indispensable to human life, it may thereby silence the internal disease, which otherwise threatens to destroy the vital organs (and to deprive the patient of life), and that it may thereby, so to speak, transfer the internal disease to the vicarious local affection and, as it were, draw it thither. The presence of the local affection thus silences, for a time, the internal disease, though without being able either to cure it or to diminish it materially. The local affection, however, is never anything else than a part of the general disease, but a part of it, increased all in one direction by the organic vital force, and transferred to a less dangerous (external) part of the body, in order to allay the internal ailment. But, as has been said, by this local symptom that silences the internal disease, so far from anything being gained by the vital force towards diminishing or curing the whole malady, the internal disease, on the contrary, continues gradually, in spite of it, to increase, and Nature is constrained to enlarge and aggravate the local symptom always more and more, in order that it may still suffice as a substitute for the increased internal disease and may still keep it under. Old ulcers on the legs get worse as long as the internal psora is uncured, the chancre enlarges as long as the internal syphilis remains uncured, the fig warts increase and grow while the sycosis is not cured whereby the latter is rendered more and more difficult to cure, just as the general internal disease continues to increase as time goes on."

Aphorism 205 (footnote):

"I cannot therefore advise, for instance, the local extirpation of the so-called cancer of the lips and face (the product of highly developed

71

psora, not infrequently in conjunction with syphilis) by means of the arsenical remedy of Frère Cosme, not only because it is excessively painful and often fails, but more for this reason because, if this dynamic remedy should indeed succeed in freeing the affected part of the body from the malignant ulcer locally, the basic malady is thereby not diminished in the slightest, the preserving vital force is therefore necessitated to transfer the field of operation of the great internal malady to some more important part (as it does in every case of metastasis), and the consequence is blindness, deafness, insanity, suffocative asthma, dropsy, apoplexy, etc. But his ambiguous local liberation of the part from the malignant ulcer by the topical arsenical remedy only succeeds, after all, in those cases where the ulcer has not yet attained any great size, and when the vital force is still very energetic; but it is just in such a state of things that the complete internal cure of the whole original disease is also still practicable.

"The result is the same without previous cure of the inner miasm when cancer of the face or breast is removed by the knife alone and when encysted tumors are enucleated; something worse ensues, or at any rate death is hastened. This has been the case times without number, but the old school still goes on blindly in the same way in every new case, with the same disastrous results."

Footnote to page 55 of "Introduction of Organon" (Boericke's sixth edition):

"... and the dynamically affected nervous power seems to unload itself in the material products."

Page 56:

"It is only by destruction and sacrifice of a portion of the organism itself that unaided nature can save the patient in acute disease, and if death does not ensue, restore, though only slowly and imperfectly, the harmony of life-health."

Page 62:

"Or if the effect upon the local affection (still recent, perhaps) was of milder character, be thereby repelled from its seat by a species of ill-applied external Homoeopathy, the local symptom which has been established by nature on the skin for the relief of the internal disease, thus renewing the more dangerous internal malady, and by this repulsion of the local symptom compelling the vital force to effect a transference of a worse form of morbid action to other and more important parts."

Page 63:

"The vital force, in order to relieve the internal malady, sometimes produces indolent enlargements of the external glands."

Page 64:

> "They dried up discharging ulcers on the legs, established by the vital power for the relief of great internal suffering, with the oxides of lead and zinc, etc., with what sad results experience as shown in thousands of cases."

Page 64:

> "All the local affections, evacuations, and seemingly derivative efforts, set up and continued by the unintelligent vital force when left to its own resources, for the relief of the original chronic disease."

It is obvious from the above quotations that Hahnemann's idea of the mechanism of the vital force is as follows:

– The primary function of the vital force is to maintain man in a state of health.

– If attacked by a morbific agent (for example infection, drugs or strong emotions), to which he is susceptible, initially there is a general reaction: in other words, a functional disturbance of the whole body ensues (for example, fever, weakness, decreased appetite, increased thirst, irritability, etc.). These general and mental symptoms will vary according to the nature of the morbific agent. They are functional symptoms of the P-N-E-I systems. These systems are deranged first.

– The vital force tries to keep the disturbance restricted as far as possible to the general level, not allowing it to produce pathological changes in the organ systems.

– When the intensity of the disturbance exceeds the level which can be tolerated by the body (for example, when the temperature is raised too high for the body to tolerate), it allows the disturbance to produce local organ effects.

– The level of the general disturbance that can be tolerated by the body depends upon the condition of the body itself and of its important organs.

In cases of children where the organs are usually in a very good state and can bear a lot of general functional disturbances (for example a heart which can bear high fever), the vital force can afford a strong general disturbance and need not divert it into local pathology. That is why among children you often find cases with a strong general disturbance but very little pathology.

The best mental and general symptoms like fears, cravings and aversions can be elicited from children. When the organs become weaker and more fragile, their capacity to bear strong general disturbances decreases. Therefore, in older people the vital force has to maintain the general disturbance at its lowest. It does so by diverting a lot of pathology. That is why amongst older people you will get many cases where there are hardly any mental and general symptoms but vast pathological changes.

- This process of shifting the disturbance to the local parts also depends on the duration of the disturbance. The body may be in a position to bear a certain intensity of disturbance, but not for too long a time.

- When such a situation is reached, the vital force will allow the disturbance to localize but only in the least important part possible.

- Even when it allows the parts to be affected, it does not allow the disturbance to take full hold of these parts. That means, it tries to keep the pathology at a minimum level.

- When it allows the disturbance to spread to certain parts, it succeeds for the time being in reducing the level of the disturbance at the centre. In effect, it sacrifices the organ for the good of the organism.

These whole dynamics seem to me to closely resemble the dynamics of a country which has to deal with criminal agents (Mafia boss). Initially, the Mafia can only produce a generalized disturbance. The government will frustrate any attempt to produce local activity, but when the general disturbance produced by the Mafia boss becomes too much for the country to bear, the government will concede the least important part of the country to the Mafia, in an attempt to lessen the pressure it is under.

To give another example, there is a dam which prevents the water contained in the reservoir from damaging the vital structures around. When the pressure of the water becomes too much for the dam to bear and it threatens to give way, then the controlling authority will divert some of the water into areas which do not house vital structures. Thus, it sacrifices these areas for the good of the state.

A more familiar scene is of a ruffian entering a restaurant. He picks an argument with the owner. The quarrel goes on escalating. When it reaches a level where the scuffle threatens to damage the valuable articles in the restaurant, the owner asks the ruffian to step outside and the scuffle between them is carried on where there is the least damage to the valuable things in the restaurant.

- The total strength of disease at any one time will be the sum of the disturbance in the centre and the disturbance expressed as local organ affections (functional and pathological).

- If the strength of the disease force is very high (the water pressure is too strong) or the body's level of tolerance decreases (the dam becomes weak), or the disturbance is diverted from a local organ (the water is displaced from the area to which it was diverted by the controlling authority) – under these three conditions the vital force is compelled to allow the disturbance to spread to more vital parts.

- Which parts will be affected depends on two factors:

1. The parts to which the general disturbing factor has predilections; for example a drug that produces colicky, spasmodic pain will naturally affect organs like the intestines or ureters;

2. The individual's inherited or acquired organ weaknesses. For example, even though the *Bryonia* disturbance has an affinity for the pleura, a person who has got a predominant tendency to thyroid trouble will develop a thyroid affection with *Bryonia* modalities.

– When the vital force concedes a local part to the disturbance, the disturbance will produce an effect in accord with the weaknesses and tendencies of that part. But even so, the disturbance will show its own peculiar characteristics.

For example, when the Mafia boss commits a crime in an area, the type of crime will depend not only on his nature but also on the local tendencies. Even though the boss may like to do drug trafficking, if there is a strong tendency towards smuggling in this area, then this is what he will do. But the manner and method of smuggling will be characteristic of him.

– If the disease progresses further, a stage will be reached where the vital force concedes parts of the mind, nervous, endocrine or immunological systems to pathology, producing in these most important parts not mere functional disturbances but manifest pathology.

– The level of the fight between the vital force and the disease force gives a clue to the strength of the vitality. If with a strong central disturbance you find very little pathology, the level of vitality is high. Conversely, with a weak central disturbance, if you find severe pathology, then it means that the level of vitality is low; and in these cases the prognosis is guarded.

– From the above discussion, we can see that there are two distinct levels of disease: 1) central or general, and 2) peripheral or local.

– By *central disturbance* we mean changes in the functions of the P-N-E-I system. These manifest themselves as mental symptoms, general symptoms and also specific changes in some parts. They will disappear along with the central disturbance or will change when the central disturbance changes. They will be directly influenced by central modalities and they will be highly characteristic symptoms. They do not represent the seat of the disease. They are among the first symptoms to come and there are among the last symptoms to go; whereas pathological symptoms are the last to appear and will be the first to disappear. These symptoms of the central disturbance will appear as concomitant symptoms to pathology (sun headaches as concomitant to eczema, or nausea as concomitant to headache) and therefore represent the central disturbance more than the local pathological symptoms. This is the reason why Boenninghausen laid so much stress on concomitants.

– It is obvious that local pathology will have some symptoms which are common to it. When the Mafia boss indulges in smuggling, some of the features of the activities will be common to whoever does the smuggling. If, for example, the local pathology is ischemic heart disease, pain in the chest from exertion is going to be a common symptom of the pathology and is hardly going to indicate the nature of the central disturbance.

— It is also obvious that since it is the central disturbance that is being diverted into local pathology, the local symptoms will be in tune with the central disturbance to some extent. You will find the local peculiarities (those which are not common to the pathology) covered by the same remedy which covers the central disturbance. A particular patient of ischemic heart disease complains of having pain in the chest worse from exertion and better from warmth and rest. The chest pain, worse from exertion and relieved by rest is common to ischemic heart disease and is diagnostic of it, but the peculiarity, namely amelioration by warmth, which is uncommon to ischemic heart disease, has to represent the central disturbance and therefore indicates the curative remedy. Thus, we can see the wisdom of Boger who considered all peculiar modalities and sensations as generals.

— This simple explanation is very useful in practice, but the discerning reader can see one flaw, which is that it assumes that vital force and disease force are two separate entities like the government and the Mafia. From our earlier understanding, we know that disease is not a separate entity but only a disturbance of the vital force. Hahnemann was fully aware of this. The vital force has a life preserving function and also the aim of fulfilling the organism's purpose. When it is disturbed, it tries to keep its own disturbance from affecting the more important organs (important regarding both life and purpose of life) from being affected as long as it can help. So, when we say that the vital force tries to keep disease in the least important parts, we actually mean that it tries to prevent its own disturbance from affecting important structures. To exemplify, we may say that it is like a disturbed government which tries as far as possible to keep its own disturbance from affecting the important organizations like army or the food supply.

Dynamics in treatment

1. If a remedy which covers the central disturbance is given, then the pathology (which is nothing but a localization of the central disturbance) will be automatically relieved and consequently disappear.

2. If a remedy corresponds by similarity only to the local symptoms, it may sometimes alleviate or palliate the local symptoms for some time. For example, if a patient's central disturbance is *Calcarea carbonica* and if his local joint complaints have the modalities of *Rhus toxicodendron* (these modalities are quite common to most cases of joint pains), *Rhus toxicodendron* will give temporary relief.

76

3. Since local pathology is only a vent (an outlet) for the central disturbance, merely removing it (by dynamic or crude Homoeopathy, Allopathy or surgery) will be against the direction of nature. It would push the disturbance back to the centre. The effect would be temporary and the vital force would strive to use the same outlet again. Such constant pushing back over time results in weakened vitality, which is then forced to transfer the disturbance to a more important organ. This process called suppression, is possible even with homoeopathic medicine if the medicine is selected on local symptoms and does not correspond by similarity to the central disturbance.

4. One of the most important implications of the above ideas is that if we take care of the central disturbance, the vital force will handle everything else. Disease is a disturbance at the centre. Our medicine should always be aimed at the central disturbance. If a person gets injured and there are local symptoms of *Arnica*, the vitality will easily take care of this. It is not necessary to give *Arnica*, unless the central symptoms too have changed to indicate *Arnica*.

Similarly, even in an acute condition (for example, a cold, sprain or emotional upset) the vital force will take care of it. We have only to see what the central disturbance is at that time and prescribe the similar remedy. Whether in an acute or chronic condition the only indication for a change of remedy is a change at the centre, or in other words a change in the indicating or characteristic symptoms. For example, if a patient who is doing well on *Pulsatilla* for his chronic condition develops jaundice, we have to examine if the symptoms on which *Pulsatilla* has been prescribed still exist. If he retains the same indications, the same mental state, the same generals and the same modalities even during jaundice, then the remedy will be the same. He may have some common symptoms of jaundice, but as long as the symptoms in the centre remain the same, we do not have to change the remedy.

It may happen that during jaundice, the original *Pulsatilla* patient develops a marked increase in thirst, a total aversion to motion and conversation, lack of appetite except for hot drinks and pain in the liver aggravated by least motion and better by lying on the right side, in this case, the original characteristics have been temporarily superseded. The whole central disturbance is different as seen from a total change in the mental state and the general symptoms, along with the local peculiarities. Only such a change can justify a change of prescription, even in acute situations.

The phrase I like to repeat often is:

The indication for a change is a change in the indications.

11

WHAT IS CURATIVE IN MEDICINE

In this chapter we shall try to understand what a remedy really is, and what it is capable of curing. This is still a matter of confusion to many, and in my seminars I could make the matter clear through the following video-recorded case. The reader would do well to follow this interesting case and draw appropriate lessons from it.

Case

This is a case of viral encephalitis in a female child of 1½ years. I got the following history.

The child was apparently normal when she developed vomiting and diarrhoea (gastroenteritis), for which she was admitted to an allopathic hospital where she was given intravenous fluids. Then she developed a mild temperature and had one convulsion. After this convulsion, she suddenly sunk into a stupor and became semiconscious. The pediatrician said that the chances of the child's survival were bleak. She was almost unconscious when I saw her and was responsive only to very deep pain stimulus. If we pinched her very hard, she would just emit a slight whine, and then go back to semi-consciousness. She had no convulsions after the first one. Her temperature was subnormal at 97 °F. They brought her to our homoeopathic hospital with all kinds of tubes around her and I think venesection had also been performed.

I had to select a remedy to meet this grave condition – from these very scanty symptoms. No other characteristic symptoms were available. The remedy I chose was *Helleborus niger*. Why did I select this remedy?

Remedy differentiation

The characteristic feature about her case was not what existed now, but how it started. In *Aconitum* or *Belladonna*, it would start with violence. In *Apis* there would be violent, shrill shrieking with head brought backward into the pillow. On the other hand, in *Opium*, there would be complete unconsciousness with constricted pupils, and stertorous breathing.

There is one other remedy that needs differentiating, and that is *Zincum metallicum*. *Zincum* and *Helleborus* are very close to each other. The difference is only one, and that is at the onset of *Zincum* there would be tremendous nervous excitement, convulsion after convulsion, then jerks, movements, twitchings and coma. So, first there is violent nervous excitement, and then, when the nerves get fatigued, comes paresis, paralysis, stupor and coma. *Zincum* would not go into this state in the manner our patient did. The central disturbance of *Zincum* is tremendous nervous excitement. Many times, even in the stage of coma, we will see jerking and twitchings in a case of *Zincum*.

In his lectures on Materia Medica, Kent describes *Helleborus* as follows:

> "*Helleborus* is useful in affections of the brain, spinal cord, the general nervous system and mind, but especially in acute inflammatory diseases of the brain and spinal cord, and their membranes, and in troubles bordering on insanity. There is a peculiar kind of imbecility or stupefaction of the body and mind; the extreme state is unconsciousness, complete unconsciousness in connection with cerebral congestion. Even early in the disease *Helleborus* lacks the wildness and acute delirium found in *Stramonium* and *Belladonna*."

Helleborus is passive. Passivity, stupefaction: "diminished power of mind over the body". A person goes into a passive state without having an active phase. That is the characteristic of *Helleborus*.

So, we gave *Helleborus* 1M, a single dose. Now, what would happen? Let us see what Kent says:

> "I have seen children, after passing through a moderately acute but rather passive first stage, lie in this stupid state, needing *Helleborus* for weeks before they received it. When it was given, repair sets in, not instantly, but gradually. The remedy acts slowly in these slow, stubborn, stupid cases of brain and spinal trouble. Sometimes there is no apparent change until the day after the remedy is administered or even the next night, when there comes a sweat, a diarrhoea, or vomiting – a reaction. They must not be interfered with, no remedy must be given. They are signs of reaction. If the child has vitality enough to recover, he will now recover."

Management of the case

This is like homoeopathic surgery. We are saying that this child is bad. Her disease is bad. It has affected the brain. We are going to give her the medicine. We want the reaction. Her vitality may be too weak to bear the reaction. That is the risk we have to take; the child may die. But she is going to die anyway. This is her only chance of recovery.

Kent says further:

> "If the vomiting is stopped by any remedy that will stop it, the *Helleborus* will be antidoted. Let the vomiting, or the diarrhoea or the sweat alone, and it will pass away during the day. The child will become warm and in a few days will return to consciousness – and then what will take place? Just imagine these benumbed fingers and hands and

limbs, this benumbed skin everywhere. What would be the most natural thing to develop as evidence to the rousing up of this stupid child?... Well, that child's fingers will commence to tingle. As he comes back to his normal nervous condition, the fingers commence to tingle, the nose and ears tingle, and the child begins to scream and toss back and forth, and roll about the bed. The neighbours will come in and say: "I would send that doctor away unless he gives something to help that child", but just sure as you do it, you will have a dead baby in twenty-four hours. That child is getting well; let him alone. You will never be able to manage one of these cases if you do not take the father into a room by himself and tell him just how the case will proceed. Do not take the mother, do not tell her a word about it, unless she is an unusual excellent mother, because that is her child and she is sympathetic, and she will cry when she ears that child's cry; she will lose her head and will insist upon the father turning you out of doors. But if you take the father aside beforehand and tell him what is going to happen, explain it to him so he will see it for himself, and tell him that if this is not permitted to go on, that if the remedy is interfered with, he will lose his child."

This is Kent's description as to what should happen after giving *Helleborus*.

I gave *Helleborus* 1M, one dose, and waited for twenty-four hours, but nothing happened. The child's condition was very critical, and I wanted a reaction immediately; so, I gave *Helleborus* CM. I didn't want to wait with 10 M and 50 M.

Within 1½ hours after giving *Helleborus* CM, her temperature went up to 103 °F, and then to 105.2 °F. This was her maximum temperature, and it remained for twenty-four hours the first time. She had a kind of convulsion along with this temperature, but after, the whole thing subsided, her response to the pain stimulus was much, much better and her level of consciousness had increased. This reaction stopped and so we repeated the remedy in CM after two days, and within an hour of the repeat, she started shrieking loudly and she kept on shrieking for twelve to fourteen hours; the temperature also steadily rose and remained the same for seventy-two hours. During the course of this temperature, her level of consciousness kept on improving. Every time we gave her a dose, the effect would last just a little longer than the previous dose, and then it would subside totally. And after each such rise and fall of temperature, her level of consciousness would just slightly improve and the symptoms which are identified with *Helleborus* started showing.

So, after *Helleborus* was given, and recovery had begun, the level of consciousness improved, the brain was less affected – only then could we see the classical symptoms of *Helleborus*, but not when we saw her in the beginning. This is a very significant point. This case is typical of *Helleborus* as it is described in the books. Symptom by symptom, observation by observation, it is a classic *Helleborus* case.

She started keeping her thumbs clenched and arms outstretched. She was constantly moaning and rolling her head. Refer to these rubrics in Kent's Repertory:

— Head, motions, rolling head, day and night, with moaning (K.R.131).

81

Her eyes were also staring at one place.

— Eyes, staring, stupor during (K.R. 266).

There was constant motion of one arm and one leg. This is the typical keynote of *Helleborus*.

— Extremities, motion, involuntary, one arm and leg (K.R. 1033).

The characteristic feature is that the other side is paralysed.

Then she started perspiring profusely, especially on the head and the upper lip. The perspiration was so much that it made the whole pillow wet. She started getting lose stools, five or six greenish stools, with increased frequency of urination. We noticed that she was very restless and was constantly moving one lower limb, while the other limb remained passive. Her nostrils were dilated, with motion of alae nasi ("Nose, dilated nostrils" – K.R. 329).

When we pinched her passive lower limb, she tried to kick away the hand with her active lower limb. The passive limb, she could withdraw but not move it actively. So, there was a marked absence of power in one lower limb with vigorous movements of the other side. We also noticed that she was not moving her eyes much; they remained still, as if she was staring. There was no vision in her eyes; if we put a hand near them, there would not even be a blink. There was also hardly any response to sound.

Now, this stage improved even further, and she became totally conscious, but she could not see and she could not hear. Slowly, her hearing came back, and then we were left with this, that she was fully conscious – she could hear, eat, sleep, cry, but she could not see.

Doubts about full recovery

We referred her to an ophtalmologist to see if there was something wrong with her eyes, but he said that they were perfectly clear. Everybody thought that encephalitis has left its mark; that she would remain blind for the rest of her life. I myself had similar doubts.

What should I do now? Should I change the remedy? Then I read in Nash:

"*Helleborus* produces this dullness of the senses that the eyes are normal, but he cannot see; and his ears are normal, but he cannot hear."

When I read this, I felt thrilled. I continued her on *Helleborus* according to the indication. Whenever the response lagged, I gave her another dose, and in this way she was treated.

I would go every two or three days to the hospital to see if the vision had come back, and for quite some time, around two-three weeks, there was no sign. Then one day, I took out my handkerchief (I would always do this to check her vision) and waved it before her eyes and, for the first time, she tried to grasp it. She could see something blurred. Slowly and gradually her vision improved until it came back totally.

What are the lessons we can draw from this case? Let us look at the pathology of *Helleborus*. What pathology does it produce and cure? Here are some choices.

Encephalitis is inflammation of the brain, and *meningitis* is inflammation of the meninges. There is a third term known as *encephalopathy*, where another organ of the body is badly damaged, for example the liver, and because of liver failure, toxins get accumulated in the brain and cause coma. So, you can have hepatic encephalopathy.

Did *Helleborus* produce the pathology?

Now, which of these conditions does *Helleborus* produce? It may seem obvious from this case that it produces encephalitis. This means that the action of *Helleborus* is not on the meninges, but on the brain substance. One could assume that *Apis*, which produces those shrill cries (cri encephalique), could be useful in meningitis. Therefore, *Apis* is the remedy for meningitis, *Helleborus* is the remedy for encephalitis, and *Opium* is the remedy for encephalopathy.

Now the question arises: Does *Helleborus* produce acute inflammation, subacute inflammation or chronic inflammation?

From our experience with this case, would it be correct to say that it produces subacute inflammation? *Aconitum* is known to produce acute inflammation, and *Helleborus* can be now said to produce subacute inflammation and chronic inflammation is produced by chronic remedies like *Sulphur*. The pathogenesis of *Helleborus* now seems to be clear that it produces and cures subacute inflammation of the brain.

But we can be happy with this for a short while only, till we find in Kent's Repertory *Helleborus* listed with three marks under "meningitis"; whereas it is given only in italics under "inflammation of the brain". What shall we do now with this information? Does *Helleborus* produce meningitis or encephalitis? It is given under both. Do you think this is a mistake? If not, then, what is *Helleborus*? What is its site of action?

There is a rubric in the Repertory, in the "Mind" chapter: "Love, ailment from, disappointed" and again *Helleborus* is listed in that rubric, in italics. Does this mean we should give it in meningitis or encephalitis which has resulted from disappointed love? Should we use it only in those cases of disappointed love? Should we use it only in those cases of disappointed love where meningo-encephalitis is the result?

This kind of thinking will lead to confusion. The fact is:

Helleborus does not produce meningitis and it does not produce viral encephalitis. Viral encephalitis is produced by a virus and meningitis is produced by organisms that cause meningitis and not by *Helleborus*. Disappointed love is not caused by *Helleborus* but by something else! *Helleborus* produces none of them. *Helleborus* produces *a state of being*, a central state, whose main characteristic is "Dullness of the sensorium". His senses become dull. His eyes are open, but he cannot see. This is the central state of

Helleborus; and wherever it may be found, in whichever patient, with whatever name of disease, whether it be meningitis or encephalitis, *Helleborus* and ONLY *Helleborus* will cure.

If it is meningitis with this dullness of the sensorium, *Helleborus* will cure. If it is viral encephalitis with dullness of the sensorium, *Helleborus* will cure. *Zincum metallicum* produces excitement of the nervous system. So, whether it is petit-mal epilepsy, meningitis or encephalitis, with excitement of the nervous system, *Zincum* will cure. If disappointed love is followed by excitement of the nervous system, *Zincum*, and only *Zincum* will cure.

Each remedy produces its own type of central disturbance

Helleborus does not produce pathology – it does not affect the brain nor does it affect the meninges; it produces a central state, a central disturbance, a dullness of the sensorium. Wherever this is found, only *Helleborus* will cure.

There was a person, following disappointed love, who was sitting in one place and staring thoughtlessly into space. His ears were normal, but he was not hearing and his eyes were normal, but he was not observing. He did not have meningo-encephalitis, but he had this state.

Then, someone who knew Homoeopathy, who knew *what is to be cured in disease*, had the conviction to give him *Helleborus* and cure him, and he recorded this remedy in the Repertory. So, you see:

If your mind is concerned with pathology, as to which remedy produces what pathology, then you will go wrong. To say: "*Aconitum* produces inflammation", is NONSENSE! *Aconitum* produces a turmoil, violence in the central state. Whether this "violence" followed fright, whether this violence is in insanity, meningitis or encephalitis, whether it is in typhoid or whether it is in a painful inflammation of one foot, *Aconitum* and only *Aconitum* will cure.

If you get a man with pain in his little toe, so severe that he says: "Doctor, do something or I will die", you will not look to see whether the site of action of *Aconitum* is "little toe". *Aconitum* has no site of action. No remedy in Homoeopathy has a site of action. It does not go and sit in some site. Potentized remedies have dynamic effect only. Their effect is central. This central disturbance is to be cured in disease, not pathology.

You can use the Materia Medica much more freely; you can open it and widen its horizons to the furthest possible degree; you can use any remedy in any condition – if the central action matches. And you will succeed.

12

THE SCIENTIFIC DEPTH OF HOMOEOPATHY
(WHAT IS HOLISTIC APPROACH)

The following (with a few minor corrections) is an interview which appeared in "The Homoeopathic Heritage" of June 1990. It resulted from a controversy initiated by the editor Dr. S.P. Koppikar, my senior colleague and good friend. The issue he raised was about the practicability of the holistic and psychosomatic approach in homoeopathic prescribing. He went so far as to suggest that prescribing on mentals and generals was just too ideal and not possible to the average (and busy) practitioner. My friend, Mr. Gunavante, was quite upset by this suggestion and felt the need to explain the standpoint of classical Homoeopathy so as to show its logic. He also wanted me to demonstrate through some clinical cases that our fundamental principles are true and sound and that we need to develop our skills to utilize them rather that find unscientific shortcuts.

This interview was much appreciated by several homoeopaths which showed me that doubts still exist about the practicability and soundness of our principles.

Interview with Dr. R. Sankaran by S.M. Gunavante, published in "The Homoeopathic Heritage", June 1990

In his editorial for February 1990 issue of "The Homoeopathic Heritage", Dr. Koppikar has raised some fundamental issues in regard to the application of Homoeopathy, which, I felt, needed to be discussed. For this purpose, I felt I could do not better than obtain the views of Dr. Rajan Sankaran whom I know well as an able homoeopathic physician as well as a thinker and teacher. Initially he felt it would be better not to enter a controversy, but on my persuasion that such a discussion is in the interest of Homoeopathy, he agreed to talk. Here is what he said.

I have found Homoeopathy to be a tremendous tool to stimulate vitality and start true curative process. However, if we aim at merely giving relief of some symptoms, we are not exploiting its potential fully. If anyone says he has found prescribing on local symptoms or prescribing remedies as "specifics" for certain conditions leads to much more curative effect than prescribing on mentals and generals, then our whole philosophy, our understanding of health, disease and cure will have to be changed. But I feel sure it need not, because that approach will not work. Many minor problems are self-limiting; they get well even without medicines. But if an acute problem is serious enough, will it remain a local complaint to be tackled with medicines which have "local" action? Will not the patient be ill as a whole, and need to be treated as a totality?

Anybody who has conscientiously practised Homoeopathy would have felt how frustrating it is to give remedy after remedy and to see nothing really happening until he finds the one remedy which is absolutely correct and fits the patient completely like a glove. Unless this whole philosophy of Homoeopathy, of totality, is grasped and practised faithfully, I am afraid Homoeopathy will not reach its true heights. It has been practised with all kind of combinations, alternations, quick changes in prescriptions and with all kinds of specific and symptomatic treatment. As soon as one hear the word "gas trouble", one tends to restrict his vision to *Lycopodium, China* or *Carbo vegetabilis*. For digestive troubles, we tend not to think beyond *Nux vomica, Pulsatilla* or *Lycopodium*. I have seen cases where, if only the practitioner had just seen a little beyond the local complaint, he would have unlocked the whole case, but he did not bother to see. He kept on giving remedies with local action one after the other, giving only temporary relief and sometimes not even that.

The principles of Homoeopathy are clear in stating that there cannot be one remedy for the whole patient and a different remedy for each of his parts. If a drug acts curatively, it will do so by virtue of its covering the mentals and physical generals as well. Only a remedy which acts on the organism as a whole can act curatively on a particular part of the body. For people with less mastery over particular symptoms of each remedy, it is much safer to rely on mentals and generals. A master might recognize a *Tarentula* cough, but most of us have not reached that stage and so we need to rely on mentals and generals. This is safer also because the provings and clinical experiences are not as complete in particulars as they are in mentals and generals. One thing certain is that if the remedy does not cover the mentals and generals (with or without our knowing it) and it merely fits particular symptoms, such a remedy often fails. We welcome any experiences to the contrary. However, whenever a characteristic particular is found, we take the trouble to study the remedy to see what its mentals and generals are, especially if no other remedy clearly fits. In this way we are able to exploit even a "small" remedy. Let me make it clear that we do not advocate ignoring the characteristic particular symptoms. On the contrary, we are only asking for a balanced view. But experiences show that mentals and generals often chiefly determine the remedy, and this conviction has proved to be extremely valuable to us.

Why were the masters successful? Probably their knowledge of drugs was so profound that they could identify a remedy by looking at a part of the individual. They could tell the difference in remedies, say, from the tongue of *Nitricum acidum* or *Fluoricum acidum*, etc., and prescribe with certainty based on local symptoms. Their identification was so good that they could select the right remedy from looking at the parts, a remedy which unconsciously covered mentals and generals; but our identification not being as good, we choose to rely on mentals and generals. Let me give some experiences, actual cases.

I was recently called to see a case which was diagnosed as pneumonitis. This lady had had a continuous temperature for the past three weeks and the temperature was not going down despite antibiotics and several homoeopathic remedies. I was taken to see her by a homoeopathic doctor who had already prescribed various medicines. There was a patch on the lungs, though the febrile symptoms resembled a malarial paroxysm. I was not able to get any characteristic symptoms of the fever or paroxysms. Therefore, I was forced to rely solely on her constitutional symptoms. She was a school teacher, and was very anxious to get back to work. She was talkative and quite humorous, was known as "the life and soul of the party". She was a very hot patient, liked to take very long walks and enjoyed going out in the open air. She would get anxious about various matters concerning her family. If we take the symptoms, "Loquacity with jesting" (Synthetic Repertory), "Ameliorated by walking in the open air" and "Hot patient" with "Anxiety", we come to *Kalium iodatum*. I gave it, two doses in 1M and 10M potencies, twelve hourly. After the second dose she had profuse perspiration. Two months have passed now, and she is in good health.

This kind of result is not exceptional. Cases treated earlier with local remedies (prescribed purely on local symptoms, which are usually quite common to any illness) usually failed. When we prescribed *Kalium iodatum* on generals such as "Loquacity with jesting", even in a case of severe leucoderma, we have been very successful, even though "White spots on skin" is not covered by this remedy. What do we mean by holistic treatment? What is the idea of giving *Kalium iodatum* in leucoderma, or a case of pneumonia or pyrexia of unknown origin? The idea of giving it is that what we are trying to treat is not leucoderma, nor is it pyrexia. The concept of disease in Homoeopathy is that disease is a total affection of the body and mind. There are no local diseases. That is what Hahnemann has emphasized repeatedly in the "Organon", that disease is nothing but a disorder of the vital force. He never says that in typhoid we have to treat typhoid, or in pneumonia we have to treat pneumonia. We have always to treat the person, that is *his disordered vital force, as represented by the totality of signs and symptoms*, not merely local signs and symptoms.

In a case of cholera, we will certainly not sit down and ask about the patient's nature from childhood. In a case of cholera, as in any acute case, what we are going to see is the present totality. When a person is dying and breathing hard, has anxiety, fear of death and restlessness, we will consider those remedies which have these symptoms in a high degree. We need not always ask whether before he developed this state he was dictatorial or mild. That is immaterial if the present picture itself is complete and clear. *Each time, what has to be treated is the present illness as a whole*. If we forget this principle and start treating parts without the remedy covering the whole, then there are two possibilities: either the remedy will not work at all, or it will work partially. If it works partially, it is going to suppress, and suppression always leads to harm. This is pure logic, and it does not change, no matter how many prescribers follow this practice.

Tell us one more case. I know you have numerous cases to draw upon.

It is not merely numerous cases, but every single case we treat is on this basis. A recent case: a lady was complaining of very severe headache, which would start and go down with the sun. They would be brought on by missing a meal. They were quite intense. She was taking around twelve tablets of Aspirin every day. I asked her why she is taking twelve tablets. She said: "Doctor, some of them are for my headache surely, but nowadays I have started liking to take the medicine. Even if I do not require them, I get pleasure out of swallowing the pills, I have some sweating after that, and get a nice feeling. If I require six tablets, I take twelve. And you also, please do not give me one or two doses a day; give me six doses, or eight." This struck me so much that I looked up the rubric in Synthetic Repertory, "Medicine, desire to swallow large doses of", and I found only *Cactus*, which also fits her headache symptoms. Her aggravation with the sun, and worse from missing a meal were also found in *Cactus*. *Cactus* 200 completely relieved her headaches.

I will give you another case. A person came with fever since over one week. Temperature was around 102 °F. He was an old man of seventy plus. He came to my clinic with his son. My female assistant was also there. He was not so neatly dressed. He sat down and said: "Doctor (in quite a commanding tone), I know that this fever is due to the cracks on my penis (he meant the foreskin). It is due to that. This is the infection that has created the fever. You treat that and I will be okay. I know that. Don't try to handle anything else." In this I could see three prominent symptoms: firstly, "Egotism", second, "Theorizing" and the third was cracks on the prepuce, which had nothing to do with the fever even though he insisted that fever was due to the cracks. When you take "Theorizing", "Egotism" and cracks on to the prepuce, you get only *Sulphur*. The way he said it in presence of the female assistant and of his son, showed a kind of "Indifference to his own personal appearance". He did not bother how it looked. It was not actually shameless behaviour but a kind of indifference to appearance which is not just the clothes. It is *Sulphur* who says: "I don't care a damn what they think of me", or "I will do what I wish to." On this basis, I gave him a dose of *Sulphur* 1M. Very soon the fever and everything subsided. You don't have to give many doses. When you prescribe like this, one or two doses are enough. Look at the state at that time. It is not that he was *Sulphur* even ten years ago. He was *Sulphur* right then, even during his fever. Any other remedy given at that time either will do nothing or it can suppress. You have to appreciate one thing, that is: *disease is a dynamic affection*; only one affection can exist at a time. If his affection is *Sulphur*, it is *Sulphur* and nothing else. A man can be only in one state at a time.

Is there any possibility that after several months he may come with a complaint about which the doctor will take a different view?

Yes, you have to change the remedy if the mentals and generals change. What do we mean by mentals and generals? By that we mean those things that are totally dissociated from pathological and pathognomonic symptoms. Now, these can be keynotes also. What is a keynote? It is something which does not relate to disease pathology. If you are going to take something that belongs to disease pathology as a keynote, you are courting trouble. But, if you are going to select symptoms that are characteristic for that particular patient, that will differentiate one patient from another, then your keynotes will be useful. Naturally, the keynotes should fit in with the mentals and generals. You cannot have a patient with a keynote of *Bryonia* and the mentals of *Rhus toxicodendron*; or a keynote of *Sulphur* and the mentals of *Veratrum*. They have to be the same. You can either approach from keynotes or from mentals and generals, but the circle must be complete. Some people find it easier with keynotes, but those who think they can prescribe on local symptoms or keynotes or on pathognomonic symptoms are badly mistaken. Naturally, if I examine a *Sulphur* patient, he might have aggravation from covering his feet at night. He may also have intolerance of hunger, as well as aggravation from standing. These are all keynotes which are written in three marks in Allen's "Keynotes". What are those keynotes? They are all symptoms that are removed from the pathological process. Thirst during fever is not a keynote.

Keynotes are uncommon symptoms. Uncommon symptoms indicate the general state, the nature of disturbance of the vital force, and hence the mentals and generals. There is no disagreement about them. But they have to fit in together. If we are able to confirm the keynotes with mentals and generals, the prescription becomes one hundred percent confirmed; and then our case cannot go wrong. We insist on mentals and generals because here there is no chance of mistaking pathognomonic and non-pathognomonic symptoms. "Egotism", "Theorizing" and "Indifference to personal appearance" can, by no stretch of imagination, be a part of the fever. By no stretch of imagination in a predominantly physical case, can a mental or general symptom be a part of the pathology. That is why reliance on mentals and generals is much safer. But if one is very good at perceiving what is characteristic and what is not, he can definitely use those local symptoms. Hahnemann said in Aphorism 153 that the uncommon, peculiar symptoms are most important. But how many prescriptions are made on this basis? If one gives *Arsenicum sulphuratum flavum* again and again for vitiligo, are we prescribing on something uncommon? But that is what many homoeopaths are doing. If we prescribe in every case of cervical spondylosis one or two particular remedies, is this the legacy of Hahnemann? And the question is asked: Was Hahnemann holistic? Certainly, he was holistic. Can we find one word in Hahnemann's writing where he said: "Do not prescribe on characteristics; do not prescribe on mentals"?

On the contrary, in Aphorism 211 he says: "This holds true to such an extent that that state of disposition often chiefly determines the choice of the remedy." In fact, Hahnemann came to his conclusions after several years of experience. Anyone who says that *Aconitum* is good for fever, *Cantharis* for urinary troubles, *Rhus toxicodendron* for joint pains, *Mercurius* for dysentery, etc., is talking of absolute pathology. He does not follow Hahnemann and ignores the teaching of the more successful practitioners who followed him.

Last month, I had a case of iridocyclitis for whom I prescribed *Iodum*. Why? Because the patient was hungry every three hours and he had a kind of anxiety that made him walk around. He must walk fast in the open air to get rid of his anxiety. He felt extremely hot. He was told that he would become blind if he does not take Cortisone. Yet, he got totally well with *Iodum* 200, I did not even care to see if *Iodum* has got any eye symptoms.

You can prescribe with absolute certainty if mentals and generals agree. Everything else is a matter of chance. That is why from Hahnemann downward, to Boenninghausen, Boger, Kent, Sir John Weir, Margaret Tyler – all these great names are known; the one true method of prescribing on totality, understanding the mind and generals of the patient, his peculiarities and the individuality of his being – only this method really has stood the test of time, because every other method is a chance.

I treated a case of fibroid of uterus with *Arsenicum album* 200, and that tumour went away. And *Arsenicum album* is not mentioned, even in single grade, for fibroid.

Why? Because the patient was fastidious, had a compulsive neurosis, was extremely anxious about health, very chilly, very lean. All the symptoms of this patient fitted into *Arsenicum album* except fibroid. If I had started with the remedies known for fibroid, this lady would never have got well. Nowadays we have the good (or bad) fortune of treating many patients coming after taking innumerable homoeopathic medicines. Sometimes they were given the right remedy, but it was quickly changed. This is what happens when we try to treat symptoms one after the other. Even if they have hit the right remedy, there is no faith in it. They prescribed on some symptoms, and when the symptom has not improved, they change. But, if they knew that *the remedy fitted the mentals and generals, they would not have changed and that remedy would have ultimately cured.*

I can give some more examples in which mentals symptoms alone led to the curative prescription. A case of pituitary tumour was taken for operation. The patient, a Minister in West Bengal government, developed symptoms of heart failure every time he was taken to the operation theatre, and hence he had to be taken home. On the basis of fear causing heart failure, Dr. B.N. Chakravarty told us he prescribed *Gelsemium*. "Cowardice", "Anticipatory anxiety", "Fear, of operation" were other symptoms. *Gelsemium* is not known to have cured tumours, but still it did when it was prescribed on mental symptoms.

Dr. Sarabhai Kapadia had a case of molluscum contagiosum. He took a full history, but could not get any characteristic symptoms. After an hour of taking the case, he saw the child scratching the head. The mother said that whenever the boy is sleepy, he does this. On the basis of Kent's Repertory: "Head: itching of scalp, sleep, when going to", Dr. Sarabhai prescribed *Agnus castus* (perhaps 1M) and the molluscum disappeared soon, though the remedy does not cover the complaint.

In his article "Trend of Thought Necessary for Comprehension and Retention of Homoeopathy" (Kent's "Lesser Writings", p. 598), Kent has given a number of examples from his practice to support his assertion: "Find the remedy for the patient and it will cure him, and the particulars will disappear though none of them were in that remedy." He says again: "Most cases of hip-joint disorder cured by me in the past twenty-five years were cured by remedies not in the hip-joint list." Further, a patient with rectal ulcer who was advised operation had the persistent mental symptom, viz. intense strain to prevent himself from self-destruction. *Natrum sulphuricum* has this symptoms, but it has no rectal ulcer recorded. A few other symptoms together with this strong mental led to *Natrum sulphuricum*, and he had no more hemorrhoids. He concludes by saying emphatically: "Guided by the symptoms of the patient you can cure inflammation of any part even if that remedy has not produced inflammation of that part."

A German journal once reported a case, I think it was Von Keller. It was a case of uterine tumour treated with *Aethusa* on the basis of two symptoms:

– Whenever the patient would close her eyes to sleep, she would get a strong feeling that she will not wake up next morning, and
– When she gets up in darkness, she feels breathless.

A case of severe cough (in a boy) taught me much about the importance of mental symptoms. The cough would not subside even after several remedies were tried. The

90

parents were getting anxious. The child was restless, very stubborn and did the opposite of what he was told to do. On the basis that *Tuberculinum* is a good remedy for persistent respiratory complaints, restlessness and obstinacy, it was given but did not work. One day when the boy was sitting in my clinic, suddenly he did something very funny: he shouted at me: "Hey, Sankaran, your medicines are useless; better give me some good medicine, else I will not come here." This, coming from a boy of five, uttered in a violent, threatening tone was shocking. I gathered from the parents that his behaviour at home was funny. He was disobedient, shrieking, mocking, quarrelsome. He was intensely restless. He threw things or destroyed them. However, he reacted to music favourably, would dance to tunes. I was not accustomed to think of *Tarentula* for cough. But after failure with "indicated" remedies, I was in a chastened mood. Maybe, I thought, when *Tarentula* covers the mind so well, it may cover the rest of the symptoms too. The response to *Tarentula* was magical in two days, whereas I had struggled over it for weeks with other remedies, and failed. Even his behaviour improved. The case illustrated to me how our mind, oriented to therapeutics, misses the right remedy.

It is worth referring to Dr. Sehgal's method of "Revolutionized Homoeopathy". He practices exclusively on mentals, whereas we include the physical generals and concomitants. The first case from which Dr. Sehgal learned was of malaria. The child wanted to vomit but could not. He was irritable and *Nux vomica* failed. Dr. Sehgal observed that the child did not want to get out of bed, and yet he did not have any complaint: "Indifference, does not complain", "Bed, desires to remain in". *Hyoscyamus* 30 cured the boy. Homoeopathy is not something mechanical. It is an art. It is an art of observation and understanding the process that is going on within man, which is disease. It is not for nothing that Hahnemann's one case which was reported was a case of warts which was cured with *Chamomilla*. Can we then doubt whether Hahnemann was holistic or not? Hahnemann was a man who laid the foundation of holistic therapeutics in the history of medicine. He was the first to link the mind with the body; the first who said that disease is an affection of the whole, not the part; the first who said treatment of skin alone is suppression. He was the beginner of holistic therapeutics in the history of medicine. We are proud that we have such a visionary as our master. Remedies for particular disease conditions (therapeutics) were advocated even in Hahnemann's time, and he was a strong critic of them. Let us use this divine tool for the higher purpose for which it was revealed to Hahnemann.

13

THE STATE AND THE PATHOLOGY

We have seen that when the central disturbance exceeds the limit which can be tolerated by the vital parts of the body, then this disturbance is diverted to the local parts and produces pathology. The type and location of pathology depends on:

– *The nature of the state itself.* Each state will choose a particular type of pathology as its favourite. For example, given the choice between producing a wart and appendicitis, *Belladonna* would choose to produce appendicitis, because here its characteristics are better expressed than they would be in the case of a wart. *Colocynthis* is much more likely to affect the intestines than produce a coryza because colicy and spasmodic pains are a very important part of its nature. If we do not take remedies, but take the characteristics of the state, a state which has violence would prefer a type of pathology that has violence with it. *Zincum* with its twitchings and chorea would normally aggravate epilepsy in preference to eczema.

So, the type of pathology depends upon the nature of the state, but this is not exclusive; there are other more important factors.

– *The inherited or acquired tendency to pathology.* Inherited tendency is genetic tendency, whilst acquired tendency is what is acquired throughout a person's lifetime. So, even though *Belladonna* would aggravate appendicitis in preference to warts, if the person has absolutely no tendency towards appendicitis, but has a tremendous genetic disposition towards warts, then *Belladonna* has no choice but to aggravate the state of the warts.

– *The level of the vitality.* If the vitality is strong, it will not allow the pathology to affect the more important parts, but will confine it to less important parts.

The type of pathology produced therefore depends upon a very delicate balance between the nature of the state, the tendency which is acquired or inherited and the level of vitality. So, you can have two types of pathology:

– *Pathology without any acquired or inherited tendency.* This happens in acute conditions especially in infections like typhoid and pneumonia, where, without any tendency to lung or intestinal disease, the virulence being very strong pathology is produced.

– *Pathology with a genetic tendency,* meaning an inherited or acquired tendency.

93

In this case again, we have two types:
- A tendency that is easily excitable and
- A tendency that is less excitable.

So, if a person has a strong or excitable tendency, this can be excited by almost any state in the person. For example, if a person has a very strong genetic tendency towards hypertension, then almost any state (whether it is *Baryta carbonica, Belladonna* or *Hepar sulphuris*) can aggravate the tendency. Even if the state is not so intense, it will still aggravate this pathological tendency, since it is so excitable. On the other hand, if the tendency is not so strong and not so excitable, then it requires intense and certain specific states to aggravate it. For example, if a person has a very weak tendency towards epilepsy then not all states can excite it; only certain states can, and even these need to be of a high intensity.

What is the importance of understanding all this? The importance is that even though we associate some remedies with a particular pathology, we need to know that if a person has a strong inherited or acquired tendency towards a particular pathology then almost any state can cause that pathology to be aggravated. We cannot then go back and say that this remedy is not capable of aggravating this pathology and therefore, we need to select one that is. For example, it usually requires a strong man to cut through a tree but if the tree is weak or already half cut, then even a weak man can make it fall. If we do not want the tree to fall, we have to remove the man who is cutting the tree. It is of no use saying: "Oh! The fellow cutting the tree is not capable of cutting it! He cannot be the culprit because he does not have the capacity." This is what we do when we find the indicated remedy by the symptoms, but then proceed to rule it out saying that it cannot produce the pathology. If the disposition, i.e. the genetic or acquired tendency is very strong, almost every dynamic disturbance can excite it and so we have to see what the internal dynamic disturbance is and direct our treatment towards it.

For example, let us take the remedy *Spigelia. Spigelia* has many neurotic pains and naturally when this state is found in a person with a tendency to headaches, it produces the typical *Spigelia* headaches, the pain that goes from the occiput to the left eyeball, producing the feeling as if they would come out of the socket. Now, this tendency to favour headaches is so strong in *Spigelia* that even if the person has a slight tendency to headache, he will definitely get severe headaches of this type. But suppose a *Spigelia* state exists in the person who has absolutely no tendency to headaches, then what happens? The state will encourage the type of pathology to which the patient does have a tendency, as for example asthma. You may find in a person with asthma the mental state of *Spigelia*, the modalities or the characteristics of *Spigelia* or indeed, the generalities of *Spigelia* but not the headache.

Take again for example *Aesculus*. It has venous congestion which, in a susceptible person, will produce typical sore and swollen piles. But, what if the *Aesculus* state is found in a person without the tendency to piles but with a tendency to conjunctivitis? In this case, you may well see swollen veins in the eyes instead of in the rectum. You are likely to miss the remedy here, because your mind is accustomed to associate *Aesculus* with piles and *Spigelia* with headache.

Also, we can make big mistakes when we use pathology alone as a guide to a remedy. We may get a case of piles with the local symptoms suggesting *Aesculus*, but this patient may have a general central state of *Spigelia*. Since he has a strong tendency to piles, he may have them, though *Spigelia* is not typically known for piles. This happens because *Spigelia* may have not have been proved in a person with such a tendency. So, we do not know whether *Spigelia* can encourage this tendency, and if so, what the local characteristics are that it can produce. Even if the local characteristics of a pathology indicate a remedy clearly, we still have to confirm if the concomitants, the mental and the general level fit the remedy too, otherwise it is bound to fail.

What is very important to note is that a given pathology can be found under several states and under several remedies, in one form or another. If some remedies are not listed against that particular pathology, it may be due to the fact that the remedy was not proved in a person with a tendency towards that specific pathology, or not used in a patient with such a condition. But if we find that the mentals, generals and characteristics fit, it is far safer to give that remedy rather than one that fits the pathology alone. Pathology should only lead us to examine the remedies and see if any one of these suits the patient. *The safest way to proceed is to select the remedy that covers the mentals and generals. Proceeding in the reverse direction, i.e. proceeding from local symptoms or starting with pathological remedies first, can be dangerous and misleading.*

One more thing needs examining and that is the prognosis of the case. Our idea of prognosis is quite different from the allopathic idea. Our prognosis differs from case to case. It is necessary to divide the prognosis into different subtypes:

–   *Cases with pathology based on a tendency which is not so excitable, or, in other words, only excitable by a specific and intense state.* These cases have the best prognosis. If we relieve the intensity of the state, then the pathology will beautifully regress.

–   *Cases where pathology is not so intense, but the state is very intense, and this intense state causes an aggravation of the pathology.* In these cases too, the prognosis is excellent. We can be almost sure of reversal of the pathology.

–   *Those cases where the pathological tendency is quite strong and which can be aggravated by almost any state of any intensity.* Here the prognosis is very poor because even if we bring down the state to a large extent, the pathology will keep on being aggravated by it.

–   *Those cases where there is pathology but there is no tendency to it,* as in acute disease. Here too, the prognosis is excellent; with the reversal of the state, the pathology will disappear.

How do we determine whether the pathological tendency is intensely excitable or not? The pathological tendency is intense if it is aggravated by a state which is not intense. If, for example, there is a weak central disturbance and the pathological condition is increasing. In these cases you find that the pathological condition will predominate.

To summarize the whole discussion: if we find that the pathology is being aggravated by an intense specific central disturbance, the prognosis is good, the pathology is reversible. On the other hand, if we find the pathology is being aggravated by a weak non-specific central disturbance – whatever the disturbance, it still aggravates the pathology – then we find the prognosis is very poor. This is irreversible because the patient has a strong tendency to the pathology.

14

MODALITY, SENSATION AND LOCATION

Modality

Disease is delusion. Delusion creates conditions, which in terms result in restriction of movement. The closer a factor is to the original situation of a remedy, the more it will aggravate the state. The further away it is from the situation of the remedy, the more it will ameliorate or be indifferent. For example, the greatest aggravating factor of *China* will be loss of fluids since this is the original situation from which the *China* state arises. One of *China*'s main condition to feel OK is: "I should not lose any fluid." Mentally, the original situation of *Lycopodium* is one when he feels he has no power. Therefore, anything concerning loss of power will aggravate him and anything concerning a gain of power will ameliorate.

So, what do aggravation and amelioration show? They show restriction, the need to be or not to be in a particular way in order to feel OK. This is directly connected to your perception of situation.

So, modalities are directly associated with the original situation, i.e. the basic delusion and for this reason they are most important. Modalities are also usually the least connected with pathology. For example, there can be an explanation for why a particular throbbing sensation expresses itself in a particular location but it will be difficult to explain why it comes at 2 p.m. That is why in medical textbooks, you will hardly find any modalities. Modalities are connected more with the state than with pathology.

Sensation

In the mind, sensations are feelings. In the body, they are types of pain or the sensations experienced. These feelings are always in tune with the basic delusion, they are always appropriate to the original situation of the state. For example, if the original situation is a ship sinking in the sea, then naturally, the associated feelings are going to be ones which help the person survive. Like modalities they too cannot be explained by the pathology. However, the difference is that they are more difficult to describe than are the modalities (what exactly you feel, you may not be sure of, but when and under what circumstances you feel it, you usually know).

Modalities and sensations have another thing in common in that they directly relate to both mind and body. Modalities usually link mind and body together since they are usually common to both. For example, a person who feels worse from movement mentally also feels worse from movement physically. Similarly, but to a lesser extent, the sensations can be related. Such a connection becomes much more difficult to observe in case of locations.

Location

With a strong tendency to pathology, a state has very little choice left in terms of the pathology to produce. One can say that the menu is very limited. Even so, it has a choice of site in the body and the radiation of the pathology, and it is definitely for a reason that it chooses one site over another. For example, in a case of leucoderma, it may show on the face or the arms, or in a case of paralysis, it may occur on the right or left side, or begin with the arm or the leg. The site chosen will be in tune with the central disturbance. The only difference between this location and the modalities and sensations, is that the individual element becomes very prominent; meaning that a paralysis of the arm of a writer or of an athlete has different significance. If the central disturbance has to do with stopping work, then the writer is likely to have a paralysis of the arm. This demonstrates that the original situation demanded stoppage of work as a survival mechanism. Whereas in an athlete, the same central disturbance will produce paralysis of the lower limb. Therefore, when we see the peculiarity or the individuality of the location in any particular illness, we have to ask what that particular location means for that particular individual, in terms of how it restricts his space or his freedom to move. It then becomes like a modality or a sensation.

The second type of location is one which is not based on pathology, for example a weak feeling in the lower limbs. In such cases, it becomes much more significant since it is directly concerned with the original situation, the conditions for feeling OK and the limitations of movement caused by such a location.

Thus, you can see that the peculiarity of the location (whether pathological or not) shows the restriction of movement, the conditions to feel OK, i.e. the adaptation to the original situation of the state. *So, location itself is a sensation and also a modality, and in reality there is no difference between these three.* All are based on the same, that is the basic delusion, and all three represent the conditions for feeling OK. To the extent that they do this, they are important, and they will do it to the extent that they are not based on pathology. Even though all three represent the same thing, you can still see that the modalities are the easiest to elicit and usually the most non-pathognomonic of the three. This is followed in importance by the sensations and finally the location. Despite this classification, we must restrain our ability to see all three as one and the same. For example, a person with desire to keep quiet, aggravation from talking and the feeling that his vocal cords are paralyzed is expressing the same thing in three ways, namely that his original situation demands that he should not talk. In fact, he may mention this as a location or a sensation or a modality, but in essence, it is one and the same.

15

CONCOMITANTS

Throughout the proving, a drug produces a number of symptoms, sensations and modalities in different parts of the body. It does this quite prominently within a few minutes, hours or days. When the symptoms are produced, further administration of the drug is stopped and pathology is not allowed to develop. It is obvious, therefore, that these symptoms are not due to pathology, but to a functional disturbance of the nervous system. For example, the dyspnoea of *Carbo vegetabilis* is not due to left ventricular failure in the provings, but it is purely nervous phenomenon.

Due to our knowledge of pathology, we interpret these symptoms in a particular way and then attribute locations to remedies, for example *Cactus* produces constriction in the chest and so we assume that it must have an action on the heart, producing ischemic disease or angina pectoris. This assumption is not logical. We know that *Cactus*, in a proving, was not proved to the point of producing pathology. So, this constricting pain is a nervous phenomenon and it is we who assume that it is heart pathology.

Similarly, the bearing down sensation of *Sepia* is a nervous sensation and not due to prolapse of the uterus (I am quite sure that the prover of *Sepia* did not get a prolapse in a few days). So, we see that the characteristic symptoms of the remedy are purely nervous sensations, but we have classified them into organs and pathologies.

I suggest that *symptoms become more important when we cannot find any organic basis or pathological explanation for them and when they occur as a concomitant to, or independent of the pathology*. These symptoms will then guide us in the selection of the correct remedy.

When taking a case, we have to look out for such symptoms which are purely due to nervous phenomenon and are in no way connected with the main pathology. A remedy which produced such phenomenon on a proving, should be very closely examined.

In a case of angina pectoris, the constricting pain alone may not indicate the remedy, but if the patient has ineffectual urge to stool with this pain, this will be a very important indication. If we understand this concept, then symptoms will have different meanings for us. For example, the spotty pain of *Kalium bichromicum* will not indicate that it is a remedy solely for peptic ulcer but we can see it in conditions where such pain is uncommon or characteristic.

The most important advantage of this idea is that it directs us to the so-called small or less used remedies, which are often considered as local ones. The local symptoms will now be open to much wider interpretation and these remedies will be used as deep acting and not merely as local acting ones. For example, *Berberis vulgaris* which has pains radiating from one point, has been used almost exclusively in renal problems. We may find great utility for this remedy where such pains are concomitant to some other condition, without the patient having any renal or ureteric calculus. Other examples of such symptoms are:

- Constriction of cardiac end of the stomach in *Phosphorus*;
- Breathlessness of *Carbo vegetabilis*;
- Constricting sensation of *Lachesis*.

There are four types of concomitants:

- *Physical concomitant to mental emotions.* For example, burning between scapula when a person is excited.
- *Physical concomitant to physical pain.* For example, during an asthmatic attack, the patient cannot tolerate light, or if the room is full of people, or he may have profuse perspiration with weakness. Throbbing of vertex during an attack of asthma is another example.
- *Mental concomitant to physical complaint.* For example, suicidal feeling during pain or becoming violent during pain.
- *Mental concomitant to mental complaint.* For example, grief with depression, but she very much likes to express herself and talk. Her loquacity is a concomitant as it cannot be explained by the grief.

Concomitants need not always be general symptoms. Sometimes, they are particular in a part of the body but have no pathological basis for their existence. My teacher successfully prescribed *Agnus castus* in the case of a child with molluscum contagiosum using the symptom "Itching of scalp when going to sleep".

16

CAUSATION

Each remedy in the Materia Medica has states caused by some specific factors which are listed as "Ailments from". These "Ailments from" come from two main sources:

- *Provings*: For examples, *Arnica* produces sore, bruised sensations, as if he had been beaten. Hence, *Arnica* is listed under "Ailments from injury".
- *Clinical sources*: It has been found that remedy symptoms occur in a patient after some stressful emotions. For example, "Ailments from grief" in *Ignatia*.

In both these cases, "Ailments from" do not come directly from provings but rather clinical applications of the remedy. Hence, in clinical practice they cannot be totally relied on in finding the remedy but at least can be used for confirmation.

A remedy has to be prescribed on symptoms and only then will it cure. Even if it is not recorded in the specific "Ailments from", it will cure provided it covers the characteristic symptoms. A remedy that covers "Ailments from" will not cure a case if the characteristic symptoms do not match. When we get a definite symptom arising from a specific "Ailments", we should examine the remedies listed against it in the Repertory to see if any of them covers the case completely. If none does, we have to leave the list and find a remedy which covers the symptoms of the case.

A study of causations listed in a remedy is very useful. It teaches us a lot about the particular remedy. For example, when we read that *Arnica* has "Ailments from blunt injury", we can understand the type of sensation that *Arnica* produces: "Sore, bruised feeling, soreness of parts lain on". Once we understand this, we will be able to use *Arnica* in many diverse situations such as typhoid fever even without a history of injury.

Whatever the constitution of the patient is, when subjected to serve blunt injury, he will most probably manifest *Arnica* symptoms. It therefore becomes his temporary medicine of that phase. It is no longer his peculiar individual symptoms that we are taking to determine his remedy. However, if the patient manifests the same symptoms, either:

- Long after the injury,
- Even without a history of injury, or
- The same symptoms from a little injury (out of proportion to the injury),

in these cases, *Arnica* is indicated not as a temporary but as a deep acting medicine for the patient.

Symptoms observed in the following circumstances will represent the central disturbance of the person, and the remedy selected for them will have a deeper and more lasting
effect when:

  – The symptoms are found without any "Ailments from";
  – They arise from a different causation (for example from grief, anger, physical
    exertion, etc.);
  – The patient's state is caused by a disproportionately minor event, such as loss
    of sleep, even for one or two hours.

In similar ways, an *Ignatia* picture without a very strong or recent history of grief
would be highly suggestive of *Ignatia* as a constitutional medicine. Thus, the "Ailments
from" in a remedy helps us in a negative way, viz. if a remedy is indicated even in the
absence of "Ailments from" in the patient, it becomes doubly indicated.

In the same way, certain situations act as "Ailments from" – like *Sepia* which has
ailments from the birth of many children. If the *Sepia* state is found in such a woman and
the state is proportional to the cause, the remedy will only act for a time and that too
provided the maintaining factor is removed. But if the same state is found in a young girl
(i.e. without a cause), *Sepia* will act on her very deeply and for a long time. Another
example, a child gives the symptoms of *Cina*, grinding teeth, itching rectum and crankiness.
Naturally, you will suspect worms. The parents tell you that they have tested his stool
repeatedly and not found any signs of worms. *Cina* becomes much more indicated now
than if there were worms. In a case of worms, these symptoms will be common, being due
to the worms themselves; but in a case without worms, these symptoms become the central
symptoms of the case (there being no local cause for them). Hence, they become indications
for the constitutional remedy.

One of the best examples I have seen is *Cocculus*. *Cocculus* has "Ailments from
loss of sleep" and nursing the sick. In fact, this means that this central disturbance of
Cocculus corresponds to a state produced when a person remains awake several nights
with watchful anxiety about a sick relative (for example, a mother looking after her sick
child). Imagine her state after four to five nights of such sleepless anxiety. The nervous
system is affected. The feeling is of great weakness, dullness, giddiness, imbalance and
nausea. This weakness is accompanied by tremendous sensitivity of the nerves, they are
"raw" and "on edge". The mental state is of great sensitivity and excitability. Sensibility
at the least noise, odours, looking at moving objects.

This state will be ameliorated by *Cocculus* in a woman who has been caring for her
sick child. But, if the same state is found in a person without the cause (loss of sleep with
anxiety, etc.), *Cocculus* will be doubly indicated.

17

SELECTION OF THE POTENCY

In Homoeopathy, the selection of the potency has been a much debated question. Many of the ideas are empirical and, from these, rules have been framed. In this chapter we will examine the basis of potency selection and, through logic, try to formulate some rules.

Basis of potency selection

We have to go back to our understanding of disease. Disease consists of two distinct parts:

- Central disturbance, and
- Peripheral disturbance.

By central disturbance we mean the general adaptation of a person which precedes localization of the disturbance. This adaptation of the whole being to a particular stress then extends to parts and organs of the body producing local disturbances, that we can call pathology. In understanding the dynamics of disease, we have to understand that the organism tries as much as possible to keep the disturbance restricted to the centre and to allow it to produce localized changes. This phenomenon can be seen very well in children when they have intense mental symptoms, such as restlessness, irritability, obstinacy or jealousy, but the local changes are very minimal. So, in most children you have a very intense central disturbance and very little local pathology.

Why does this happen? Let us consider the opposite state. In old people we do not find such an intense central disturbance, instead, we see very severe local pathology. You see cancers, hypertension and so forth, but very little central disturbance, namely very few mental and general symptoms. This phenomenon can be explained by stating that the central disturbance belongs to the whole being and it affects all the organ systems in a functional way so that the heart beat faster, the respiration becomes rapid, the blood pressure increases, etc. When the vital organs like the heart, lungs or liver cannot bear the intensity of the disturbance, then the organism will keep the level of the central disturbance to the point where it can be borne by the vital organs without any adverse effect. For example, when the stress of a microorganism like bacteria affects the system, the first response is a generalized one. There may be loss of appetite, malaise, weakness, aversion to being disturbed and high temperature. When the temperature reaches 104 °F, 105 °F or 106 °F, then vital organs like the heart cannot work fast, and the high temperature itself can damage the organism. So, the central disturbance is restricted at that level, the temperature is not allowed to rise, and the disturbance is diverted to some local part such as the lungs, kidneys, or joints (producing, for example, pneumonia, glomerulonephritis or arthritis, respectively). So the level of central disturbance is determined by the amount of stress the vital organs of the body can tolerate at a particular time.

When we understand this, then it becomes simpler to understand that in children, where the vital organs are in good shape, where the heart can bear a lot of stress, where the lungs can breathe much faster and where the body can stand much higher temperatures, the vital force can afford to keep the central disturbance at a very high level and the local disturbance at a low level. That is why we see many mental and general symptoms in children and fewer local ones.

Application of this idea

The potency (power) of a medicine consists in its ability to produce a central disturbance, the higher the potency the more intense the central disturbance it can produce. So, when we select the potency we have to select it at the level which is just above the level of the central disturbance of the person at that time. If the potency selected is much lower, then it will have very little effect and therefore have to be repeated quite frequently. If the potency selected is much higher, then it may produce a level of disturbance greater than the one the body currently has. Since the level of disturbance of the body may be just the one the organs can tolerate, producing a much higher disturbance could lead to a bad aggravation and may be harmful. Therefore, *the selection of potency has to be based on the intensity of the central disturbance (which is represented by the mentals and generals).* The intensity of the mentals and generals is seen by the extent of clarity of their expression. *If the mentals and generals are clear and intense then the potency has to be high,* if you want a quick response.

I have heard that if there is gross pathology we cannot give a high potency. Many people advocate this as a cautionary rule. I do not subscribe to such rules. If the central disturbance is high it means that the organs are in a position to tolerate a high potency. Therefore, if you give a high potency in such a case, it would not be harmful even if the pathology was marked.

Based on this understanding I have given high potencies in cases with severe pathology without noticing any aggravation of the pathology. Of course, in these cases, the mentals and generals were quite marked. However, in case of doubt, it may be better to start with the potency that is just one step lower than the one we actually want to give, and then increase it later after we have seen the effect.

Potency and delusion

We have already seen that a higher potency produces a more intense central disturbance, i.e. a more intense mental and general disturbance. When such intense mentals and generals are produced, the delusions become quite specific and marked. So, when we talk about 6th, 30th, 200th, 1000th, 10 000th, 50 000th, 100 000th potency, what is happening? If we look at a remedy, say *Nitricum acidum*, we see that it has anxiety about health, malice, anger, irritability, hatred of persons who offend, unmoved by apology.

All this comes from the situation of a person who is fighting a court battle, or someone who is having a long-standing feud and whose survival depends upon his being obstinate, hateful, malicious and unresponsive to apology.

In low potencies *Nitricum acidum* produces anxiety in the prover. This is unasso-ciated anxiety, free floating anxiety with some irritability. When we go to the 30th potency, the anxiety becomes a little more specific. He feels anxiety about himself, and some hatred appears. In the 200th potency, the anxiety about health becomes a little more marked. As we go higher, 'say, to 10 000th, it becomes clear to him that he has hatred for persons who offend, and is unmoved by apology.

As we go higher to the 50 000th potency, the delusion that he is fighting a court battle, that he is engaged in a long-standing war in which he cannot yield, comes to him quite clearly. So, one can say, as potency increases, the delusion becomes clearer and the original situation of the state is more clearly revealed.

Application

When the remedy we select for a patient is not well indicated, when the picture is not clear or when you prescribe on something broad like general anxiety and irritability, it is necessary to give a low potency of the drug repeatedly, and hope for some change, as the selected remedy will produce a state of undefined anxiety and irritability.

As the person's mental state becomes clearer and clearer and we feel sure that the remedy is well indicated (and we are even able to find the exact delusion), then we go to the higher potency immediately, provided, of course, that the central disturbance is intense. However, if the central disturbance is intense, but the remedy we find is not the exact one, we have to use a low potency because the higher potency of the non-indicated remedy will not touch the case. If, for example, the man who has the state of *Nitricum acidum*, with the delusion of a court battle (this is his specific delusion), is given a remedy like *Lycopodium* which also has anxiety and irritability, then you give it in 30th or 6th potency. If you give him *Lycopodium* 10M or 50M, it will produce the specific delusion that he does not have the capacity to reach his goal, and so he will reject it straight away. His system will just reject *Lycopodium* 10M because it is producing an exact message in the delusion that he does not have the capacity to reach his goal, and when such an exact message is given and this is not the message inside the patient, it will be rejected. If you give *Lycopodium* 30th or 6th, however, he will feel OK in his anxiety and irritability. This message is accepted because it is not specific. As the indication becomes more and more specific, you can go higher and higher in potency, but if your remedy selection is very broad-based, then you have to use lower potencies. This probably is the reason why the biochemical remedies are prescribed in low potencies, even in decimal potencies. As there are only twelve of these remedies, they cannot be specific, the effect is going to be very broad-based, and so the lowest potency four times a day has some effect.

Change of potency

After giving the indicated remedy for a few months in a chronic case or a few days in an acute case, sometimes even a few hours, we are able to bring about a change in the condition of the body itself where the vitality increases. The body is now able to tolerate a higher central disturbance than the one it was able to before treatment. The level of central disturbances goes up a fraction with every amelioration or peripheral pathology. In chronic cases, therefore, my experience has shown that after six-seven months or sometimes after one year or even two years, the same potency does not hold good any longer and I have to increase it. This means that the level of central disturbance which can be tolerated has now risen. Usually, in one or two years, we find that the peripheral pathology has regressed considerably.

The risk in "local" prescribing

We can prescribe on the local symptoms and local modalities; for example, a person has a *Calcarea carbonica* constitution, but has joint pains with the modalities of *Rhus toxicodendron*, i.e. worse by fast motion, better by continued movement, better by heat, etc. These are common symptoms of the joint problem – they are pathological symptoms, and not symptoms of central disturbance being expressed locally. In this case, if we give *Rhus toxicodendron* in any potency, especially a high one, there will hardly be any effect on the whole person (because it does not match the whole person), but it will have an effect on the joint because it has the modalities of *Rhus toxicodendron*. It produces, therefore, local homoeopathic effect. By ameliorating the joint, it will relieve the patient temporarily but it is harmful in the long run, because, if we keep repeating *Rhus toxico-dendron*, we will find no amelioration in the mentals and generals, which shows it is not the remedy for the patient. Even this effect on the joint is temporary and therefore, frequent repetition will be needed.

As you keep on ameliorating the joint with high potencies, the body has no choice but to take the joint problem and push it into the deeper organs or systems of the body. We have seen that the organism tries to keep disease in the least important organ, but if we do not allow the disturbance to localize there, it has no choice but to push it to more important organs, because it cannot afford to increase the level of central disturbance. By pushing it into more important organs, we are causing a suppression. So, if you keep on repeating a high potency for a long period of time based on the local modalities, the result will be suppression.

To summarize from the above, the rules of potency selection are:
– The higher the central disturbance, the higher the potency;
– The clearer the mentals and generals, the higher the potency;
– The closer we get to the exact remedy of the patient, the higher the potency called for.

A small controversy

When in my seminars I suggest that after treatment the central disturbance may increase in level, with reduction of peripheral pathology, the listeners are confused. The confusion is that according to Hering's law of the direction of cure, cure proceeds from the centre to the periphery and I was seen as suggesting that in the process of cure, the direction is from the periphery to the centre.

I wish to remove this confusion. There is no contradiction between my ideas and Hering's law; in fact, my ideas are based upon Hering's law. Let us understand Hering's law first. It states that in cure, the disease travels from more to less important organs, from above downward, from within outward and in the reverse order of appearance. Hering here referred to pathology.

When disease comes, the central disturbance occurs first. Hering did not mean that initially you will get an affection of the little finger and then it will start producing mental symptoms. He meant that the central disturbance occurs first, and then the body tries to keep pathology at peripheral level. The body first tries to keep disease at the level of the finger joints, then at the level of the lungs and then at the level of the heart. This is the direction of the disease in pathology. The central disturbance is there initially and then, because the central disturbance cannot tolerate the stress anymore, i.e. the level is increased beyond endurance, it localizes the effects in joints, and then spreads to the lungs and then localizes in the heart. When cure takes place, disease takes the reverse order, first it will leave the heart, then the lungs and then the joints. This is what Hering meant.

It is unfortunate that Hering's words about the progress of pathology have been understood wrongly as applying to the entire affection of the organism. Masters like Stuart Close and H. A. Roberts have emphasized that functional disorder precedes development of pathology. Does this mean then, that the central disturbance (functions of mind and body) are first disordered and then follow disorders of the body (periphery)? Hering's law explains developments at this point.

Disease always proceeds from the central disturbance to the periphery. In pathology, it proceeds from the periphery towards the centre; this is the idea. In a curative direction, disease first abates from an important organ that is affected pathologically, and the last disorder to go will be that of the least important organ affected; only then will the central disturbance be relieved. When you have a patient of *Lycopodium*, he will first have lack of confidence, i.e. the central disturbance cannot be contained, he will develop eczema or asthma. When cure takes place, his asthma will go first, the eczema second, but lack of confidence will be there throughout. If lack of confidence goes, then there is no basis for the eczema or asthma. Without the central disturbance, there cannot be peripheral pathology, because peripheral pathology is only a diversion from the central disturbance. Now, as the level of health improves, the body becomes strong enough to tolerate a greater central disturbance (this takes place over a long period of time). It is not that I gave him *Lycopodium* and his eczema disappeared and his lack of confidence increased. This does not happen; if the asthma disappears, his level of lack of confidence remains the same; and when the eczema disappears, his level of lack of confidence also remains the same.

How do we know? Because the same potency is working, the same potency is effective, and at a certain point, the potency stops working and a higher potency is required. This shows that the central disturbance has gone up and when this happens, it means that the body has become stronger and it can tolerate better. This does not take place immediately in a *chronic case* but over a period of one or one and a half years. In *acute cases*, it will take place more quickly: the weakness of the system gradually reduces, and its ability to tolerate the central disturbance is improved. You can then give higher potencies 1M, 10M or 50M within a few days. You can increase the potencies because the system gets stronger more quickly in an acute condition. It is like water in a reservoir which is marked with a danger level. The water should not rise above the danger level; otherwise the surrounding important structures will be flooded. Hence, when water comes to that level, a little water is diverted (let off) to the less important areas somewhere in the periphery and then, when that area gets full, a somewhat more important area is filled up with water. But, when the danger mark is raised, there can be more water in the reservoir.

Difference between crude and potency

The crude remedy produces a peripheral disturbance and the potentized remedy produces a central disturbance. The mental symptoms that are produced by the crude remedy are either:

– Direct effects on the brain, as caused by hallucinogens like opium, etc., or
– A generalized, non-specific mental agitation or dullness as a result of physical distress or weakness caused by the drug in its toxic form.

The crude remedy has very little dynamic effect and most of its effects are nothing but local, toxic effects, the sum total of which resembles its general disturbance. A potentized remedy, on the other hand, has no local effect. Its action is seen in the form of a delusion of a situation both physically and mentally.

We can, therefore, understand that a crude dose of *Arsenicum* will produce local effects like diarrhoea, gastritis and changes in skin, hair, etc., with restlessness, agitation in the mind and irritation of the nervous system. Potentized *Arsenicum* however, would produce a delusion of a situation in which there is fear of death, fastidiousness, thirst, etc.

The higher the potency, the clearer the delusion. In sensitive persons a delusion is followed by generalized disturbances and later by local effects. Those who are not sensitive to the delusion (who for some reason are non-reactive to such a suggestion) will not show any reaction from a potentized drug, whereas one will react to toxic or crude doses, because the crude dose is a direct assault on the local part and is not dependent for its effect on producing a delusion. Therefore, given in crude form, a drug can only make the pathology worse.

The potentized drug, on the other hand, does not usually produce any damage if given in a single dose since it is just like asking a person to imagine a situation. Unless the picture is so horrid and the person too fragile, such an imagination cannot cause harm if given only once.

18

REPETITION OF THE DOSE

I think it is fairly obvious that the ideal time to repeat the dose would be when the effect of the previous dose is exhausted.

We shall discuss three aspects of this question:
- How do we know when the effect of the previous dose has been exhausted?
- What will happen if we repeat before the dose has exhausted its action?
- What will happen if we do not repeat even after the dose has exhausted its action?

How do we know that the dose has exhausted its effect?

For this, we have to first understand what the effect of the dose is. This effect of a dose (of the correct remedy) is to reduce the level of central disturbance. This means that the patient feels better on the whole, his mentals and generals are ameliorated, he feels more comfortable, his conditions for himself and others have gone down and he has more space to be in the moment both physically and mentally. After a period of time, when we see that the level of central disturbance has reverted back to its original position, he again feels the same way as before. This means that the dose has exhausted its action.

We must distinguish between an "apparent" return to the original position, and a "real" return. It is possible that the return to the original position as reported by the patient is not real but apparent, meaning that the person was and is ameliorated but due to an immediate exciting cause the state has been temporarily aggravated and now it looks as if it is in the same (original) position. In this case we have to wait for the exciting factor to go away and then judge the level of the central disturbance. This is like when we want to know the blood pressure, we take it at a time when the patient is not excited so as to avoid factors of instability. So, we take it, usually, first thing in the morning after sleep. But suppose the patient suddenly gets anxious as you measure his blood pressure, you will see that there is a marked change. This cannot be relied upon as we have ignored a factor of instability at the time of recording. In the same way, we have to keep the standard conditions in mind when measuring a man's central disturbance. Unless we judge the effect of the dose under (unchanged) standards of circumstances, we may reach wrong conclusions about the state of his mental disturbance.

For example, when a man is depressed because his boss has fired him, we should allow his depression to settle down; and, after a few days or weeks, we can assess him.

If that time we find the central disturbance to be the same or higher than earlier, then this is the time for repetition of the dose.

Why does the dose exhaust its action?

We have already seen that disease is an out of proportion or an unsuitable reaction. Out of proportion reactions occur because of the phenomenon of aggravation when under an exciting factor (*phenomenon of excessive reaction*). Unsuitable reactions take place also because of a root of disease. It is these two factors that tend to bring back the state to the original level.

The second reason why the dose exhausts its effect is that when the central disturbance is lowered and the patient's condition is somewhat ameliorated, the body draws back a little of the peripheral disturbance into the central disturbance, and then the level of central disturbance touches its original level. The cases that will not require repetition are therefore:

- Cases with no pathology, or
- When the central disturbance was caused by an acute exciting factor which has passed away.

For example, a person who is subjected to sudden fright is now in a state of *Aconitum*. You give *Aconitum*, and it will not be necessary to repeat. There is no exciting factor and therefore there is going to be no automatic aggravation of the state. Further, there is no root and therefore the chances of the state getting excited are even less. In such a case, repetition will not be required, but when there is an exciting factor, repetition is necessary because, as long as there is stress, the state will tend to go out of proportion automatically. Or, if there is root, as in a chronic case, depending on the excitability of the root, the state will get excited from factors which are innocent for other people. That state will aggravate itself and the central disturbance will reach the same level again.

After a remedy, as we start reducing the central disturbance, the excitability of the root will also decrease and as this happens it will be less affected by outside factors. It will be less excitable and therefore aggravated to a lesser extent.

How long does it take the dose to exhaust its effect?

- If the exciting factor is very strong and it is still persistent, the dose will exhaust itself very quickly.
- If the root is very excitable, even minor exciting factors will strongly aggravate the state and therefore, the effect of the dose will be soon exhausted.
- Aggravating factors in the environment and in the situation also cause the dose to exhaust itself quickly.
- A strong pathology will also cause the dose to exhaust quickly.

All these circumstances will require frequent repetition of the dose. The matter of the repetition should be determined by when the dose really exhausts itself and therefore one cannot make a standard rule to apply in all cases.

If we repeat high potencies frequently, the following possibilities arise:

– Where the potency is equal to or lower than the central disturbance, such a potency is not capable of aggravating the central disturbance since it cannot produce something more intense than the existing central disturbance. It is therefore not capable of producing much harm, given the fact that the body is already able to tolerate the central disturbance. It may be worth repeating the lower potency frequently to speed up the cure, but only when the previous dose has exhausted its effect. You can also gradually step up the potency until you get an aggravation, then stop. Do not repeat the potency that causes the aggravation, especially in cases which are not in a position to tolerate such aggravations.

– If you repeat a potency higher than the central disturbance, the body which could tolerate the higher stimulus, may not be able to tolerate prolonged high stimuli and this can lead to:

  – the death of the patient, or

  – the body diverting this increased central disturbance into the preexisting peripheral pathology, thus aggravating the pathology, rendering the case more difficult to cure.

So far, we have talked about repeating the dose of the correct remedy. If the remedy is wrong, repeating the dose may lead to suppression and the pathology could be pushed even deeper, since the remedy will act locally.

Whether the potency is higher or lower than the central disturbance will be decided on the intensity of mentals and generals. In our assessment of the central disturbance, the following criteria could be helpful:

– If the aggravation is sharp, the potency is higher;

– If the remedy acts quickly, it is likely to be very near the central disturbance, or higher;

– The longer the duration of action, the closer the potency is to the central disturbance, provided there is no exciting cause, since an exciting cause will exhaust the action of the remedy faster.

The effect of the dose is instantaneous. It is one impact that the dose gives but the effect of this impact can last for a long time. The aggravation is momentary, but if we keep on repeating these momentary aggravations for a long period of time, it can be harmful in some cases.

Sometimes, we may be too cautious to repeat, despite repetition being needed. The central disturbance was better but now it has come back to its original level, but we just wait and wait. In such a case, the central disturbance will do two things:

- It will excite the root, making it even more prominent.
- With time, it will again go back into the peripheral pathology. What came out of pathology will go back into the pathology and so, your good work will be spoiled.

For these two reasons, we have to repeat the dose when its action is exhausted.

19

ACUTE PROCESSES

An acute disease has an exciting cause, comes suddenly, has a rapid course and end in either death or recovery. Strictly speaking acute diseases are states of being which last for a limited period of time. Often, however, we are tempted to call such processes as infective hepatitis, pneumonia or coryza, or acute diseases though these are pathological processes and not states. Two observations can be made in such cases:

- During the acute process the state of the patient has not changed from the one he had earlier; or
- In the acute process, the state has changed.

We have to ask what the significance of each of the above types is. It is obvious that if the state has changed, it needs to be treated by another remedy. If the state remains unchanged, then we may require either to wait and watch, repeat the dose or go higher in potency, depending upon the intensity of the state.

Usually, an acute process is caused by an acute exciting factor, for example psychological, physical, biological or chemical. It is necessary to examine the intensity of the exciting factor and we can do this by asking what percentage of people will be affected in the same manner by that factor. A causative factor can be called a factor of epidemic proportion, if it is intense enough to affect almost anyone in the same manner.

We have seen two types of acute processes:
- Where the state is changed;
- Where the state remains the same.

We also have two types of exciting factors:
- Of epidemic proportion;
- Of non-epidemic proportion.

	Epidemic cause	Non-epidemic cause
Change of state	A	B
No change	C	D

Each of these types has different significance as far as the prognosis is concerned.

113

Type A: There is a change of state from an intense cause of epidemic proportion. What does this mean? It is like saying there is an epidemic affecting a large number of people and this man is one of them. He has average vitality and an averagely intense chronic disease state. He reacts to this particular exciting factor by a change of posture to suit it. For example, when there is a war, all doctors, farmers, lawyers, become soldiers until the war ends. This change results from intensity of the exciting factor which necessitates that reaction for survival. Now, the question arises – if this is a survival mechanism, why do we need to treat it? Why does the soldier state require treatment if the doctor becomes a soldier in a war as a survival mechanism? If the reaction was suitable to the cause, then why does it need treatment? The answer is simple. It is that under an exciting factor, the state aggravates itself and blows out of proportion. As long as the war continues, the man will not just remain the soldier, but will keep on getting more and more intense as a soldier, much more intense than is needed and this can kill him.

Homoeopathic medicine brings back the reaction to the proportion required, i.e. to the optimum intensity, thus saving lives in acute conditions even when the state is suitable. This, we have already discussed in the chapter on "Out of Proportion Reactions".

Type B: Change of state from a non-epidemic cause. For example, a doctor becomes a soldier at the merest threat of war, a minor injury brings out an *Arnica* state, or a slight loss of blood brings on a *China* state.

Two conditions are required for this to happen:
– There was a silent disease or an excitable root of that state already in existence;
– The state which was dominating earlier was not equipped to meet this exciting cause.

For example, in a *Calcarea* person, the slightest fright can cause a *Stramonium* state because a *Calcarea* state is not equipped to handle a situation of terror. A healthy man is equipped to face it but a *Calcarea* state has to change. Likewise, an *Arsenicum* state or a *Hyoscyamus* state is capable of facing that terror but not *Calcarea*.

This can frequently be seen in acute asthmatic attacks where patients may require a remedy like *Arsenicum* in the acute and some slow remedy like *Baryta carbonica* in their chronic phase.

Type C: State unchanged even when the exciting factor is epidemic (intense). For example, a person gets 40% burns and remains in the same state as earlier, or there is a big injury and the person remains *Phosphorus* and does not become *Arnica*. During the acute pain of the injury, he still likes sympathy and wants to be touched (opposite of *Arnica*). This means that this chronic state is so intense that it tries to manage all acute crises without changing the state. His conditions are so strong that they cannot be changed. The doctor, even during war, remains a doctor when everyone else is becoming a soldier.

Type D: No change of the state in non-epidemic cause. This means that his state is able to manage this exciting factor without needing to change.

If after some time of homoeopathic treatment a patient who has been in the same state even during acute troubles, develops a change of state from a not so intense cause, this is a good sign. It shows that the strength of the dominating disease has gone down and this has allowed other states to come up.

For example, a man has both the doctor and soldier state within him and the doctor state is very intense (even during war he remains a doctor). You keep treating him and now he becomes a soldier with the threat of war; this means that the strength of the doctor state has gone down and now the soldier state is excited. He may come back to the doctor state once the threat is over, but during the exciting factor, you could see the soldier state coming up. So now you will be cautious that after further treatment, the soldier state may come up even without an exciting factor, and alternation of soldier and doctor treatment may be required until he is cured.

Satellite and distinct states

Question: What is the difference between a state of *Stramonium* produced in a *Calcarea* person as you mentioned earlier and the person with two distinct states of *Calcarea* and *Stramonium*?

Answer: The former I call *satellite* and the latter I call *silent state*. What is the difference between a satellite and a silent state?

A satellite state is dependent upon another state for its existence. The chance of a satellite state coming up are less and less as the original state goes down. As he becomes less of a *Calcarea*, there are fewer chances of a *Stramonium* state coming up in him if the *Stramonium* state is a satellite. The reverse is true if the *Stramonium* state in him is a distinct state. Here the less *Calcarea* he becomes, the greater the possibility of the *Stramonium* state coming up. A satellite is like a branch of a tree. When you cut down the tree, its branches will also be cut, but the other tree will become more prominent.

Usually, a satellite remedy is a regional remedy. It shows in a specific region and with a special purpose, with not such prominent mentals and generals. It comes up because the main remedy is not able to cope with that specific region.

At that time the original mentals and generals of the previous remedy will be suppressed, and the satellite will take charge of the whole but it will concentrate on a part. If a *Calcarea* patient lifts a weight, he gets a sprain with the typical *Rhus toxicodendron* modality. At that time the original *Calcarea* state will be suppressed and the patient will be hoping about seeking relief from the pain. There may not be any mentals of *Rhus toxicodendron* except probably some restlessness. If left to itself or with some balm or analgin this pain will disappear. If the *Calcarea* state is taken care of later, the chances of his spraining occurring so easily will also diminish. Similarly, *Calcarea* will have other satellite spheres like glandular inflammation of *Belladonna*, or fear and fright of *Stramonium*.

115

A remedy is called a satellite only if the state is excited by something that normally cannot excite such a state; for example, a bit of dust causes a lot of wheezing.

A patient can be cured without even once using a satellite remedy. The whole satellite state can be relieved with time or local treatment, but if it is a distinct state, it cannot be cured without a medicine or with local treatment. It will persist until the right medicine is given.

Also, we must always examine if what we think of as a satellite remedy does not fit the entire case even after the acute crisis is over. Many times we have prescribed *Nux vomica* for an acute complaint only to find even the chronic one improved drastically, which means that in fact the main symptoms of the case were also covered by *Nux vomica*. It is for this reason also that we like to avoid prescribing the satellite medicines, because, for all we know, one of them could inadvertently be the right medicine for the whole case and we would be left with the mistaken impression that it was just a satellite medicine. Therefore, when in doubt it may be advisable to use local measures, rarely even allopathic medicines such as pain relievers or bronchodilators to tide over the acute crisis, so that we are at least sure which medicine is working or not working.

The satellite will be in some way the opposite to the main remedy (otherwise it will not be a satellite). It will possess at least one quality intensely which the main remedy does not have. The acute inflammation of *Belladonna*, the acute terror of *Stramonium*, and the tremendous amelioration by motion of *Rhus toxicodendron* are all features which are opposite to mild, slow, indolent *Calcarea carbonica*. Also, one must remember that even though we call these satellites, even though they are dependent upon the main remedy, they are full-fledged diseases in their own right and any disease which lasts for too long is bound to develop its own root.

When such a root is developed, you will find that now you have a full *Rhus toxicodendron* picture with the mentals and generals of the remedy; then it is no longer a satellite. It becomes a disease in its own right and can be transmitted as such to the next generation along with the root of the main disease, so that in the next generation the satellite becomes a separate disease and this time an exciting factor will bring about a full-blown picture of that disease which will not subside without the indicated remedy.

Example 1

A man of 24 years presented with infective hepatitis with high Bilirubin, SGOT, SGPT. He had many symptoms common to hepatitis, such as nausea and decreased appetite, but his cravings and aversions remained unchanged. His state of mind was also the same. He was a very mild person, answered by nodding, was social, affectionate and did not like any quarrels. During the hepatitis, I saw no change in his state from what it was before. I gave *Pulsatilla* and he recovered beautifully. He required no other medicine even after his recovery from the hepatitis. In such cases where there is no change of indication in the acute condition, you will find a very strong state.

116

Of course, at this time there will be symptoms of the acute stress factor. For example, in a case of injury a person will have pain and swelling, but what we have to see is the mental and general state. If the mental and general state has changed, then a change of remedy is required. If it has not changed, despite the fact that all the local symptoms have changed, it still does not require a change of remedy. That is why I say: *the indication for change is the change of indication, i.e. change in the indicating symptoms.* If the indications on which you have based your remedy are changed, then and only then will you change the remedy.

Example 2

I am treating a man with diabetes and chronic myeloid leukaemia. His remedy is *Arsenicum album* and for the past three years he has required nothing else. He has had several acute crises – a severe tooth infection and cellulitis – which were also tackled by *Arsenicum album*. He wrote in the form: "I have consulted several doctors, all have spoiled my health." He could think of nothing else but his health. If his blood count went up by 400, then he would calculate that if every three weeks it went up by 400, then at the end of one year, it will be up by a certain number and he will die. He was very cautious and mistrustful. He had very little space for others.

After three years of *Arsenicum album*, he had significant relief from his anxiety with concurrent relief of the diabetes and control of the leukaemia. At about this time, his sister who was also my patient, had some problem in her own life and came to seek my advice. I was a bit rude and strong with her because I felt it was required. She complained to her brother about this and it made him so angry that he came to my clinic and he could not speak, he was trembling and even said that he would like to strike me. You must remember that he was better with my treatment and I was the only physician in whom he had some trust. If he antagonized me, it might not be good for his health. He regarded me with respect and knew that my intentions were good. But to my surprise, he went into an intense *Staphysagria* state from an exciting cause which in my view was not so intense. *Staphysagria* helped him beautifully and he was again back in an *Arsenicum* state. It was a good sign. The *Staphysagria* state is in no way dependent on *Arsenicum*. This root or silent disease existed in him. Since the *Arsenicum* state had gone down, this allowed the *Staphysagria* to come out.

If in a chronic state there is an acute phase, for example headache and vomiting, but the general state remains the same or is a little better, do not touch the case. You need interfere only when the state inside has gone up in intensity or has changed. If the person says: "I am better but yesterday I went out, so I got headache", leave him alone. But if he says: "For a minor reason, I have a severe headache", you are to reevaluate the case. You may have to give another remedy or the same remedy in a higher potency.

Example 3

A man of 36 was brought by his relatives for treatment of acute schizophrenia. He was violent and had to be tied up in our hospital, since he was attacking everybody. The

117

history was that he was an artist who was poor and had got married to a very rich man's daughter. This woman had a congenital deformity of one arm and therefore could not find a suitable groom. Her father decided that the best option was to find a poor man for her and support him in coming up in life. After the marriage, there was a lot of domination of our patient by his father-in-law. One day, after a serious insult, this man became openly abusive and violent and developed this acute condition. The symptoms of the case fitted into *Hyoscyamus*, which in 10M potency, after a few days, brought him out of this state. I then studied his case again and found his remedy to be *Staphysagria*, since *Staphysagria* his known for its suppressed anger and suppressed violence as well as its control. It is such a person who, when provoked beyond a limit, needs to become expressively violent and lose control, which is precisely the state of *Hyoscyamus*. One can say that here the *Hyoscyamus* state depended upon the underlying *Staphysagria* state.

Eight months after this, the patient had a minor relapse of the *Hyoscyamus* state, which was again promptly brought under control with *Hyoscyamus*. He has been on *Staphysagria* since then, and in the past six years he has remained quite well, despite several exciting factors.

In summary, treat the state that exists at the present moment. If it is out of proportion to the cause, then treat it, but if it is in proportion , leave it, do not treat it. Treat the state with the remedy for that state.

I like to give this example – if someone is setting fire to your house, catch him and stop him rather than inquire who has sent him!

20

THE HOMOEOPATHIC APPROACH
TO DIABETES

There are many diseases for which, these days, people recognize the superiority of homoeopathic treatment. Among such diseases are recurrent colds, asthma, skin diseases, rheumatic disorders, etc.

However, there are some diseases for which most people think modern medicine is better. Diabetes is one such disease. In this chapter, I wish to share with you some facts about diabetes; where modern medicine stands and how Homoeopathy differs. I am using diabetes as an example to show the difference between the two systems in their approach to any pathology.

The old idea

If you ask an allopathic general practitioner what diabetes is, he will tell you that it is increased blood sugar and that it is caused by deficiency of insulin.

He will explain that there is an organ called the pancreas which produces insulin. When we eat, various carbohydrates, sugar and starch are digested in the intestines and simplified into glucose. This glucose is absorbed into the bloodstream and carried to various parts of the body. Glucose is the fuel or energy for various organs and cells in our body. But, for glucose to go from the bloodstream into the cells, insulin is essential. If there is not enough insulin, then glucose cannot enter the cells in the proper amount. Thus, it remains in the blood and the blood glucose level rises. When the glucose level rises beyond 180 mg/dl, the kidneys are given instruction to throw out the excess sugar and so we find sugar in the urine also.

The old idea was that diabetes is basically a disease of the pancreas, that the primary problem is the deficiency of insulin, and the treatment consists in controlling the blood sugar level. The normal blood glucose level ranges from 80 to 120 mg/dl and the prevailing idea is that the blood sugar must be tightly controlled. This control, according to general consensus, could be achieved by three means:

- *Diet*: Diabetics are advised a diet low in starch as a counterweight to the deficient action of insulin; no rice, no potatoes and no sugar.
- *Pills*: When diet fails to control blood sugar level, diabetics are put on oral antidiabetic tablets. These (oral hypoglycemic) pills are meant to reduce the

blood sugar.
- *Insulin*: When even the tablets fail, direct supply of insulin through injections is advised and is supposed to bring about good control.

Change in viewpoint

As explained, it was commonly believed that diabetes is due to lack of insulin. This was the idea until the time when there emerged certain methods of finding out exactly how much insulin there is in the blood. When these methods were discovered (i.e. radio-immuno assay), it was found to the great surprise of the investigators that in the majority of diabetics, the amount of insulin in the blood was normal and even sometimes more than normal. Therefore, diabetes could be classified into two types:
- *In which insulin is lacking*: Type 1 diabetes or juvenile diabetes, which usually occurs at a young age.
- *Where insulin was normal*: Type 2 or maturity onset type diabetes, which begins usually after the age of thirty or so.

Regarding maturity onset diabetes, since no deficiency of insulin is found in most cases, it was suggested that probably there is a defect in the insulin receiving power of the tissues, that the number of insulin receptors is less. This is still a speculation.

A very significant discovery

The first thing any doctor advises on seeing a diabetic is tight control of blood sugar. He will say: "If you don't control the sugar level, you will develop complications." The only acute complication of high blood sugar is coma. See what Harrison ("Textbook of Internal Medicine") says:

> "Maturity onset diabetics develop not ketoacidotic coma but hyper-osmolar coma, which develops at a blood sugar reading of 1000 to 1600 mg/dl."

Thus, coma is very rare in the adult who has developed diabetes. It is the juvenile diabetic who can develop coma when the insulin intake falls short of the requirement. Even in these cases, the incidence of death due to coma is only 1% if treated correctly.

So, diabetologists are not so worried about coma. The worry is about *chronic complications* of diabetes. These are changes in the eye (retinopathy), changes in the kidney (nephropathy), changes in the nerves (neuropathy) and changes in the heart (ischemic heart disease). The basic cause of these complications is a change in the blood vessels which occurs in diabetics. This is called *microangiopathy* and can be assessed by measuring the thickness of the capillary basement membrane.

It was presumed that these changes occur because of high blood sugar. Therefore, it was thought that by controlling the sugar level, these changes would not occur. However, certain significant discoveries were made that upset this idea. The first was made by a renowned diabetologist named Siperstein.

Siperstein found that these changes of microangiopathy occurred *even before the blood sugar actually developed*. He measured the capillary basement membrane thickness of potential diabetics, i.e. those people who are very likely to develop increased blood sugar after the age of thirty-five to forty. When he measured their basement membrane thickness, long before they developed this increased blood sugar, he found that it was already thickened.

The significance of this discovery

Siperstein's discovery meant that microangiopathy, which was until now considered to be a complication of blood sugar, occurred long before the increase in blood sugar. Siperstein speculated that perhaps microangiopathy is the fundamental trouble in diabetes and high blood sugar itself is a complication of microangiopathy. The question, which comes first, microangiopathy or sugar, is like asking which came first, the chicken or the egg. This question is hotly debated in the diabetes circle of the world today, i.e. are complications like retinopathy, nephropathy and heart disease caused by high blood sugar or not?

Other scientists started finding evidence that blood sugar control may not be related to these changes. For instance, Knowles found that in large number of juvenile diabetics, the complications occurring in controlled diabetes on the one hand, and uncontrolled diabetes on the other, were the same. Then again, it was found that in certain races, the complications are more or less similar, though blood sugar may fluctuate. Also, in diabetic twins, complications are almost the same though their blood sugar may be totally different. This means that these complications are probably inherited separately along with the blood sugar, and that they are not dependent so much upon the control of blood sugar. It is generally acknowledged that these changes in diabetics do develop despite tight control of blood sugar. The best that the diabetologists can say is that controlling the sugar probably slows down the rate of these changes, but even this is not very certain.

Let us consider the different forms of treatment now in vogue for reduction of blood sugar and control diabetes. The first is diet control.

Diet

Previously, doctors used to advise a typical diabetic diet low in starch. The moment high blood sugar is detected, a doctor would immediately advise: no rice, no potatoes and no sugar.

Now, they found that *those diabetics on this typical diet have the highest rate of heart disease in the world, whereas African and Asian diabetics, who have never seen a dietitian or a physician in their life, seem to have little incidence of coronary heart diseases*. This means that a diet which is given to reduce sugar in order to prevent heart disease, causes heart disease. That is why now a very high starch diet has been recommended and found to be most successful in preventing heart disease.

It has been found that in maturity onset diabetics, reduction of weight cures diabetes. Therefore, in obese diabetics one must be strict in diet. In diet, it is necessary to cut the total number of calories.

The diabetic pills

The next method of controlling blood sugar is the use of oral hypoglycemic agents. These diabetic pills were subjected to a clinical trial in America: the University Group Diabetes Programme, which involved medical departments of leading American universities. They put 205 patients on placebo and 205 patients on the pills for an eight year period. To their surprise they found that among those taking the pills, heart attacks were three times more frequent than among those taking placebos. They had said that blood sugar must be controlled otherwise it will lead to heart attacks, and they found that the very pills which control the sugar cause heart attacks. It is like saying that "the diabetic pills control the sugar but kills the patient." The U.G.D.P. recommended that at least some varieties of the pills be banned. Most authorities today do not recommend the pills but use them only as a last resort if diet fails and insulin therapy is not possible.

Is insulin the final answer?

Let us go now to the most dramatic treatment of diabetes, i.e. insulin therapy. In the body, insulin is manufactured by the pancreas. When the sugar level in the blood increases, as after a meal, insulin is also secreted more. Thus hypoglycemia (low sugar) and hyperglycemia (high sugar) are prevented. At present, in insulin therapy of a diabetic, such adjustment is impossible. Therefore, there are likely to be periods of hyperglycemia and hypoglycemia. Hypoglycemia can cause permanent neurological damage, among other effects. It can also cause coma and death. Besides these, it can cause the Somogyi effect which leads to more severe hyperglycemia.

It is a matter of debate whether high sugar (below the coma level) can cause complications. But it is certain that low sugar is very dangerous. Therefore, fewer and fewer physicians now insist on tight control of blood sugar.

Now we use human insulin. There are some impurities in the insulin available today, which can have their own side-effects. Zinc which is used in insulin preparation can, as homoeopaths know, cause its own symptomatology. Hyperinsulinemia (high insulin level in the blood) is known to cause vascular changes and it is suspected that at least some of the vascular complications in diabetics could be due to insulin therapy.

What is diabetes?

Is diabetes increased blood sugar or is it vascular changes? Which is the cause and which is the effect? What is the cause of diabetes? Is it inherited? Is it due to lack of insulin? What should the diet be? Are diabetic pills to be lauded or banned? Is insulin therapy as dramatic as it was made out to be?

These are the problems diabetologists face today. No wonder Joslin, the pioneer among diabetologists, confessed that really we cannot answer the question: What is diabetes? In order to understand this question, let us look at a few facts.

In the Pima Indian race of the United States, diabetes is common but heart attacks are rare. In the same country 75% of diabetics die of heart attacks.

Natal Indian and Black South Africans have similar diets with respect to the proportion of carbohydrates, proteins and fat, but vascular complications are rare in the South African with diabetes, while they are common in the Indian.

Thus, we can see that the diabetes of the Pima Indian is different from that of the American, and that of the black South African. Diabetes is not one disease, but it is different in different patients. Even in the ultimate stage of diabetic coma, we can find that one diabetic is different from the other in response to therapy.

Diabetes is different in each patient. The cause is different. The effects are different. The course is different. Hence, the treatment must be different in each individual patient.

The limitations of allopathic treatment

The authorities on diabetes now realize that the insulin level is normal in many maturity onset diabetics. They speculate that there may be some lack of the insulin receiving apparatus, but they have not found any way to correct this. They found that the diabetic pills are doing more harm than good, so they switched over to insulin, but they find that this cannot give perfect control, and that insulin has its own side-effects. Finally, after so much struggle when they managed to control the sugar, they found that *all the chronic changes of diabetes are taking place despite the control!*

The homoeopathic approach

Kent, the master homoeopath, said a century ago what modern medicine claims to have discovered recently. He said: "The person who says diabetes disease is insane in medicine, talk of a species of diabetes."

In Homoeopathy, we do not fall into the trap of arguing what is diabetes – the sugar or the vascular changes. We say both are a part of the diabetic process.

Each patient has a specific constitution. By this, we mean that each person has a specific individual body, mind and disease. That is why different people get diabetes at different times, of differing severity, with different complications, and with varying response to the same treatment. In Homoeopathy, we try to find a medicine to suit the mental disposition, the physical attributes, as well as the various complications of the patient. That is why a homoeopath will select a different remedy for different patients with diabetes.

For a homoeopath, diabetes is not the thing to be treated, it is the man suffering from it. Recent findings in modern medicine emphasize the psychosomatic factor in diabetes. It has been repeatedly verified that stress is a primary contributor to the diabetic process. If stress is removed, there is a significant improvement. Stress, as we homoeopaths know, comes from our false perception of reality, that is what we call disease. Each diabetic has his own individual disease state that is aggravating his diabetes, besides other things. The homoeopath aims to identify the disease state and treat it with the similar remedy. When the disease state is removed, the diabetes loses its grip like a creeper without a stick.

21

TREATING THE PRESENT STATE

The body and the mind have both possibly gone through several states in the past, each of which has left a mark. It is also possible that these states now exist in a silent form alongside the dominant state. In the body, the signs of such states which existed in the past can often be seen. For example, the presence of the typical warts, corrugated nails and a hairy body give ample evidence that at some time the person was in a *Thuja* state. However, at present these are not the prominent symptoms. Right now, the person has tremendous restlessness, thirst for sips frequently, loss of weight and severe burning in an eruption which is better from warmth. The present symptoms indicate *Arsenicum album*, despite the fact the *Thuja* signs still exist. However, they are neither *active* nor *predominant*, and therefore not the *present* state of the person. Our totality should be the *totality of the present*.

It is reasonable to assume that a similar thing takes place in the mind too. Here again, we may see remnants of past states. In the former *Thuja* person, the fixity of ideas, the sense of brittleness, etc., may still be found, although in a less prominent form. If we ask leading questions in this direction, we may elicit positive answers, not so strongly, but they will nevertheless be positive. Combined with the physical remnants like warts, we may be tempted to consider this a *Thuja* case if we do not see that the symptoms we have taken into account are not the one that predominate at present. What dominates is the tremendous anxiety with restlessness, the mistrust, the fear of being robbed and the fear of death, symptoms which are much more in tune with the predominant and present physical state. Together they make the totality of the present state, to which we have to direct our treatment.

Does this mean we have to keep changing the remedy every minute since moods keep changing? No, a remedy is not selected on the mood. The mood is often dependent on the situation. From the mental symptoms which are prominent at the moment, we have to identify those features which are unsuitable or out of proportion to the situation. The totality of these features will indicate the basic delusion or, in other words, the false perception of the present. This is what needs to be treated. *So, we have to see what it is in the person that is not adapted to the present situation.* When we are able to see this, it will become clear that the state does not change as often as we think; the changes are only superficial and the basic state (which comes from the basic delusion) remains the same, even though there may be different expressions depending on the situation. For example, a patient who was formerly in the *Calcarea carbonica* state, with its desire for security, its many fears, timid nature, stubbornness, etc., and physically with features like obesity, desire for sweets and eggs, sweating on the scalp, etc., will have some of these features in a less intense form even when he goes into a state of *Stramonium*. At this time, however, these will not be the prominent features. Now, we will see violence, terror, the cornered feeling, the desire to escape, etc. The patient will come and shriek: "Doctor, this cold is killing me, do something about it immediately." He may still answer in the positive for obesity, timidity or desire for sweets, but these are not the prominent or predominant features now. If we fix our mind on *Calcarea carbonica* we shall see only that, but if we set our minds on the patient, we shall be able to see the present state which is *Stramonium*.

This understanding should make us cautious, especially with patients who have had multiple states in the past. They are likely to answer positively to leading questions about any of these states. So, we must be careful to observe what is predominant now, without classifying the patient into some idea of a remedy.

The question arises, what would happen if, instead of treating the present state, we give a remedy that suits the previous state (which may still be there in a silent form)? There are some who may feel that in not so serious circumstances, this would also benefit the patient, and that the state that you treat (even if it is silent) would respond and get less intense.

Though still open to this idea, I feel that it is not too logical. For example, if a person is in a *Stramonium* state of terror and has a silent *Calcarea carbonica* state in the background, what would happen if we give him the latter remedy?

It would be like asking a person who is terrified: "Why are you timid, why do you need security?", instead of asking him: "Why are you terrified? Why are you so mortally afraid?" To the former question, there would be some hint of response as if it strikes a chord somewhere in the distance, but this effect is not going to be so beneficial to the patient, even in terms of diminishing the silent state. It is as if this is not the right question for the moment, and so it is likely to be dismissed without producing any appreciable effect anywhere.

I feel, therefore, that we have to concentrate only on the present state. The way to do this is to be an unprejudiced observer of what is happening in the present and of what is not adapted to the present situation. Such unprejudiced observation is a fundamental requisite of good case taking.

Part II

The Mind

22

IMPORTANCE GIVEN TO MENTAL STATE

Local peculiarities, general symptoms and modalities indicate the central disturbance as much as do the mental symptoms since they all come from the same source, which is neither mental nor physical, but deeper than both.

The mental symptoms, however, form a pattern which can be easily associated with delusions. To identify such a pattern with physical symptoms is somewhat difficult. Physical symptoms seem discrete. If one or two aspects of the mental symptoms of a patient are not covered by the remedy, we can still view it from other aspects, since the patterns of the remedy can be seen. Cross references can be made. We can confirm the feelings through several ways with the use of dreams, hobbies, etc. Such a confirmation is not easily available with physical symptoms. Mental symptoms are available from each and every expression of the patient, since each expression can logically be broken down into its component parts. In this way, expressions which are not given in provings can also be utilized.

Since psychological causations are prominent nowadays, mental adaptation will almost always precede physical adaptation. Usually, mere observation can help us to understand the mental state, even without the patient saying anything. Such observation is useful to elicit physical symptoms too, but its use is more limited.

It is a valid argument that mental symptoms, especially in patients who have had too much intellectualization, can be confusing, and in such cases one needs to rely more on physical symptoms. But in cases of manifest pathology, the mental state is clearly non-pathognomonic and one does not have to decide (as with physical symptoms) which mental symptom can be explained and which one cannot be. It depends upon when the individual practitioner feels more comfortable – when dealing with the mental state or when dealing with the physical state. Both are doors to the same house. One might even say that both are sides of the same coin. We may choose to identify the coin from either side. The wise man is he who chooses to look at both sides of the coin before finally identifying it, no matter which side he begins with. Experience tells me that the identification of the mental state is a skill which, if mastered, can be very gratifying. Therefore, in this section, I shall concentrate upon the understanding of the mental state and its various aspects. The next section will be concerned with techniques of eliciting the mental state. The idea of these chapters is not to tell the reader to concentrate on the mind alone. Rather I have chosen to concentrate on the mind because I find that it is accuracy which is needed in eliciting physical symptoms, but to elicit the mental state requires a special understanding and skill which develop with practice.

23

COMPONENTS

Some time ago, I conceived the idea of studying a remedy as being made up of various components, and its symptoms and expressions as combinations of these basic components. I also started understanding patients in a similar way. This idea has proved very useful in practice.

Only later on did I understand that behind the components of the remedy and the patient lies the delusion of the situation which necessitated these components. This understanding made the idea of components much clearer and put them into perspective. However, the utility of identifying the components of the remedies and of the patients did not diminish. It remains our first and most vital step towards a systematic understanding of the various facts which ultimately make the whole picture.

In this chapter, I have traced the origin of this idea, through the pictures of various remedies to show how different combinations of components produce different characteristic symptoms. I have also taken two symptoms from the Repertory, namely "Clairvoyance" and "Anticipation, ailments from", in order to look at the difference between a basic symptom and an expression which may occur from different basic feelings. In both instances, I have explored certain remedies with a view to showing how components blend into each other to form symptoms and how these symptoms are expressed in practice. Finally, we will look at the practical utility of this idea through actual clinical cases examples.

The key to understanding the mind

In Aphorism 212 of the "Organon", Hahnemann writes:

"There is no potent medicinal substance in the world which does not very notably alter the state of disposition and mind in the healthy individual who tests it, and every medicine does so in a different way."

The idea of remedy-essence and its limitation

In trying to explain the mental state produced by a drug, some homoeopaths talk of a central point of the drug. Various names like "core", "primary disturbance" and "essence" have been used to denote this central point. Using one feature as the centre, they explain all other symptoms as resulting from that feature. For example, the hurried nature of

Lycopodium is explained in the following way: *Lycopodium* has lack of self-confidence as the central theme, and since he is anxious about completing his job, he is hurried. To take another example, since the central theme of *Aconitum* is fear of death, this can explain the symptom "Predicts the time of death". This kind of explanation assumes that a drug can produce disturbance of only one feature, and all other disturbances result from that one disturbance.

This idea is very useful since it identifies the most important feature of the drug. But it may not be possible to explain all other symptoms in this way. For example, one may point out that *Arsenicum album* has "Fear of death", so why does *Arsenicum album* not have the symptom "Predicts the time of death"?

Temperament as combination of traits

We know that a drug causes a certain state of disposition. We could use the term "temperament" to denote this in a person. Let us first understand what temperament means. How do we describe the temperament of a person? Is it enough to say that the person is intelligent? Obviously, this cannot identify the person. But if we say that the person is intelligent, hurried, lacks confidence and is irritable and anxious, will these components not describe his disposition and also identify him? Thus, "temperament" is not limited to one mental trait, but is a combination of several mental traits. The dictionary defines temperament as *a characteristic combination of physical, mental and moral qualities constituting a person's character*. Again here, the same meaning is implied, i.e. a person's character is not composed of a single trait, but is a characteristic combination of qualities.

In the same way, when a drug changes the disposition in a proving, it does not change one trait alone, but brings about changes in several traits at the same time. The sum of these changes represents the change in disposition brought about by that particular drug.

Common single trait with differences in other traits

Many times a single trait may be common to many remedies, but we can differentiate between these remedies because the other traits will be different. For example, "Increased sexual desire" is a trait in many remedies like *Fluoricum acidum, Lilium tigrinum, Hyoscyamus, Staphysagria* and *Bufo rana*. Let us see how this feature is modified by the other traits of each remedy to form characteristic symptoms.

In *Lilium tigrinum*, the two other prominent traits are "Hurry" and "Religiousness". Because of very strong religious affections, *Lilium tigrinum* considers her sexual desire as something sinful, which therefore needs to be repressed. Since this remedy increases the speed of a person ("Hurry"), the easiest way of doing things is to keep busy with some occupation, and so we get the characteristic symptom, "Has to keep very busy to repress sexual desire" (Phatak's Materia Medica).

Fluoricum acidum is similar to *Lilium tigrinum* in its high sexual desire, but its other components are opposite in nature. See the rubrics: "Adulterous" and "Indifference to business affairs" (Phatak's Materia Medica). Phatak also gives the symptom, "Responsibility, inability to realize" in his Materia Medica. He has no problem in spending all his time impertinently looking at women, with lascivious thoughts. So, the characteristic symptom of *Fluoricum acidum* reads: "Stand on streets ogling at women as they pass by".

The components of this symptoms are:
- Sexual desire increased;
- Indifference to loved ones;
- Delusion, must dissolve marriage;
- Cheerful;
- Buoyant;
- Lascivious;
- Warm-blooded.

Staphysagria has a totally different set of components. He has increased sensitivity to hurt, with a tendency to brood and suppress emotions. He is very timid and cowardly, and has feelings of guilt. He cannot express his increased sexual desire directly for fear of being hurt, and out of a sense of shame and because of his self-respect, he cannot ogle at women. He, therefore, suppresses his desire and we get the characteristic: "Dwells, sexual matters, on". There is also a prominent tendency to masturbation.

Hyoscyamus has other traits: foolish and shameless behaviour. It is a loss of sanity. Therefore, he exhibits his increased sexual desire in a very foolish, shameless way through lewd talk, exposing genitals, etc. One other prominent feature of *Hyoscyamus*, namely loquacity, combines with these components to give the characteristic symptom: "Speech, prattling, lies naked in bed". (Components of this symptom are: "Shameless", "Foolish", "Loquacity", "Insanity", "Obscene talk".)

In *Bufo rana*, there is childish lack of control with the increased sexual desire. A mature mind can exercise control and postpone pleasure. If we like something, we see whether it is wise to have it and also decide how much is good for us; as for example, when we get the urge to eat ice-cream. But in *Bufo rana* this control is lacking, he cannot postpone pleasure and so behaves in a very childish, immature way. Whenever he gets an urge, he must fulfill it immediately. The same thing happens with his sexual desire. As soon as he gets the urge, he must fulfill it, and he goes off alone and masturbates. *Bufo rana* has early physical and sexual growth with lack of maturity of the mind. This combination gives it the individual symptom: "Seeks solitude to practice masturbation".

In this way we see that, though all these remedies share a common trait, namely "Increased sexual desire", they differ widely in their other traits. It is this difference which gives them their individuality and also gives them their characteristic symptoms. Thus each one's temperament is a combination of traits.

We describe people by parameters

If we want to describe any object, how do we do? We describe it by certain attributes. We may talk about its size, its colour, its texture, its utility, etc. We have to describe all its attributes. Just by describing its colour alone, we cannot identify an object.

Similarly, to describe the nature of a person, we use certain attributes. We talk about his intelligence, then we quantify his irritability, then we have to mention whether he is fearful or bold, and so on. We are to study a man by these parameters.

We can compare a person to a key. If you compare two keys, you may find both the keys have the same number of projections, but the difference between the two keys will lie in the relative length and shape of each projection. It is a peculiar combination of the different lengths and shapes of the projections that gives individuality to the key.

The parameters like irritability, fear, etc., are like the projections of a key. All of us have all the projections, but the length of each projection in each of us differs from others, and it is the characteristic combination of these lengths of projections that characterizes our disposition.

Let me now roughly indicate which parameters we have to look into when studying a remedy or a person. I am describing the parameters in sets of two opposite qualities; the intensity of the parameter in a person can lie anywhere between these two extremes.

The parameters

Irritable	:	Mild
Fearful	:	Bold
Sadness	:	Cheerful
Sharp	:	Dullness
Hurry	:	Slowness
Moral	:	Amoral
Lascivious	:	Low sex desire
Overconfident	:	Diffident (lack of confidence)
Rigid, firm, determined	:	Irresolute
Hypersensitive	:	Insensitive
Company, craves for	:	Company, averse to
Affectionate	:	Indifferent
Memory, sharp	:	Memory, weak
Impulsive, violent	:	Slow reaction
Loquacious	:	Silent, taciturn
Egotism	:	Humility
Industrious	:	Indolent
Fastidious	:	Unclean, untidy
Jealous	:	Totally not jealous
Ambitious	:	Ambitionless

Musical	:	Aversion to music
Changeable	:	Unchanging, fixed
Consolation ameliorates	:	Consolation aggravates
Anxious regarding health	:	Indifferent regarding health
Theorizing, planning	:	Imagination, lacking in
Strong-willed	:	Weak-willed
Obstinate	:	Yielding
Cunning	:	Lack of guile (simpleton)
Weeping easily	:	Never weeps
Expressive	:	Reserved, secretive
Clairvoyance	:	Total absence of clairvoyance
Childish	:	Precocious
Travel, desires to	:	Averse to travel
Despair	:	Hopeful, optimistic

It is important to realize that all the parameters are found in all remedies. Fears are to be found in all remedies and so are anxiety, sadness, etc. It is only the types and the degree which will differ from remedy to remedy.

Characteristic symptoms are formed by a combination of components

It is very interesting and useful to study the characteristic mental symptoms of remedies. We have already seen how characteristic symptoms are formed by the combination of components, for example, by examining the symptom: "Has to keep very busy in order to repress her sexual desire", we were able to identify the four components required to produce this symptom, viz. "Hurry", "Religiousness", "Guilt" and "Increased sexual desire". This method of identifying components of a characteristic symptom helps us to understand a remedy, and such an understanding helps us to differentiate it from other remedies.

Let us examine a very characteristic symptom of *Natrum sulphuricum*: "Loathing life, must restrain herself to prevent doing herself injury". In fact, this symptom is found in *Natrum sulphuricum* alone. I examined this and analyzed which components are needed to form this symptom:

– Loathing of life; she is so depressed that she does not want to live any longer;
– Impulses to injure herself; in other words, suicidal thoughts.

In the Repertory, *Natrum sulphuricum* is mentioned under both "Sadness" and "Suicidal thoughts". The question that occurred to me here is that as *Aurum metallicum* also has these components in the same degree, why does it not have the symptom: "Must restrain herself from doing herself injury"? To answer this, let us understand what this symptom really means. "Must restrain herself" gives the idea that she has to use all her self-control. The same idea is expressed by the rubric: "Injure, must use self-control to prevent shooting himself". Another rubric is: "Injure himself, fears to be left alone, lest he should". The person gets depressed, feels life is not worth living and has suicidal

135

impulses. What kind of person will be scared by such an impulse? It has to be a person who is really weak-willed, who feels he may not be able to control himself, a person who has to use all the will power he has, in order to control that impulse. This gives us the idea of a timid, irresolute, anxious and a very, very weak-willed person. If *Natrum sulphuricum* has this symptom, then it must be weak-willed.

With this in mind, I referred to these rubrics in Kent's Repertory: "Anxiety", "Timidity", "Irresolution" and "Confidence, want of self". To my surprise I found that *Natrum sulphuricum* is present in none of them. Sure of my idea of the traits of *Natrum sulphuricum* however, I then went to Hering's "Guiding Symptoms", where I found prominently mentioned: "Spirits, low, extremely timid and anxious. Mind enfeebled". Also, from Kent's Repertory: "Fear, suicide, of".

Aurum metallicum shares two traits with *Natrum sulphuricum*, namely "Loathing of life" and "Suicidal thoughts". But *Aurum metallicum* is the very opposite of *Natrum sulphuricum* in the last feature, i.e. *Aurum metallicum* is very strong-willed, whereas *Natrum sulphuricum* is weak-willed. The strong will of *Aurum metallicum* is indicated by the symptom: "Delusion, has neglected his duty and deserves reproach".

From this symptom not only do we see the heightened scruples of conscience but also we are able to see the firmness with which *Aurum metallicum* makes the decision, "I have done wrong and must be punished." This kind of firmness and strong will is characteristic of *Aurum metallicum* and is the very opposite of *Natrum sulphuricum*. It is for this reason that when *Aurum metallicum* gets suicidal thoughts, he does not have to fight with himself as *Natrum sulphuricum* has to. *Aurum metallicum* will make a decision and act. He will ask himself: "Do I jump or not?" If the answer is, "I jump", he just jumps.

Single symptoms represent peculiar combinations

"Single symptom" is the term used to denote a symptom for which there is only one remedy. Study of a remedy's single symptom is very useful because many times it represents a particular combination of components of that remedy, a combination not found in any other remedy.

To give an example: a single symptom of *Kalium carbonicum* is: "Company, desire for, yet treats them outrageously". In this, three of the main components of *Kalium carbonicum* have come together. The first is the desire for company: he wants company, and is dependent on it, he is aggravated when alone, he must have support and he always likes to be with people who support him. Other remedies also have this desire for company and support, for example, *Calcarea, Phosphorus, Pulsatilla* and *Stramonium*.

The second component of *Kalium carbonicum* is: "he treats them outrageously", indicating that he can be irritable with the person on whom he has called to keep him company. This shows discontentment with the person on whom he is dependent.

The third aspect is: "Quarrelsomeness"; this means that when he is discontented, he cannot keep quiet, he has to quarrel. With these three components, *Kalium carbonicum* becomes unique. A person normally depends on people, most commonly on his family members (in fact, we can give a wide definition to the word "family": a family consists of those people who are interdependent on each other). *Kalium carbonicum* is very anxious about the security and integrity of his family unit, and so worries a lot if there is any threat to it (for example, ill health of one of its member). But, at the same time, he is never content with any of them. That is why we find in Phatak's Materia Medica: "Quarrels with his family" and "Quarrels with his bread and butter". In other words, he quarrels with those on whom he is dependent. The rubric should really be: "Quarrelsome (only) with his family", "Impatience (only) with his children" (Synthetic Repertory).

The trouble for the physician begins when the *Kalium carbonicum* patient starts considering the physician as a family member. Then, he will truly depend on the physician, will never ever leave him, but each time he comes, he will quarrel and insist that he is not better. The best way to test the dependence in a very discontented person is to say to him: "Since, according to you, I have not been able to do anything for you, it is better you consult another physician." Immediately, the *Kalium carbonicum* patient will say: "Oh no, doctor, you alone must treat me. I will not go to any one else!"

A *Kalium carbonicum* patient who manifests these traits very prominently will open the follow up with: "Doctor, I am not in the least bit better. In fact, I am feeling worse; pains here and pains there." When you go into her previous complaints, you will find that some of her most troublesome symptoms are better. She will not say this on her own, and will admit it with great reluctance, only after asking and then will hasten to add: "That symptom is better, but another has come", or "It may come back again." This kind of dependence, discontentment, quarrelsomeness, anxiety and irascibility forms the components which make up the mental disposition of the *Kalium carbonicum* patient. They also give us the two single symptoms: "Company, desire for, yet treats them outrageously" and "Quarrelsome with his family".

One of the well-known single symptoms of *Nitricum acidum* reads: "Hatred of persons who have offended him, unmoved by apologies". Which components are required to make up this symptom? If you understand all the components, your idea of *Nitricum acidum* will be much clearer. First, we can see "Hatred"; second, "Offended easily"; third, "Rigidity of thinking"; fourth, a marked "Obstinacy"; fifth, you feel a "Hardness", and this is confirmed by referring to the rubrics: "Contemptuous" and "Consolation aggravates".

These are the components that make up a *Nitricum acidum* patient. For example, you will see hatred even for persons who do not offend. You will see that the person hates not only some people but also the way some things are. You will see the rigidity and obstinacy even in other areas, especially in rigid views about health and his disease (since *Nitricum acidum* also has a very strong anxiety about health). The hardness, you will see expressed in other situation too. All these components come together to form the single symptom in all *Nitricum acidum* patients. We may get only some of the components. This is why we will be at an advantage if we clearly appreciate how single symptoms are formed.

137

To illustrate the blending of components and the formation of symptoms which characterize remedies, let us study one component, namely "Clairvoyance". We shall examine the remedies listed under this rubric.

Extrasensory perception

These remedies act on the intellect, producing a kind of clear perception, a hallucinogenic effect. The person feels very clear in his mind, as if he sees things which normally cannot be seen. If we look in the Repertory we shall find certain symptoms which are common to the "Clairvoyant" remedies.

Presentiment of death

One of them is presentiment of death. A presentiment of death is due to the same clairvoyant feeling, an increased perception as if death is approaching. It is an internal feeling that cannot be explained by eyes or ears, nor in the mind through either logic or intellect.

Absentminded

These clairvoyant remedies, because of their clearness of perception, are engaged in their own thoughts, absorbed in their thoughts so that they become very, very absentminded. *Anacardium* is one of the most absentminded remedies. *Nux moschata* is also one of the most absentminded remedies. He makes purchases, leaves them and goes away, and makes mistakes in speaking. When we examine *Medorrhinum*, we find that he loses the thread of conversation and we ask him: "What's happening?" He says: "I have got pain in the abdomen." Here, he stops, wanders and repeats: "I have got pain in the abdomen." He says the same thing over again. Never give *Medorrhinum* an acting part in a drama! He will forget the next line, he stands there and says: "Oh! My darling", and he forgets what is next; he just keeps standing there and he is lost.

These remedies with extrasensory perception have this kind of absence of mind, this kind of loss of memory, that they lose the thread of conversation. They lose their way in well-known streets; it is the kind of absence of mind where they are in a dreamy state, like a person who is on drugs. He can see things that we normally cannot see and feel things that we cannot feel. In *Nux moschata*, this symptom is very prominent. He acts as in a dream, automatically, as if he were sleepwalking. He does his daily routine as if he is in a dopey, dreamy state. This is not especially a characteristic of *Nux moschata*. Most remedies in this extrasensory state, in this state of clear perception in the intellect, have got these symptoms in common: the presentiment of death, the absence of mind, the dreamy dopey state.

Happy feeling

There is also a happy, ecstatic feeling. In *Medorrhinum*, it is described as a happy feeling. In *Nux moschata*, it is described as a ludicrous feeling. Ludicrous means he finds everything funny. In *Cannabis indica*, it is described as a heavenly feeling. So, all these remedies with this clearness of perception produce states of happiness.

Things seem strange

Another symptom in the Repertory is: "Delusions, strange, familiar, things seem". That means he goes to well-known streets but he does not recognize them. You will see many clairvoyant remedies here. In this state of intellect, this dreamy state, he feels as if all these things which he is familiar with look strange, funny or unfamiliar. This is the opposite of déjà-vu. In the déjà-vu phenomenon, strange things seem familiar. This means, for example, that he goes to America, to a particular city and a particular street for the first time in his life, and he feels: "I have seen this before! I have been here before!" He is talking to somebody and feels that the conversation has happened earlier. The opposite is found in *Medorrhinum*. Something he knows, he thinks, looks strange. This happens in the remedies that are given there, so it is not peculiar of *Medorrhinum*, but to the group of clairvoyant remedies.

Times passes too slowly

One of the other symptoms that most of these remedies seem to feel is that time passes too slowly. Again if you look in the Repertory, you will see almost the same remedies. In these clairvoyant state of clear perception, thoughts happen so fast, they run into each other so fast that each minute seems like an hour. Time passes too slowly, there are too many thoughts in too short a time with clear perception. This is the opposite of the state of *Cocculus*, where the person has no thoughts, he is just absorbed. Time passes too fast, but he does not know how it has passed. These are opposite states, an active mind and a dull mind. An active mind has clear perception, too many thoughts, all rushing in, and a short space seems as if it were too long.

Sense of duality

A sense of duality is characteristic of these remedies. For example, the symptom "Sees double or more than one person" is common to these remedies. *Petroleum* sees too many people in the bed. *Medorrhinum* and *Staphysagria* have the feeling that somebody is behind them, while *Thuja* feels that someone is beside him. Almost all these remedies have the feeling, as if there is someone beside them. The rubrics are: "Delusion, sees people behind him" or "beside him".

Common symptoms of the clairvoyant remedies

These are the common symptoms of a group of remedies that have a specific action on the intellect, producing an increased awareness of perception. *Medorrhinum* has all the symptoms of this group. Refer to these rubrics in the Repertory and see how beautifully almost the same group of remedies comes through.

How can we differentiate these remedies from one another? If you start differentiating on the basis of intellectual symptoms, you will end up nowhere. If you just look at the fact that the fellow loses the thread of conversation, he loses his way, he feels somebody is behind him, you will find almost the same remedies are there.

The emotional concomitant will differentiate

The differentiating factor lies not in the common symptoms of this group but in the concomitant. A remedy produces a certain action on the intellect, which is common to other remedies, and it produces a certain action on the emotions. The action on the emotions is the concomitant to the action on the intellect. This will differentiate the remedies.

A common mistake is made while selecting symptoms of the mental state. There is a tendency on the part of the homoeopath to take several expressions of the same basic symptom (parameter); and then, of course, he will find the same group of remedies coming through in repertorization. This is not correct. For example, if you take "Clairvoyance", it is not necessary to take the other symptoms in the patient associated with this clairvoyant state, i.e. "Absentminded", "Time passes too slowly", "Sense of duality". Instead, it is important to find the basic parameters from other spheres (concomitants).

Emotion blends with intellect

You will notice that the symptoms of intellect and emotion blend easily. The way the action on the intellect blends with the action on the emotion, and produces a new symptom, a combination-symptom, is quite fantastic. Actually, the two symptoms exist individually, but they blend with each other to form a combination which is characteristic. In *Aconitum*, the tremendous fear of death is the emotion and clairvoyance is the intellectual symptom. They combine into one: "Predicts the time of death". This means two things: he has got the ability to predict and he has got the fear of death. Two separate symptoms come together into one which becomes the characteristic of *Aconitum*. Let us study three other remedies in this way, namely *Phosphorus*, *Cannabis indica* and *Medorrhinum*.

Phosphorus: intimacy with clairvoyance

Phosphorus has clear perception, everything seems strange and he can prophesy and feel things which others cannot feel. One strong emotion of *Phosphorus* is amativeness, a desire for intimacy, for closeness with somebody else, a feeling of intense sympathy. The difference between *Causticum* and *Phosphorus* is that *Causticum* feels anxious for others, while *Phosphorus* feels the anxiety of others. A *Causticum* mother says: "Oh, don't go, don't go, you will get ill." She is anxious for the child, anxiously cautious, but she does not understand the child's feelings. She feels something might happen to him, he might not come home, he might get killed, the train might run over him, all imaginations – anxious for others. Whereas *Phosphorus* feels the feeling of the other person, and he expect the same from them. So, in *Phosphorus*, there is this feeling of intimacy, this feeling of closeness, a tremendous love. When you combine clairvoyance with the feeling of intimacy, there will be a very strong feeling of love. When he is with somebody, he will feel waves pass between them, he will feel all the vibrations, and he will say: "Yes, I can feel intimacy, I can feel love. I know this person is feeling a lot for me, the air is electric with feeling."

So, the extrasensory perception, the clairvoyance of *Phophorus* is generally expressed as a feeling of tremendous intimacy. He may say: "I knew as soon as I walked into the room, the vibration was there between us, even though we had never met each other before." There is the desire to be magnetized and magnetic waves travel. Another way the clairvoyance of *Phosphorus* is expressed is in the anxiety he feels for another person. One of my colleagues, for whom I prescribed *Phosphorus*, had the feeling three times that his father was having a heart attack, and each time within one hour of getting this feeling, he received a telephone call telling him that indeed his father had a heart attack. This kind of feeling for another person is very typical of *Phosphorus*.

Cannabis indica: joy with clairvoyance

A strong emotion of *Cannabis indica* is heavenly, ecstatic pleasure. It is the most beautiful feeling in our Materia Medica.

Ecstasy! It is known that hallucinogens produce this ecstatic feeling. When the patient describes, she will talk and talk all about beauty. She looks at the shadow, this shadow falling here, at this pattern on the wall, and the moment she looks at it, she imagines that it is a palace and that these are the sculptures of a palace... that fan over there is the canopy of the king, and that is the throne... all of you here are the courtiers. *Cannabis indica* is right there in the middle, enjoying the whole thing, and there is song and dance, and she is lost, completely absorbed in such thoughts. This is an expression of the clairvoyance of *Cannabis indica*. One patient told me: "I just sit down, and suddenly I am transported to a beautiful place with trees, grass, lakes, mountains and I am running up and I am going down." So, ecstasy, heavenly pleasure, is an emotion associated with clairvoyance, and gives this kind of extrasensory feeling.

Medorrhinum: fears misfortune

What is the emotional symptom of *Medorrhinum* that is associated with the clairvoyant feeling? The emotion is "Fear of misfortune". If you read this symptom in the Synthetic Repertory, you will see that *Medorrhinum* is the only remedy which is underlined by Dr. Pierre Schmidt. It is not in the other books in this way, but I have seen it in my practice, and Pierre Schmidt confirms it, so it must be true. Imagine how the clairvoyance and the fear of misfortune together produce the symptom: "As if something is going to happen – I can feel it! I can get the vibration! I can feel something is going to happen!" He is always anticipating and may have presentiment of death. Allen's "Keynotes" gives this symptom: "Anticipating, feels matters most sensitively before they occur and many times correctly". Whether it is correct or not is a different matter, but the feeling is as if something is surely going to happen, a sensitive feeling, an internal feeling, an inexplicable sensation inside. This can also be seen in the Synthetic Repertory in the rubric: "Prophesying, disagreeable events", in which *Medorrhinum* is the only remedy listed.

Anticipates events

Let us examine the rubric: "Anticipation, ailments from". Now, this is not a component or a parameter. It is an effect or expression, and each remedy in this list appears in

141

the rubric for a different reason. All these remedies have this type of anxiety. What I want to point out to you, as I did with the rubric of "Clairvoyance", is that each of these remedies is different. We are taking five remedies, namely *Medorrhinum*, *Lycopodium*, *Silicea*, *Ambra* and *Psorinum*.

Medorrhinum has "Fear of misfortune"

The feeling of *Medorrhinum* is the feeling of apprehension, as if there is going to be some misfortune. Something bad will happen, something evil, something very unfortunate. Children usually like to go in a car, but this child says: "Father, don't drive fast, there will be an accident. The police will catch you and put you in prison." It produces tremendous anxiety before going to an examination. *Medorrhinum* will feel that something will happen on the way, may be the car will break down. When a time is set and he has to catch a bus, or keep an appointment, he gets very tense. Fear as if something is going to happen, an alive fear, tremendous apprehension, if a time is set.

Physical signs of anxiety

The signs of *Medorrhinum* anxiety are classic. The first is *restlessness of feet*. The feet are in constant motion if he has to sit down. The two other remedies which share this are *Rhus toxicodendron* and *Zincum metallicum*. Another sign is *constant biting of nails*, they are great nail-biters, and the third expression of the *Medorrhinum* anxiety is *constant washing of hands*. It is obsessive compulsive behaviour: bites his nails, washes his hands, shakes his feet.

Lycopodium lacks self-confidence

In *Lycopodium* there is no fear of misfortune, it is absent in this rubric, whereas *Medorrhinum* is present in three marks and is underlined. But *Lycopodium* is present in three marks in the rubric "Cowardice". *Lycopodium* is not scared that some misfortune will happen, but he is scared that he will not be able to do the job. For example, he is not scared that the car will break down before the examination, but that he will not be able to do the examination properly. *Lycopodium* has the feeling that he will not be able to do a job. He lacks confidence but characteristic of this is that once he starts doing it, he regains confidence, and then he goes through it with ease and comfort. Initial hesitation, followed by ease and comfort, and then he masters the job. So *Lycopodium* is scared that he will not be able to do something, even though he has the capacity to do it. Now, this is important – even though he has the capacity to do it.

It is not that *Lycopodium* is a very capable person, or intelligent one: there are stupid *Lycopodiums* and intelligent *Lycopodiums*, capable *Lycopodiums* and incapable *Lycopodiums*. But the symptom is: he is scared that he will not be able to do what he is capable of doing.

Suppose he is a boy aged ten, not a brilliant child at school, not very intelligent, and not coming first, but he is capable of doing some things, just as everybody is capable. This child is capable, for example, of jumping from here to there, but he is scared that he will not be able to jump. He is scared that he cannot do what he is capable of, whatever that may be. We are not saying that *Lycopodium* is a great man and he is a great achiever. No. He can be a great achiever or a small achiever, but he always fears before doing something. If you push him, he will do it with ease and comfort. *Medorrhinum* is afraid of things that might happen to him from outside and *Lycopodium* is afraid that he cannot do it, that he is incapable.

Lycopodium deals in abstractions

There is another difference in the intellectual symptoms of *Medorrhinum* and *Lycopodium* which is very prominent, and this is that *Lycopodium* has increased ability to deal in abstractions. In Clarke and in Allen's "Encyclopedia" – intellectual symptoms, the same is given: "Increased ability to deal in abstractions whereas he mistakes between plums and pears. Says plums when he means pears." Instead of saying: "I ate a plum", he will say: "I ate a pear." So, he makes mistakes in ordinary, everyday things. However, he has increased ability to deal in abstractions. An abstraction is something which is derived from facts, but is not a fact. *Lycopodium* has got easy ability to abstract from something. He will generalize very easily, he will look at many facts and from those facts, he can easily construct theories. If you leave him in the sharemarket, he will have a fantastic time, and he will tell you that this is the trend of the market, and this is going to happen, and that is going to happen. He is very clever in making abstractions. But, in ordinary everyday things, he makes mistakes.

Medorrhinum is the opposite. *Medorrhinum* has inability for abstractions. So, *Medorrhinum* can easily add up some figures but *Lycopodium* will make mistake doing this, but has ability for logic like Geometry. If you ask him to analyze the political situation of the country, he will analyze it well, but he will not remember the names of the politicians.

Silicea is concerned with image

Silicea looks like *Lycopodium* because it also has lack of self-confidence. But, in *Silicea* it is not whether he is capable of doing the action that bothers him, but it is his image that must be protected at all costs. So, anything that threatens the image, the rigid image of *Silicea*, is going to cause anticipatory anxiety. The feeling is: "Am I going to do well? And if I fail, what will others think about me? What will their impression of me be? My image will be spoiled." That is why *Silicea* is very bashful, shy and nervous, especially before meeting people or before appearing on the stage in public.

This is the difference between *Lycopodium* and *Silicea*. *Silicea* is afraid to appear on the stage and *Lycopodium* is afraid to speak. "Whenever I go on stage, I get very self-conscious, I get scared, and I get anticipatory anxiety." I can cite as an example the case of a businessman who made donations to social institutions, and when he made donations, naturally, he was called on to the stage. They had to force him on to the stage and he walked looking down and then he sat and spent the whole hour not raising his head. I asked him: "Suppose you don't have to say anything, and you don't have to perform?"

He said: "Even then, the situation is the same. Just the thought of all those people looking at me, and what they are thinking about me, that itself is enough." So, *Silicea* is not as much bothered about his capacity for action as he is bothered about what other people think about his image, especially about whether his image is going to remain intact, not only with other people but with himself. That is why you find *Silicea* in the rubrics: "Egotism", "Conscientious about trifles" and "Timidity, when appearing in public".

Ambra is embarrassed

Here I would want to differentiate *Silicea* from another remedy which is very close. This remedy is *Ambra grisea*. *Ambra grisea* and *Silicea*, *Carbo vegetabilis*, *Plumbum* and *Gelsemium* are the main remedies in the rubric: "Timidity, when appearing in public". The main idea of *Ambra grisea* is a tremendous sense of embarrassment. Remember that there are elements of all remedies in all of us; we have all felt embarrassed at some time or other, but *Ambra grisea* feels it intensely: he is very, very conscious, acutely conscious of the slightest thing he does.

The embarrassment is more when it comes to personal habits like passing stool and urine. One constipated patient, when asked if he used anything made of aluminium, said: "No sir, no aluminium, all steel." The next time he came, he brought a paper-wrapped object. It was an aluminium mug. He said: "I use it in my toilet, is it OK?" The mug he used to clean his bowels was right on my table! It is the opposite in *Ambra grisea*, who, at any mention of stool, urine or belching, is acutely embarrassed.

There is a symptom: "Company, aversion to, presence of strangers, people intolerable to her during stool". I think this is true for most of us. I don't recall having seen anybody sending out invitations: "I am going to pass stool. I request the pleasure of your company with family and friends." So, what is the meaning of this symptom? Some say, if the *Ambra grisea* patient is immobile and in the ward of an hospital, he will find it difficult to pass stool in the presence of others. Does this mean that we have to wait until the *Ambra grisea* patient is in the hospital before we can prescribe for him? What this symptom ("Cannot pass stool in the presence of others") means, is that he cannot even have somebody in the next room when he is passing stool. It means that the sounds he makes in the toilet embarrass him so much that he cannot bear the thought of somebody standing in the next room and hearing him. He has to clear the whole house before he passes stool. He has to see that there is nobody around.

This is the kind of embarrassment. *Ambra grisea* cannot bear the thought of going to somebody else's house, he is afraid he may get an urge for stool. There is a rubric: "Anxiety from ineffectual desire for stool", when he gets the urge for stool he gets anxious. That is the kind of anticipatory anxiety that *Ambra grisea* has. It is quite close in some respects to *Baryta carbonica*; both have: "Timidity", "Bashful" and "Stranger, presence of, aggravates". But *Ambra grisea* has this very acute embarrassed feeling which *Baryta carbonica* does not have, and *Baryta carbonica* has tremendous irresolution which represents a feeling of lack of capability which *Ambra grisea* does not have.

144

Psorinum has despair

Another remedy that comes very close to *Medorrhinum* in the fear of misfortune which causes anticipatory anxiety is *Psorinum*. In *Psorinum* the feeling of misfortune is associated with despair. In *Medorrhinum* it is an internal feeling as if something bad is going to happen, which makes him anxious, hurried, impatient and restless. In *Psorinum* the feeling is: "Whatever I do, it is certain to be a failure". He feels that nobody likes him and he is sad, anxious and depressed. There is absolute despair. Further you do not find the restlessness of *Medorrhinum* in *Psorinum*.

Two types of mental symptoms

From the above we can see that mental symptoms are of two types:

– Basic parameters and their combinations. Examples of basic parameters: clairvoyance, fear, anger. Examples of combinations: "Predicts the time of death", "Company, desires, yet treats them outrageously".

– Expression of the parameters or their combinations. Example: "Anticipation, ailments from" is a rubric where you can see remedies coming in for different reasons and under different circumstances. This rubric does not represent a basic feeling or a parameter, but is a common expression to different components.

We can always ask: "Why does a person have anticipatory anxiety?", and find a satisfactory explanation. For example, we said *Lycopodium* has anticipatory anxiety because of lack of self-confidence. If a *Lycopodium* patient did not have lack of self-confidence, he would not have anticipatory anxiety. So, the anticipatory anxiety in *Lycopodium* is only an expression of, and is completely explained by one of its basic parameters, viz. lack of self-confidence. Similarly, we see other remedies come into this rubric for different reasons.

For example:

Baryta carbonica has anticipatory anxiety because of feeling of incapacity.
Ambra grisea has anticipatory anxiety because of an embarrassed feeling.
Medorrhinum has anticipation because of fear of misfortune.
Staphysagria has anticipation because of sensitivity to hurt.

Hence, "Ailments from anticipation" is neither a basic parameter nor a combination of parameters, but it is an expression of these. Basic parameters can be found again and again, but their expressions may not always be found; and even if they are found, they differ from person to person.

Difference between basic parameter and expression

If I ask you to name an object which is cold, hard and colourless, you will immediately say "Ice". If I ask you why it cannot be a glass kept in the freezer, you may be puzzled for a while. But soon you will say: "A glass is not cold unconditionally. It is cold only when it is kept in the freezer." We can see that the basic parameters of ice are "coldness", "hardness" and "colourlessness". These are unchanging. Even in a hot room, ice will remain cold. "Coldness" is thus its intrinsic quality, whereas for the glass, "coldness" is not the basic parameter. So, we can see that:

- Basic parameters are unconditional (like the coldness of ice). They cannot change and cannot be explained;
- Expressions are conditional (like coldness of glass);
- An object is more readily identified by its basic parameters.

How to differentiate

In order to determine whether a symptom is a basic parameter or its expression, keep on asking the question: "Why does this symptom exist?" If we get an answer to this which is complete and satisfactory, then it is an expression. We have to question the explanation too by asking the above question again and again, until we come to a point at which there is no satisfactory answer. That will be the basic parameter, and whatever the patient has said before will be the expressions.

For example, if a person says: "I like company", we must ask him why. If he says: "I don't know why, but I just like company", then we have reached his basic parameter, namely "Desires company". But if he says: "Because I am frightened of being alone", then we have to ask again: "Why?" He may say he does not know, in which case his basic parameter is "Fear of being alone". He could also say: "I am afraid of being alone because I am frightened, I may get a heart attack and die." Then his basic parameters would be "Fear of impending disease" and "Fear of being alone".

Search for basic parameters

It is the basic and innermost feelings (emotions) we must search for and not limit ourselves to their expressions. If you are sure that these basic parameters are found in the remedy, you can prescribe it, even if it does not have the precise expressions of the patient.

Just see how many additions of remedies have been made to the rubric: "Ailments from anticipation" in the Synthetic Repertory. Before this Repertory came to our hands, we would have missed so many remedies if we had taken this symptom as eliminating, and not prescribed on the basic parameters. From the given examples you would have observed how useful it is to split up the rubric "Ailments from" into its basic components. For example, "Ailments from, death, parents or friends, of" could mean "Fright", "Guilt" or a combination of these. We must carefully consider what the patient says, ask him "why" again and again, until we are able to accurately analyze the components.

Basic parameters are proving symptoms

Basic parameters are often proving symptoms. It will be difficult to add to the list of drugs for these parameters unless more drugs are proved. Expressions are often clinical

146

symptoms, and so the list of drugs for each of them can grow with clinical experience. It is therefore safer to rely on basic parameters, using expressions only for confirmation. For example, "Jealousy" is a basic parameter, and its own expression may be "Sarcasm". In proving, this expression, viz. "Sarcasm" of the remedy which has jealousy, may not yet be known.

In the Repertory many rubrics contain remedies for which the symptom is basic and also remedies in which the symptom is an expression of a more basic feeling. What we have to remember is that the remedies for whom that feeling is basic are more certain to be included in the rubric than those remedies for whom that symptom is merely an expression of another basic feeling.

Basic feelings are more reliable

In practical terms, we select the rubric which represents the expression, we are likely to miss the remedy, but if we select the rubric that represents the basic feeling of the patient, is less unlikely that we will miss it.

Most of the additions of Gallavardin to the Synthetic Repertory are expressions and do not represent basic feelings. For example, "Revolutionary" (*Mercurius*) or the addition of a somewhat large rubric like "Adulterous".

In provings, due to the acuteness of the effect, basic parameters such as "Fear" and "Anger" stand out clearly and sharply, and are recorded as such, even before the prover has the opportunity to find various expressions for those feelings.

Master the components

Components are like letters in a word. Individually, they mean little, but together they make sense. Initially, we have to spell out the letters (division of symptoms into components) but later it becomes quick, unconscious and automatic. We cannot reach this state unless we pass through the stage of spelling out the letters.

If you can see it, each thought, each act, each pastime, each profession, each gesture and indeed every single thing is constructed out of components like letters in a word.

The component idea in practice

One of my favourite early examples was the observation that *Aurum metallicum* patients like to hear bhajans. Bhajans are Indian religious songs, which are sung with exact meter and with a lot of devotion. Persons who like listening to bhajans have three component qualities:

– Religious affections;
– Music ameliorates;
– Exactness.

147

These three in combination are found only in *Aurum metallicum*, and *Aurum* patients are almost the only people I have found to be markedly ameliorated from hearing bhajans.

Another observation is of children who, whenever they see a dog or cat, pick up a stone and throw it at the animal. This can be possible only if the children have the following three components:

- Fear of dog or cat;
- Destructiveness;
- Impulse to throw things.

This combination can only be found in *Tuberculinum* and I have invariably found these children to require *Tuberculinum*.

Let us take the symptom "Jesting, fun of somebody, making". This symptom has a number of components, namely:

- The person is witty;
- One has to be mischievous to make fun of somebody;
- This is an element of pride and contempt for others;
- It may be a feeling of jealousy which inclines a person to make fun of others;
- Loquacity (vivaciousness) is also a trait in one who tries to jest at the expenses of others;
- One has also to be quick witted, quick to act.

These components clearly characterize *Lachesis*. *Hyoscyamus* is jealous and mischievous, but not witty nor quick to act. *Coffea* is jealous and witty as well as quick to act, but not mischievous.

Analyzing a symptom into components

Here is an illustrative case from my colleague Dr. Jayesh Shah, who has been utilizing this idea in his practice. A girl of nine developed symptoms of diarrhoea accompanied by severe headache. The diarrhoea was somehow brought under control with Allopathy, but the headache did not respond even to heavy doses of pain killers. Jayesh observed something funny in the case. The child was painting frantically, producing picture after picture. She was painting for fourteen to sixteen hours a day during the severe pain and at a very rapid pace. She said painting was the only activity she liked. Jayesh tried to study the symptom in various books, but "Desire for painting" could not be found anywhere.

Firstly, he felt it could be taken as "Ameliorated when busy". He wanted to confirm this and so asked whether any other activity would give relief. To this she said: "No". Then, he thought, may be it has to do with physical activity involving movement of her hands. He asked if writing or knitting gave any relief, and the girl said she had tried knitting without relief. Finally, he asked her if drawing with a pencil afforded any relief, and once again he got a negative reply. So, what exactly was this painting doing to her?

Jayesh then realized that each picture she had drawn was in bright colours, so he questioned her about her reaction to colours and she said she liked them very much.

That is when the component idea came to his help. He reasoned that painting must be a combination of some features and if he could split it up into its components, then he might find the remedy. Painting, he reasoned, is combination of three components:
- Busy mind;
- Busy hands;
- Colours.

So, he took the following rubrics:
— Mind busy (Synthetic Repertory);
— Industrious;
— Hurry;
— Mind, colours, charmed by (Synthetic Repertory);
— Extremities, restlessness, hands (Kent's Repertory).

From these he came to the remedy *Tarentula hispanica*.

On going through Phatak's Materia Medica, Jayesh found that *Tarentula hispanica* not only has: "Must keep hands busy" and is "Sensitive to colours", but also has: "Violent crushing headaches as accompaniment to other complaints" (these are called synalgic pains). *Tarentula hispanica* gave prompt relief.

Here is another simple example. Describing their eight year old son, his parents gave a typical example of his behaviour. They said that just the previous day he looked out of the balcony of their second floor apartment and saw that on the first floor, a boy was leaning out of his balcony with his head jutting out. Our patient just picked up a pebble and dropped it on the head of the boy below him and vanished.

This one typical description of the boy can be reduced to the following components:
- Mischievous;
- Destructiveness, cunning;
- Restlessness/Fidgety (the need to do something);
- Throws things away.

From these we can see that the remedy is *Tarentula hispanica*, and again *Tarentula hispanica* helped the case.

All components of a remedy need not be found in a case

From the above two cases of *Tarentula hispanica*, it should be clear that every case of a remedy need not manifest all the traits of that remedy, not even the so-called characteristic ones. A remedy should never be ruled out because the patient does not manifest one or the other feature of it. We have to select the remedy which covers all the prominent traits of the patient even if the patient does not fit in with our idea of that remedy. What I want to point out is that whatever traits do exist in a case can combine to form very characteristic expressions. The question we have to ask when we see such peculiar or striking features is: "What are the components required to form this feature?"

As an example, I will give another from Dr. Jayesh Shah's cases. It illustrates that when a patient gives a definite symptom, it is worth breaking it down into its components and examining the remedy which has them. A child of three, whenever approached by a stranger, either slaps him or spits on his face. The symptom "Spits or strikes at strangers approaching" is not available in this form in our Materia Medica. Jayesh analyzed that in order to have this peculiar tendency, the child must have the following components:

- Striking;
- Fear, approached, of being; children cannot bear to have anyone come near them;
- Fear, strangers;
- Spitting, faces of people, in;
- Timidity.

The only remedy having these components is *Cuprum metallicum*.

Another case:

A lady, aged 59, complained of arthritic pains and backache. She said she did not have much pleasure in life and was fed up with it. She was the only child of very strict parents. The parents themselves were not a happy couple. She was very repressed as she had never been allowed to do what she wanted to. After marriage, her relations with her husband were not very happy. "No one showed me much affection", she said. Her only son died in an accident at the age of three and a half. She still broods over her loss. During the interview she was excited, fidgety, fumbling hands and pricking nails. She had to keep herself occupied with such things like knitting and needle work. She liked watching television, but only quiz programmes. Even while watching one of these, she had to keep her hands busy knitting. She started from the least noise.

What are the components of this case?
- Forsaken feeling;
- Restless hands;
- Occupation ameliorates;
- She watches the quiz programme at the same time does knitting, i.e. she likes to be (or is better when) busy mentally as well as occupied physically;
- Brooding over the loss of her child;
- Depressed, low-spirited; has nervous anxiety.

The remedy is *Kalium bromatum*. The first three components are found in the Repertory, the fourth in Phatak's Materia Medica on *Kalium bromatum*, and the fifth and sixth are given in Hering's "Guiding Symptoms".

In the physical sphere also combinations of components can give rise to the characteristics of a remedy. Take the single symptom: "Cough of students", with *Nux vomica* against it. This could involve a combination of aggravating factors for cough such as:

- Loss of sleep;
- Stimulants, i.e. coffee;
- Reading aloud;
- Sedentary habits;
- Mental exertion;
- Excitement.

In this example, we can see how a combination of mental and physical factors combine in producing a characteristic single symptom.

Components blend into each other

It will strike you that though a person is made up of various components (as is a remedy), these components do not stand out separately, but blend together to give a special flavour. In cooking, various ingredients contribute to the taste though we do not perceive the ingredients as distinct from each other. Together they form a particular dish which we are able to identify. From this analogy, one can also understand that though two dishes may have several identical ingredients, the addition or substraction of an important one, such as salt or sugar, can make the taste of the two dishes totally different.

For example, you may have a person who is very religious, conscientious and industrious. He looks like *Aurum metallicum*, but you find in him an extreme irresolution about trifles. This one component in a marked degree would change the indication to *Baryta carbonica*. Therefore, the whole flavour of the person has changed from a rigid *Aurum metallicum* to an irresolute *Baryta carbonica*.

Component idea in practice

This idea enables us to understand symptoms and expressions of the patient in terms of their components and hence in terms of their repertorial rubrics, making it easy to come to the remedy, since the expressions as such may not be listed in the Materia Medica. It is important to confirm that the components we are identifying from that expression are not isolated or accidental symptoms of the patient (i.e. which may have occurred in response to some bad situation) but which represent his innermost personality (basic symptoms), and can be confirmed from other events in his life and other aspects of his case. Here I give some successfully treated cases as illustrations.

Case 1: A six year old male. Whenever he sees a cockroach, he stamps on it and makes it into a pulp.

Components:
- Destructive;

- Violent;
- Kill, impulse to;
- Moral feeling, want of;
- Fear of cockroach.

Belladonna

Case 2: The child, when asked to go out of the consulting room with his father, drags his mother (who is sitting in the room) with increased strength. He holds on to her and pulls her, stamps his feet and shrieks.

Components:

- Gestures, stamp the feet;
- Clinging;
- Shrieking.

Stramonium

Case 3: A man aged seventy comes and sit with his son (my female assistant is also in the room) and says: "Doctor, I have fever. I know it is due to cracks in the penis. Treat it and the fever will go."

Components:

- Egotism;
- Theorizing;
- Indifferent to personal appearance. (He does not care what others think about him.);
- Cracks in penis.

Sulphur

Case 4: A five year old boy: restless, stubborn, disobedient; stamps feet if his wishes are not fulfilled. Severe chronic cough. I was talking to his mother when suddenly he said loudly: "Hey, Sankaran, why is my cough not stopping?"

Components:

- Speech, abrupt;
- Speech, threatening;
- Abrupt;
- Threatening.

Tarentula hispanica

Case 5: Lady patient. Her son says of her: "My mother keeps sharply reminding me from 11 o'clock to give her medicine dose at 12."

Components:

- Particular about time ("Fastidious, rest, cannot, when things are not in their proper place");

- Anxiety about health;
- Carefulness;
- Critical;
- Suspicious;
- Restlessness.

Arsenicum

Case 6: Boy, six years. Whenever he sees anything in anybody's hands, he snatches it and won't give it back.

Components:
- Avarice;
- Jealousy;
- Greed;
- Envy;
- Impulsive;
- Violent;
- Courageous;
- Obstinate.

Nux vomica

Case 7: Boy, ten years. Mother says he vomits before exams. Question to the boy: "Are you scared of school?" Answer: "Why should I be scared of school? I have no reason to be scared of school, and I get irritated when I am asked again and again if I am scared of school."

Components:
- Precocity;
- Ailments from anticipatory anxiety;
- Egotism, ailments from;
- Anger from contradiction.

Lycopodium

Case 8: Lady, thirty-six years. Developed shoulder pain (arthritis) after the death of her neighbour of the same caste. She is not communicative with others in the building.

Components:
- Childish;
- Strangers, presence of, aggravates;
- Bashful;
- Delusion as if beloved friend is sick and dying (so much dependence on a friend).

Baryta carbonica

Case 9: Angrily, a patient complaints: "Other people are saying bad things about me."

Components:

– Suspicious;
– Delusion she is being criticized;
– Delusion she is being watched;
– Quarrelsome.

Hyoscyamus

Case 10: A forty-five year old male patient said: "Doctor, I have had this cough for the last nineteen days. It is absolutely dry. I went from one doctor to another and took all kinds of medicines and nothing helped, absolutely nothing helped. So I threw away all the medicines and said I won't touch them again and I have come to you."

Components:

– Anxiety about health;
– Absolutely cannot think in between. Thinks of things as black or white (hatred, sympathetic) as too good or too bad. Either you are a very good friend or a very bad enemy;
– Hatred for persons who offend, unmoved by apology;
– Obstinate.

Nitricum acidum

Case 11: A child with cough, cold, vomiting and diarrhoea. His mother gives the following history: During pregnancy, her husband had some enemies. So every time he went out at night, she would be scared that something would happen to him. She lost a lot of weight and became extremely restless. Her sense of smell became acute and also she felt everything very dirty and wanted to clean up.

Components:

– Anxiety about others;
– Restlessness at night;
– Restless, anxious;
– Delusions about criminals, delusions sees thieves at night;
– Emaciation;
– Fear at night;
– Fastidious;
– Washing, cleanliness, mania for.

Arsenicum album

The child did well on *Arsenicum album* (based on the remedy of the mother during pregnancy).

Case 12: A man aged sixty was suffering from gout. He said: "Doctor, this is all emotional. That Guru of mine keeps making new courses to teach yoga and meditation, so that when the students finish one course, they go on to the next course. Then he goes away and leaves all the responsibility on me and I have to handle everything.

Components of the patient:

– Conscientious about trifles;

– Delusion that he has neglected his duty (duty conscious);

– Forsaken, feeling;

– Industrious.

Aurum metallicum

Components of the Guru:

– Ambitious;

– Flies from his own children (flies from his creations);

– Dictatorial, power, love of;

– Delusion of being in two places at one time;

– Dictatorial;

– Impatience.

Lycopodium

24

DELUSIONS

There is one large but little used portion of the "Mind" chapter in our Repertory. This is the section on "Delusions". Delusions are feelings which are not fully based on facts, but they are feelings nevertheless. The difference between delusions and feelings is that delusions are exaggerated, more fixed and often expressed in terms of images.

The idea of using delusions came to me when I found that the rubrics: "Unfortunate feeling" and "Delusion, unfortunate, he is" have the same remedies listed in Kent's Repertory. This led me to think that "Delusion, unfortunate, he is" is nothing but a feeling that he is unfortunate. I started studying the "Delusion" rubrics and tried to understand what each delusion means in terms of feelings.

Understanding a delusion

One of the commonest delusions known to student of Materia Medica is the delusion of *Thuja* which reads (Phatak's Materia Medica): "Fixed idea, as if he is made of glass". After reading this symptom, I was sure that one day some patient would come and say: "Doctor, let me tell you a little secret. I am made of glass. In fact, I was born in a glass factory!" After all, if the symptom is recorded in the Materia Medica, I thought at least one patient must have it. But no one came with this symptom. Even in the literature, I hardly came across a case in which this symptom was found. When I asked a few homoeo-paths, they said that they felt this must be a sign of insanity and therefore it can be found only in insane people.

However, from my present understanding that delusions are often only exaggerations of normal feelings, I have been able to use this symptom in many cases to prescribe *Thuja*. What feeling could that be which can make us feel as if we were "made of glass"? I think it is a feeling on the part of a person that he is fragile. It is a feeling of being delicate, a brittle feeling, that one has to be cautious, otherwise something could break. Pierre Schmidt gives in the Synthetic Repertory the symptom: "Frail, sensation of being". Frail means "delicate", or "easily harmed". Also refer to the rubrics in Kent's Repertory: "Delusion, body is brittle" and "Delusion, body is delicate". In some degree many people have this feeling at some time or other. That is why they are careful when climbing down the stairs, or crossing the street, or when walking on a slippery surface. This is a normal caution and a normal feeling of fragility, but in *Thuja* such a feeling is exaggerated to a very marked degree. It is expressed by the prover as a feeling "as if he is made of glass". These are the words used to express such an exaggerated fragile feeling.

How this delusion is expressed by patients

One *Thuja* patient reported that she was scared to go in a crowd. When asked why, she replied that she was afraid that someone may fall over her or step on her feet and cause her injury. Typical is the way another *Thuja* patient shakes hands. He extends only the tips of his fingers forward, and even that with great caution, and his arm is tense as if he would have to withdraw it at any moment. It is a feeling as if the other person shakes his hand too hard, he may not be able to bear it. Another expression of this feeling is to be seen in the patient who says: "Doctor, I hope your medicines are not too strong for me." Sometimes at the second visit, the visibly anxious *Thuja* patient reports: "Doctor, I took your medicines and they produced a lot of palpitation; I got scared and immediately stopped the medicine." The feelings which she gets is as if one more dose could permanently injure her system. I see this as yet another expression of that delicate, fragile feeling.

This fragile feeling can extent to particular organs also. Thus, a patient may get a feeling that his heart is fragile and if he exerts just a little bit more, it will break down, or if he eats a little extra fatty food, his heart will not bear it and will stop working.

In *Thuja*, this fragile feeling is combined with another prominent feature, and that is *fixity of ideas*. This fixity of ideas is nothing but an exaggerated rigidity of thinking. To some extent all of us are rigid in our ideas; for example, we may have a notion that all villagers are dull-headed. Such ideas remain fixed, but when we come in close touch with several villagers who are intelligent, and observe that the facts are quite contrary to our beliefs, we will alter our ideas. But a *Thuja* patient remains fixed in his idea, even if faced with very strong proof to the contrary.

There is an anecdote about a lady who told her doctor that there was a cat in her abdomen. The doctor tries to explain that it was not possible, but she insisted that she knew she had a cat in her abdomen. In order to pacify her, the doctor told her he would operate on her and remove the cat. He took her into the operation theatre, anaesthetized her and made a scar on her abdomen. When she came back to consciousness, he pointed to the scar and said he had removed the cat. She asked him to show her the cat. The doctor went out and somehow got hold of a cat and showed it to her. "Oh!", she said, "this is a white cat. The cat I have in abdomen is black!" Such are the fixed ideas of *Thuja*!

More expressions

When fixity of ideas is combined with a feeling of fragility, then there is a fixed idea of fragility. This is commonly seen in a patient who, despite undergoing several stress tests and even angiography, and despite all the results being negative, will still feel that his heart is delicate and he must be very cautious or it will stop working. He will go from one doctor to another to get his idea confirmed and he will not fully believe a doctor who gives a negative report.

Another example of this frail feeling is the patient who says: "Doctor, I avoid all sour things entirely; I know if I eat even a little sour, all my joints will start hurting."

When you ask the patient if she had eaten sour and observed such an effect, she will say: "No, I never eat sour things because I know I can't bear it." Here you get the combination of fixed ideas and frail feeling.

At this point, an important lesson that we must keep in mind is that all these feelings are within us, only they are found in an exaggerated and more persistent form in disease. Unless we are able to recognize these feelings in ourselves, we canhot claim to have fully understood them in a remedy or in a patient. In other words, the feelings of a remedy or patient are not some strange feelings of a particular kind of people, but modifications of the feelings that exist in all of us. When we read a delusion, we must perceive what kind of feeling in us, when exaggerated, can lead to that delusion. Is there anyone who has not felt trapped, or inferior, at some time or other? Remedies can be better understood by experiencing their feelings. On studying the chapter on "Delusions" further, I found that many of the delusions have very few remedies, sometimes only one or two. On studying these remedies, I found that many expressions of the remedy are explained by that single delusion. The delusion is often the main feeling expressing itself in a variety of patterns.

For example:

— Delusion, walks on his knees;

— Delusion, legs, cut off, are;

— Delusion, laughed at.

These are all delusions of *Baryta carbonica*. What did the prover mean by this? He meant that he had an unreasonable (fixed) idea; the feeling of a person who walks on his knees with his legs cut off. He feels like a person who is one foot shorter than the rest of the world, handicapped, and that he is looked down upon, laughed at and ridiculed. This is one of the main feeling of *Baryta carbonica*. Once one understands this main feeling, several other features of *Baryta carbonica* are explained.

A case example

The following is an interview with an eighteen year old girl who came with the problem of several pimples on her face.

— Since when are you having these pimples?

— More than a month.

— Now they come and go?

— It was even more than this. They keep coming.

— What other complaint? Pain or burning?

— Yes, itching, no pain. Some pus – after bursting, with blood. No pain.

— (Examines hands.) Any reasons? Why since more than one month?

— Not going now. Previously they would suppurate.

— Any cravings?

— Everything.

— Anything special?

159

— Flower and rice. (Cauliflower.)
— Salt, sweets?
— Little sweets, salty – I like.
— Appetite?
— No appetite – must have food on time.
— Thirst?
— OK.
— Hot or chilly?
— Hot and chilly.
— Sweat?
— Less.
— Periodes (menstruation)?
— Otherwise normal, 2-3 days early. Now, scanty.
— How do you sleep?
— Sleep on back.
— What do you do?
— I was studying and temporarily working in Indian Airlines as office assistant.
— How is your nature?

No reply – smiles.

Again questions.

— I'm mild, sometimes very angry. I don't strike but don't speak for one or two hours. A small child comes and I become OK. I forget my anger.
— What else about your nature? Do you weep?
— If someone says something, I cry.
— On which matters do you get angry?

No reply for a long time. Just concentrating.

— (Repeats question.) Give an example.
— Somebody reprimanded me.
— Does your face become oily? (Sudden physical question to test reflexes.)
— Yes, very oily. (Quick reply.)
— You like company or to be alone?
— I like to be alone, don't like noise – like silence. No problems to remain alone the whole day. (Spontaneous reply.) Always silent and do some work.
— Like to remain in one place or move about?
— Remain in one place. Do not like to go out anywhere.
— What else you like to do?
— (No reply for a long time. Then says:) When my work is over I just sit alone.
— (Question repeated.) You like to talk?
— I like silence.

160

— Do you get dreams?

— Very rarely.

— Tell me about your dreams.

— (Silence.) How can I tell?

— Good or bad dreams? Bad dreams what? Dreams of water?

— Yes. But why do you need to know all this?

— Tell me your dreams. I will get you well.

— How can that be?

— We select medicine on this basis.

— Dreams of water, trees, quarrels.

— Tell me one thing. How are your menses?

— First two days, very dark menses.

— Do you feel fresh on waking?

— Sometimes I feel a burden on my head on waking.

— Is there itching in the daytime or night?

— It is at daytime.

— Are the pimples related to menses?

— Yes, more before menses, and all the time since the last few months.

— Cravings in food?

— I like cauliflower, radish, raw vegetables, these I like very much. But if I don't get them, it's OK.

— Sleep on your back, side or stomach?

— On back.

— You like windows open or closed?

— Closed – my mother shouts (noise).

— Do you suppress anger?

— I never tell anyone. I feel like saying, but I never speak.

— How do you like sweets?

— I like little – not too much.

— What is your name?

— Shahnaz.

— I am giving medicine for ten days. Tell me how you are after ten days.

From the above interview I could see the following:

–   The girl was extremely reluctant to talk about her emotions and gave the impression that she was not used to talking about herself to anyone.

–   The question she asked ("Why should I tell you all this?") indirectly meant: "Why are you taking interest in me (since no one else has ever done so)?"

–   The basic feeling is one of having no one to whom she can tell her feelings, or no one who cares to know about them. This is a feeling of being friendless.

- This was confirmed by all her behaviour and activities (like not going out, etc., despite her being in the prime of life).

So, I choose "Friendless feeling" as the main theme in the case and took the symptoms:

- Delusion that she is friendless;
- Unfriendly humor;
- Forsaken feeling;
- Ailments after anger, vexation.
- Company, aversion to;
- Food and drinks, vegetables, desires;
- Introspection;
- Sensitive to noise;
- Talk, indisposed to, desire to be silent, taciturn;
- Thoughts, thoughtful;
- Dreams of forest (many trees) and water;
- Face, eruptions, pimples, menses, before, aggravates.

She is a very closed person, will not speak out to anybody, and prefers to be alone. Symbolic dreams of trees and water. From these rubrics I came to the remedy *Magnesium muriaticum* which not only removed the pimples, but made changes in her attitude.

Feelings and reactions

Feelings and reactions make two components of the same person's state of mind. We feel and hence we react. In reactions we have a choice which we exercise depending upon our circumstances, training, culture, etc. Thus, the range of reactions to the same feeling may be wide, but the feeling itself will be basic and unalterable. We can say that feelings are involuntary and uncontrollable but reactions are to some extent controllable and modifiable. Thus, it is easier to rely on feelings much more than on reactions. Feelings are felt in all spheres of a patient, in all the relationships he establishes with himself, his family, his society, his doctor, his illness, etc. We have to observe and uncover them, perceive them.

For example, a girl who had been taking my treatment for pimples for a long time, came to me and said: "Doctor, why am I not getting better? You don't want me to make me alright?" I asked: "Why should I not want to make you alright?" She answered: "You must have some kind of grudge against me. Other patients are getting better, why am I not getting better?"

The feeling behind her statement is: "You have the capacity as a doctor but you are not treating me properly because you don't like me as much as others." You have to look at the feeling behind this statement.

When I examined her life from the past, I found that she was from a large family. She was engaged when she was eighteen years old, but the engagement was broken for some reason. She had a sister, one year younger, who was more beautiful and was always given more attention. That sister had got married and had a child now. Our patient had had to struggle to get her proper value recognized in the family since childhood. So, she needed to be quarrelsome out of jealousy.

I gave her *Calcarea sulphurica*, which helped her a great deal, based on the following rubrics:

— Lamenting, appreciated, she is not;

— Quarrelsome;

— Jealousy;

and on physical symptoms that were present in her case.

This feeling of jealousy, that I was giving more attention to other patients, made her quarrelsome and complaining with me. She behaved as if I was her father giving more attention to other patients than her, just as it was happening in her house. The way she spoke with me showed her feelings and her attitude to her situation. Here we can see that the feeling that she was not appreciated, that she was not valued, made her react in different situations in a particular way. Her reaction was perfectly in tune with her feelings. Thus, we can say that a delusion makes the rest of the symptomatology meaningful and congruent.

Not all delusions are equally important. We have to differentiate between two types of delusions.

Which delusions are more important and why?

When we defined disease, we said that disease is the inability of a person to react appropriately to his situation. For example, a man chased by a dog behaves as if it were a lion. This is his delusion and so he reacts in a way which is inappropriate to the actual situation. Thus, his delusion is his real disease. If this delusion goes away, then he will react normally, i.e. he will see the dog merely as a dog and drive it away. The delusion is the person's viewpoint of the situation. It explains most of his reactions. It is his false perception of the situation. Expressions like violence, laughing, anger, weeping, etc., can be common to many situations, but the feelings behind them will be different in each case, and the choice of the remedy will depend on the feelings which trigger these reactions rather that on the expressions themselves. The remedy which has the exact delusion will be the only one that will be able to cure the patient.

Here, I shall introduce two new terms: *incidental delusion* and *basic delusion*. By *incidental delusion* I mean the false perception of the patient in a specific situation, which is temporary, and will pass off when that incident is over. For example, when starting a troublesome car, I am afraid of what may happen if it breaks down on the way. I have an abnormal fear that is out of proportion to the situation; it would be appropriate in a person going into the middle of a jungle. This delusion (of the city being a jungle) is temporary and hence incidental. The reason why this delusion occurred in this specific situation is because of a deeper delusion namely a feeling that I may not be able to cope, since the problem may be beyond my capacity. This false perception of myself in relation to the situation and the resulting diffidence is the basis for the incidental delusion of being in a jungle.

The delusion that I am in a situation which may be beyond my capacity to handle, forms the basic delusion and will be the basis of several different incidental delusions. However, the basic delusion will remain the same at all times, and will be expressed in several ways such as feelings, conditions of OKness, hobbies, manner of speaking, and recurrent dreams. We have to try to find the basic delusion of the patient.

The key to the case lies in observing all the expressions, how the person walks, talks, comes to the clinic, narrates his complaints, etc., and then understanding the feeling behind all these expressions, the feeling that makes him react in that particular way. We have to find out in which way he perceives his situation. If we can find out as we saw in the cases of *Calcarea sulphurica* and *Magnesium muriaticum*, and now in the case below, then we can get to the centre of the case, and the remedy selection becomes accurate.

Just as we saw in the chapter on "Components" that we have basic parameters and expressions, similarly in delusions we have basic delusions and incidental delusions. This basic delusion will explain each and every feature of the case and will form the basis of varying incidental delusions. From whichever direction you approach the patient, you will come to a stop at this basic delusion; such is its quality.

Case example

A male engineer, forty years of age, came with the complaints of pain in the stomach and malena. He came from a family of doctors and all the investigations had been done. A Barium meal taken ten years earlier has shown duodenal ulcer for which he had taken allopathic treatment.

He spoke of his physical problems, the numerous investigations done in great detail, giving precise dates and details of treatment taken. He said: "Although all investigations are now normal, I still get acidity from even the most simple foods. I am very careful about what I eat. I eat only boiled food, and for many years I have avoided all fried and spicy things. But there is always the fear that the malena will start again. Whenever it starts, it starts suddenly. Everybody in the family takes the same food as I do, but only I am suffering."

"I was an ambitious person. In the early stages of my career I worked very hard. I was not particular about food and I neglected my health a lot. I ate out and didn't care about when and what I was eating. Now I have become cautious. My health problems have come in the way of advancement in my career. I have now reconciled myself to my fate and given up all ideas of advancement. I feel I can't do what others can do; I have got a handicap. If I go to Madras or Bangalore, I carry my lunch with me. When I went to Japan I was always searching for milk. I had to refuse all the drinks and other luxurious things."

"The main fear is that it should not become malignant. The doctor said that a duodenal ulcer never becomes malignant, but I still have this fear. Everybody tells me to eat everything but I get into trouble if I eat everything. The doctor says there are no restrictions, just avoid the foods which give you a problem, but everything gives me a problem."

"I can't concentrate on my work. I have lost my memory and confidence. I don't feel like working. I am constantly thinking about my health. I want to get back the billion dollar health at any cost. Without health you can't do anything. A poor man, if he is healthy, can at least enjoy good sleep. So, I keep telling my son and daughter not to worry about their grades, but to take care of their health. I want to live happily, that is all."

— What do you attribute your problems to?

— I kept neglecting my health. When there were symptoms, I should have done something about them. I came up very fast, I was a very good student, precocious and ambitious. I could have taken up medicine or engineering. But as I was good at maths, I became an engineer though my family profession is the practice of medicine. I would have done better as a doctor. At least, I could have looked after my health."

In this case all the expressions of the patient:
- His lack of interest in his work,
- His feeling that he cannot fulfil his ambition,
- His regret at not becoming a doctor,
- The advice to his children,

stem from the central feeling that in pursuing his ambition he had neglected his health, which accounted for his suffering now. I took the rubrics:
— Delusion, that he has ruined his health;
— Fear, that he has ruined his health.

Both these rubrics have *Chelidonium* as the only remedy. Taking the other rubrics:
— Anxiety of conscience, as if guilty of a crime;
— Remorse;
— Thoughts of disease;
— Delusion that his disease is incurable;
— Loquacity;
— Work, aversion to, mental;
— Indolence;
— Concentration difficult;
— Forgetful.

I confirmed this prescription. Incidentally, this delusion that he has ruined his health is not found in any Materia Medica but only in Kent's Repertory.

165

It is interesting to note that this man was not *Chelidonium* from birth. He was ambitious, precocious and industrious, indicating *Lycopodium*. His ambition made him neglect everything to come up in this competitive world. In the process, he neglected his health to such an extent that he went into the *Chelidonium* state in order that his health gets more attention.

In this case, we can see that wherever we knock, whatever approach we take, we keep coming back to the basic feeling – that he has ruined his health. This feeling, though justified to some extent, is vastly exaggerated in the present context and hence becomes his basic delusion. This represents his view of himself and his situation and from this stem all his feelings, reactions, conditions and compulsions.

It is not always that we can find the rubric readily in the Repertory. Often, we have to search among various rubrics – including the ones under "Fears", "Sadness", etc. Indeed we may have to search in the whole "Mind" chapter to find a remedy with the same delusion, or its equivalent feeling.

Even if we do not find such a rubric, our perception will deepen through understanding the basic delusion of the patient. As we have seen in the chapter "Health and Disease", disease is nothing but the basic delusion of the patient. Hence, by understanding what this delusion is, we go straight to the crux of the problem.

25

AURUM METALLICUM AND
THE IDEA OF COMPENSATION

The idea of compensation first occurred to me after treating several cases with the remedy *Aurum metallicum*. One of the first cases is given below.

Case

Mr. D., aged fifty-eight came on 23.11.82 with the following complaints:

– Since one year, he has pain in the chest on walking fast, on ascending stairs and especially on walking after meals. Relieved by rest, relieved by pressure. Perspires during the pain. The ECG shows ischemic heart changes.

– Formication of soles. Numbness of feet up to ankles.

– Diabetic – last count: 304 mg%, post lunch.

– High cholesterol – last count: 283 mg%.

Important symptoms: Likes bitter food, warm food, hot drinks and sweets. Stools not satisfactory. Urine: once a night. Sweat scanty. Early baldness.

Originally, he was living in Bombay. He was posted to Delhi where he was promoted as chief accountant, and was given the responsibility of handling a lot of money, something which he was not accustomed to. He became tense and since then, he has the chest pain. Now he is transferred back to Bombay and is not so tense. He likes company, feels lonely when alone. He is very religious and must say his prayers daily. Music soothes him.

On examination: Cold hands. Vertical furrows on the forehead. BP: 140/90.

Observations: Very neat in appearance. Punctual. Has his medical papers very neatly filed. Goes for check regularly. Speaks humbly. Not loquacious.

How I looked at this case

When I studied this case, one definite thing that struck me was that his troubles were aggravated after he was given responsibility which he was not used to. After searching in various Repertories like Kent's, Boenninghausen's and so on, I found the rubric in my own backyard, that is in Phatak's Repertory. The rubric on page 292 is: "Responsibility, unusual, aggravates" and the remedy is *Aurum metallicum*. At this time I only knew the traditional Materia Medica picture of *Aurum metallicum* – that is a depressed, melancholic, suicidal personality. Clarke in his "Dictionary of Practical Materia Medica" says:

> "Melancholy, with inquietude and desire to die. Hopeless, suicidal, desperate, inclined to jump off heights; to dash himself into a chair, sad, feels that all is against her, life is not desirable and the thought of death alone gives pleasure – great anguish which even induces a disposition to suicide."

Phatak in his Materia Medica says:

> "Intense hopeless depression and disgust for life, suicidal anguish. Peevish at least contradiction. Brooding melancholy, future looks dark."

There was no suicidal tendency or depression in my patient, I therefore doubted if *Aurum metallicum* could be his remedy. However, when I considered his other symptoms and looked them up in the Repertory, I was surprised to see that *Aurum metallicum* covered almost all of them:

- Industrious;
- Religious;
- Conscientious about trifles;
- Music ameliorates;
- Chest angina;
- Ascending aggravates.

Since the symptom picture came to *Aurum metallicum* in spite of the absence of the traditional Materia Medica picture and the fact that *Aurum metallicum* did not cover his cravings, I decided to give him *Aurum metallicum* 200 and 1M over a period of a year in weekly doses. Gradually, as you can see, his complaints improved and he became almost totally well.

Condition in December 1983:
- Cholesterol: 253 mg%.
- Blood sugar: 141 mg% (post lunch).
- Heart pains much less. Can walk and climb much more.
- Numbness very occasional; much reduced in intensity.

In early February 1986 he had no chest pains, no numbness, blood sugar and cholesterol were normal. He is now settled in an ashram giving free service as an accountant.

So, *Aurum metallicum* cured him completely, and from this case emerged a beautiful picture of *Aurum metallicum*. I started using this picture in other cases with good results. I found that these patients were very conscientious, responsible, duty bound and very affectionate. They could develop almost paternal feeling for others. I developed from these cases a vivid picture of the remedy.

The first thing you will notice in an *Aurum metallicum* patient is that he is neat in appearance, conservatively dressed in an old fashion, sometimes with a religious mark on his forehead. He is punctual in his appointments. His case form is very neatly and completely filled out. He brings all his medical reports properly filed in sequence. On going through these records we find that he has been checking up on his health very regularly. He has taken the medicines scrupulously, not missing out a single dose. He describes his ailments correctly, datewise, and talks confidently, not too much and not too little. In his work, he is very meticulous, careful about even the smallest of things, a perfectionist, will work late, check the last file, count the last penny; he is duty conscious and will never rest until he has completed that day's work. He is very much trusted and valued by his employer and colleagues, since he is extremely hardworking, highly responsible and honest.

He is sincere. He sticks to his limits. He is not ambitious. He does not want money, power or fame. He is happy to have done his duty. He values appreciation, but that is not the aim of his work. Generally, he is mild but he will get angry when others are neglecting their duties. He has a strong sense of right or wrong, and the wrong doings of others provoke his anger. He is thus *censorious*, critical and sets very high standards for himself, as well as for others. He will be very punctual and will expect you to be punctual too. If you delay him in your waiting room, he may burst in and demand that you keep the time. He can be *quarrelsome* and *reproachful*. This creates a lot of mental tension which can lead to hypertension, heart disease, psoriasis or even myocardial infarction and cancer. Despite his sickness, he carries on with his work and gets sicker.

Aurum metallicum patients have a fixed idea about what their duties are. This generally depends on the way they have been taught by their parents. For instance, one person might be given to understand that after the children are married and settled, his duty is over. So, until that task is completed, he works hard and is very caring, etc. But once the marriages are over, he relaxes totally and he may not be industrious, etc. If at this stage you ask him: "Are you tense or worried?", he will reply: "Why should I be tense, now that all my children are settled, all my responsibility is over. Now I just spend my time praying and helping others." You may be surprised that this hardworking, busy, hurried man is now totally relaxed and is listening to music, as if he had no care in the world.

An *Aurum metallicum* patient may have been taught that after he has fulfilled his responsibilities towards his family, he should turn to religion or social service, so he devotes his time to religion or helping others. He helps others more from a sense of duty than from sympathy or anxiety for others. Religiousness also arises out of sense of duty. Some fixed time of the day is devoted to religious prayers. He is not philosophical. He does not question what he is doing. He is very much inclined to religious music which gives him tremendous relief. He also reacts well to classical music.

He can be proud but not egoistic. He is justifiably proud of his integrity and sincerity, of his uprightness. He often talks and answers in questions.

Aurum metallicum can be mild but revengeful also; this depends on parental upbringing. We had a typical *Aurum metallicum* patient whose father was mild but whose mother was a very strong lady. She set the example that a person must not forgive someone who has harmed him, one must obstinately fight and take revenge until justice is done. This patient was once taken to court by his neighbour for some offence he had not committed, so he created an alibi and had his neighbour beaten up by a couple of roughs. Then he was satisfied. He even made friends with the neighbour later on. His mother was of such a nature.

We have so far seen what we could call the "parent" side of *Aurum metallicum*. I am using the term "parent" as meant in Transactional Analysis, a system founded by Eric Berne, and exemplified by Thomas Harris in his best-seller, "I'm OK, You are OK".

Transactional Analysis analyses a person's mind in three components: the Parent, the Adult and the Child. The Parent is the tape of our parents' instructions, prejudices, beliefs and attitudes. It differs from person to person, depending upon his society, nation and ultimately his parents. "To tell a lie is a sin", "Beware of strangers", etc., are statements coming from the Parent part of us. A person in whom the Parent part dominates is not able to objectively look at reality. He views everything through the eyes of his own parents and he has a strong sense of right and wrong, and he likes to correct everyone else who is wrong. He often lands up parenting other people. For instance, if you ask him: "Where are my keys?", he will retort: "Why don't you keep them in one place?" An objective Adult statement like: "I don't know", or "Let's find out", etc., are rare from a person in whom the Parent part is dominating.

So, we see a very strong Parent in *Aurum metallicum*. This strong parental influence can be seen in the fact that *Aurum metallicum* hardly lives in the present. He plays back his parental tapes and judges everything on what his parents have given him to understand. "The world is going to the dogs", "All politicians are thieves", etc. Such attitudes are common, though often unexpressed, in an *Aurum metallicum* patient.

There is also an equally strong Child tape in *Aurum metallicum*, but it is more hidden than the Parent part. By Child in Transactional Analysis, we mean the tape of our own childhood with the anxiety, fears, sadness, guilt, disappointments, despair, rejection and also the joyous moments. We feel sad when someone rejects us, guilty when we are selfish or tell a lie. Taking the same example, if you ask the person in whom the Child part is dominating: "Where are my keys?", he will react with: "Why do you always have to keep blaming me?" Developing strong attachments is also a quality of the Child part of us.

Aurum metallicum can develop a very strong attachment to another person often much younger than himself. Such a parent-child relationship, I have seen him develop with a person of the opposite sex, or it could be with his own child. The attachment is so strong that he must see the other person every day, hear that person's voice, etc. The affection goes side by side with expecting the other person to obey and to act according to his wishes. Such relationships probably represent the *Aurum metallicum* need to be parent to someone else. It is when the other person rebels, in other words, refuses to be parented anymore, that *Aurum metallicum* becomes heartbroken. He experiences many emotions: indignation, mortification, anger, tremendous depression, sadness, forsaken feeling, disappointment and he feels that life is not worth living. He can become suicidal at this stage, he totally withdraws and becomes highly irritable.

When viewed side by side with the intellectual level of *Aurum metallicum*, this emotional nature seems paradoxical. You find on one hand an intelligent, hardworking, sincere, honest, religious person and, on the other, the same person getting attached and then depressed and suicidal. The rubrics in the Synthetic Repertory are:

— Ailments from disappointment in love (page 20);
— Sadness and suicidal from disappointment in love (page 719).

I treated many such cases in two years and found on analyzing them, that conscientiousness was topmost amongst the symptoms, whereas suicidal disposition figured at the bottom of the list – only one patient had it (see table with detailed analysis of the symptoms in those cases).

Analysis of symptoms of 19 cases of *Aurum metallicum*
(The figure indicates the number of cases in which this symptom was found)

– Conscientious	18
– Music ameliorates	12
– Religious	10
– Religious, insanity	1
– Religious, melancholy	1
– Anticipatory anxiety	9
– Responsibility aggravates	9
– Anger with trembling	8
– Thinking of illness	8
– Brooding	6
– Industrious	6
– Anxiety of conscience as if guilty of a crime	5
– Contradiction, intolerant of	6
– Sympathy	5
– Company aggravates	3
– Aversion to company	5
– Company ameliorates	4
– Consolation, aversion to	1
– Consolation ameliorates	4
– Anxiety about others	4
– Hurried in genera	3
– Hurried, eating	5
– Hurried, talk	1
– Hurried, walking	2

– Hurried, work	2
– Hurried, reading	1
– Fear of looking down from high places	4
– Fear of being alone	1
– Fear of quarrels	1
– Fear of dark	2
– Fear of death	2
– Fear of robbers	3
– Fear of disease	2
– Fear of snakes	1
– Fear of future	1
– Fear of sudden noises	4
– Fear of thunderstorm	1
– Fear of something unknown	1
– Fear of heart disease	1
– Fear of air travel	1
– Fear of animals	1
– Fear of dogs, cats	1
– Memory, poor	3
– Memory, poor for places	1
– Memory, poor for names	5
– Memory, poor for faces	1
– Memory, poor for what is read	2
– Mildness	3
– Anger, sudden	1
– Anger, violent	1
– Anger, suppressed	2
– Anger, throws things away	2
– Anger, injures himself	1
– Anger, from contradiction	1
– Anger, with indignation	1
– Ailments from anger	1
– Sadness, cloudy weather aggravates	2
– Sadness near sea	1
– Starting, sudden noise aggravates	1
– Suicidal thoughts	2
– Suicidal thoughts, pain aggravate	1
– Weeps, when alone	2
– Forsaken feeling	3
– Indignation	3
– Slow in eating	1
– Envious	2
– Sentimental	2

– Censorious	1
– Decides quickly	2
– Indifference	1
– Indifference to business	1
– Indifference to affairs of children	1
– Weeping	3
– Weeping during sleep	1
– Weeping from anger	1
– Weeping from sympathy	2
– Dwelling	1
– Grief, suppressed	1
– Loquacity	3
– Cheerful, when praying	1
– Cheerful, in cloudy weather	1
– Cheerful, in thunderstorm	1
– Delusions, God	1
– Praying	1
– Impatient	4
– Fastidious	2
– Egoistic	2
– Remorse	1
– Anxiety aggravated by sudden noise	1
– Moody	1
– Sadness before menses	1
– Suspicion	3
– Jealous	2
– Ambitious	1
– Mistakes in talking	1
– Mistakes in writing	1
– Thoughts intrude upon mind working	1
– Thoughts wandering	1
– Concentration difficult in conversation	1
– Presence of strangers aggravates	1
– Ailments from disappointment	1
– Ailments from shock	1
– Ailments from shame	1
– Anxiety about health	1
– Anxiety about money matters	1
– Dictatorial	1

–	Superstitious	1
–	Obstinate	2
–	Affectionate to an unrelated person	1
–	Malicious	1
–	Somnambulism	1
–	Talking, during sleep	1
–	Moaning during sleep	1
–	Defiant	1
–	Injustice, cannot tolerate	1

I wanted to see how prominently the increased sense of responsibility and heightened consciousness are mentioned in the provings.

I started reading the proving pictures carefully and realized that depression and suicidal tendency come from the feeling of having neglected his duty and the feeling of having committed a crime. The picture given in the provings is as below. I have extracted from Hering's "Guiding Symptoms" and Hahnemann's "Materia Medica Pura":

> "Moroseness; he is indisposed to talk. He sits apart, all by himself in a corner, wrapped up in himself, as if in the deepest melancholy, but the slightest contradiction excites the greatest heat and anger, when he quite forgets himself, at first quarrelling and much talking afterwards with few remarkable changeability of mind, now impulsive, rash, now very mercy, now sad, anxious longing to die, soon after, laughing aloud. Very much given to feel offended, the slightest thing which he thought offensive affected him deeply and caused him to resent it. Peevish dejection, he thinks nothing will succeed with him. Discontent with his circumstances, blames his fate or himself for it. Remorse about his incapacity to do things fast enough. Restless and undecided with a feeling he was neglecting something for which he must incur reproach. Self-condemnation, self-reproach, self-criticism, continuous feeling of doing everything wrong. Imagines he has forfeited the affections of others and this grieves him to tears. Intense hopeless depression and weary of life. Melancholy, he imagines he is unfit for the world, he is unworthy of life. Looks on the dark side and constantly thinks about committing suicide. Thoughts of death give the maximum pleasure. Broods over the thoughts that he has neglected his duty and that he deserves reproach and he is not worthy of salvation. Desperate, desires to jump from a height. All the time a dark, hopeless mood, frequently anxiety and despair, life is a burden to him."

I asked myself why there was so much difference between the clinical picture and the proving picture. One thing that was apparent was that both pictures came from one source, i.e. "Increased scruples of conscience" (Clarke).

174

Since both suicidal and neglected duty feelings came from this increased scruples of conscience, why should one aspect come out more in the provings and the other in the clinical picture? Both are part of *Aurum metallicum*, but in the prover, the *Aurum metallicum* state comes on suddenly. A normal healthy person, seeing his life from the *Aurum metallicum* perspective, with the increased scruples of conscience, feels that he has hopelessly neglected his duty. He is totally depressed, thinks that he has done wrong, that he has lost the affection of his friends and that he deserves reproach; death is the only escape now.

On the other hand, the chronic *Aurum metallicum* patient would never have neglected his duty due to his heightened scruples of conscience. The suicidal disposition being harmful and unpleasant, he has compensated for. In the provings, there is no time to compensate.

This thought made me quite aware that probably many symptoms of our state are in a compensated form. For example, the *Aurum metallicum* patient would retain his sense of duty, morality and industriousness in a direct form, but his depression, he would compensate for by saying something like: "Why should I be sad that my son has not come up in life? After all, I have done my duty. I have done everything I could, I have fulfilled my responsibility. Now, if his fate is not good, how am I responsible?", or : "After all, I have to live and fulfil my responsibility. I can't just run away once I have taken this up. I have to finish it, there is no escape." Or, in a stressful situation he might say: "Doctor, I wish death would come, but now, how can I die, I have so much to do?"

These statements to himself are his attempts to keep away his suicidal feelings that come to his mind; to mask the real state within. This process, I term compensation. We have already seen how much difference the process of compensation can make between the Materia Medica picture and what we see in patients. In the next chapter, we will study the process of compensation in more detail.

26

COMPENSATION

Compensation involves our covering up by an act of will some elements of our nature (without there being a change in these elements). This cover-up is needed if the situation is not intense enough to require a change in the elements, and a mere cover-up will serve the purpose. In such a case, the mind has the capacity to, and does, adjust itself. Thus, compensation is a *voluntary act* counterbalancing something in our nature. It is a process of effort which, to a large extent, is uncomfortable, because it involves a struggle against our basic nature.

Compensation is seen in all of us and we have to compensate for different elements in different situations. For example, take a person with a strong element of restlessness who cannot sit in one place. When this man has to attend a lecture, he has to make an effort to check his restlessness. As a compensation for it, he sits with legs tightly interlocked and reminds himself constantly that he must not move.

The process of compensation is very interesting and has far reaching implications in Homoeopathy. If we understand the workings of this process, it will make a vast difference in our understanding of patients.

A person is at his easiest in a situation where he needs to compensate the least.

In situations where a person has to control himself a lot, he is most compensated. Normally, we choose situations where we have the least need to compensate. For example, the physically restless person will choose a profession not of a clerk but of a postman, salesman or sportsman, where he needs to compensate the least. A person with an urge to travel (*Tuberculinum*) will choose to become a travelling salesman, so that he need not compensate for this aspect. Most of the situations we choose are those in which we have to compensate the least, yet, even in these situations, there are always elements which go against our basic nature.

The man who has chosen the job of a salesman can travel a lot, but he also has to keep accounts. To prepare a statement of accounts he has to sit and concentrate, and keep everything in order. This goes against his nature, so he must compensate for (control) his urge to be on the move when he has to write accounts. Similarly, in every situation there are some elements which are in tune with our basic nature and others for which we need to compensate. We can see this in the relationships between a man and his wife, society, friends, religious group, etc.

Suppose *Lycopodium* marries *Pulsatilla* by choice. *Pulsatilla* is very affectionate, yielding and mild. The dominating *Lycopodium* likes this part of her nature; he does not have to compensate. But, at the same time, she is also very dependent on him, making him shoulder increased responsibility which he does not like since, by nature, he prefers to avoid responsibility. So, either the wife has to compensate by not demanding so much responsibility, affection, sympathy and attention from him, or the husband must compensate and start giving her sympathy and affection and being responsible. Both have to compensate to some extent. This is also called adjustment. Having to compensate is not comfortable for him, but looking at the advantages he gets out of this relationship, he does so.

Similarly, though the *Rhus toxicodendron* person does not like to sit through the lecture yet, since he gets other benefits, he compensates. *In all relationships, man has to compensate in some way.*

Why is knowledge about compensation so important? When we are taking the case, the uncompensated symptoms are easily brought out, but the compensated ones are much more difficult to trace. The *Lycopodium* man cares for his wife out of compensation. Should we take "Caring" as his symptom? If we do so, we will go wrong because that is not his *basic nature*. We have to prescribe for his basic nature. In fact, we must be able to see that the real symptom is just the opposite.

We had a case of a couple, both *Pulsatilla*. *Pulsatilla*, as we know, is a mild and irresolute person. The beauty was that the husband was more intensely *Pulsatilla* than the wife. So, in their relationship, the wife had to take all the decisions. When I asked the husband: "Does your wife take decisions slowly or quickly?", he said: "Quickly", because she was the one who took the decisions and had to do it quickly, even though it was not in her nature, for if she did not take the decisions, none would get taken because this man was a high grade *Pulsatilla*.

The husband saw her as very irritable, stubborn and decisive. But, as I saw her, she sat in front of me and asked: "Doctor, what shall I do? Tell me." She was very mild and yielding in my presence, but in his presence, she could not afford to be so. Either she is really a *Lycopodium* who is pretending to be *Pulsatilla* in front of me or she is *Pulsatilla* and must appear as a *Lycopodium* to him. How do I make out what is the truth? I had to ask myself: "Which situation demanded greater compensation on her part?" I am not dominating in my clinic and yet she was much more mild in the clinic than she needed to be. In her husband's presence she was dominating as she needed to be; there, she was acting very much in proportion to the situation, and whatever is in proportion, or appropriate to a situation is more likely to be compensation (unless the situation has been created by her).

In my presence she was bending too low: "Doctor, please tell me what I should do." Almost begging. This is not compensation. Compensation is useful and appropriate to the situation. A person compensates only if the situation demands it and this situation (when speaking to me) did not demand it. There was no need for her to be so mild and begging. Therefore, she was uncompensated, whereas in her husband's presence, she was compensated, because her husband was so intensely *Pulsatilla* that she had to compensate for her own *Pulsatilla* state, in order that the family survives. Otherwise, both will start crying and no one will take decisions!

So, compensation is:

– An act of will (i.e. voluntary);
– It is against some aspects of one's nature;
– It requires an effort; and
– Usually it is needed for facing the situation.

I remember treating many patients with *Nitricum acidum* who had not a whit of maliciousness, which is one of its well-known features. Initially it surprised me that the prescription was effective although I has prescribed the remedy because all the characteristics fitted *Nitricum acidum* alone. When I pondered over the nature of the patients, I felt they were so calm, overly non-violent, mild and gentle people. Now I realize that these people were coming from a religious group which has non-violence as one of its principles. Maliciousness, cruelty and violence are taboo and are:

– Not useful in this situation;
– Not approved by their society;
– Positively harmful to their image and their life in that society.

So, these people, by their extreme mildness and charity (opposite feature) are compensating for inner malice. The almost manic intensity with which they are charitable is indicative of the force required to keep the malice in abeyance.

Another form of compensation in their case could be the diversion of malice towards socially approved forms, for example a war against poverty, or even, at a personal level, they might say: "This disease bothers me so much, I will see to it that it is completely destroyed." So, the malice will show itself in socially approved patterns and we should have the ability to perceive it in the person. We can have this vision if we understand the social context, and consider which features will be compensated for, and what the possible avenues are where these features in uncompensated form will meet with social approval.

If we examine a *Nitricum acidum* person in another situation, for example a man who is engaged in a very important court battle, where he is morally justified and where it is a question of survival (original *Nitricum acidum* situation), in such a case we will find the malice and unforgiving attitude in an uncompensated form. On the other hand, if in such a situation the person remains very forgiving and gentle (where aggressiveness is approved of and needed), then we shall seriously doubt if our prescription of *Nitricum acidum* is correct.

Overcompensation

If a component is very intense or is considered to be very bad in the society in which the patient lives, or the patient is extremely sensitive to its presence, then overcompensation takes place. This means that a pattern of behaviour will be voluntarily developed which is exactly opposite to the patient's real nature. For example, if your nature is very cruel, and you belong to a religion which considers cruelty as the most grievous sin, then you need to cover up your cruelty so completely that you choose to become a saint. So, overcompensation takes place when the situation you are in is very much against your basic element; it will involve a great effort and usually makes you feel uncomfortable.

How do we find uncompensated symptoms?

We need to ask the following:

- What is the situation the patient has chosen for himself? There must be a lot of uncompensation in that.
- What are the things in the situation he is happy or comfortable with? Those will be in tune with his uncompensated state.
- What are the features which, despite knowing that they are not good in that situation, he still cannot help? These will be his uncompensated symptoms.
- What are the things in his nature that are socially frowned upon, but still he cannot avoid. These too will be uncompensated features.

Signs of compensation

When a patient acts according to the demands of the situation, this may not be his basic symptom. You have to examine whether he would act in the same way in a place where there was no need to do so. If a person is working in a busy office, for example, he has to be very particular about keeping his papers in order. This cannot be considered as fastidiousness, but if he is very particular at home (where he can afford to be careless), we can say fastidiousness is his basic nature. This is uncompensation. But where he has to do an effort to be neat and clean because the situation demands it, this is compensation. So, we have to probe deeply into this aspect. Before taking a symptom as a basic symptom of the case, we must see whether:

- The situation demands it – it is likely to be a compensation;
- He is comfortable with it – it is uncompensated;
- His behaviour relates to a situation which does not demand it – it is uncompensated.

Separating compensated symptoms from uncompensated ones is of great value in case-taking. We will be able to do this exercise if we look at ourselves and examine which things we do with an effort. In this way we will come to know our own uncompensated nature as well as our uncompensated actions.

Nature of compensation

Compensation is a voluntary act and it arises as a defence against involuntary feelings or urges. What gives the clue that a person is compensating, it is the need for him to resort to an act more often than is normal. For example, when a person tells you spontaneously and repeatedly: "Doctor, what is the use of getting offended? Everybody behaves according to his own nature. I never let these things affect me. When someone offends me, I think it is better that I should ignore it rather than say something further and create a conflict. So, I always forgive and forget." Not only does he say this once, but gives us countless occasions when he was offended and let it pass. When we look at this kind of statement, we should ask ourselves why this theme of forgiving and forgetting is such a big issue. What type of man is it who constantly has to remind himself to forgive and forget? It can only be a very sensitive person and one whose very natural tendency is to be malicious and revengeful (*Nitricum acidum*).

Compensation and change of state

We can look at a *Calcarea carbonica* woman for example, one who has been *Calcarea* right from childhood. *Calcarea* is a state coming from a particular situation of being protected where there is a threat from outside, and the person is not capable of facing it. She confines herself to the house and is afraid to go outside. She seeks protection, security and shelter. By compensating she will be able to go out, take some risks and have some courage, but she will have to use extra effort or energy to do these things. This type of effort shows that it is a compensation. As long as a favorable, protective situation continues in her life, she will continue to be in the uncompensated state. But the moment the situation changes, she enters the compensation phase. When even such compensation is insufficient, there is a change of state.

For example, we know that the *Calcarea* situation is one where a person is in protected surroundings, and is not capable of facing an external threat. He just seeks the security within his home. So, as long as the person has some protection at home, he can afford to view to situation comfortably. He can remain in a *Calcarea* state, some of whose features will be compensated and some uncompensated. But when the situation changes and he loses the security of his home, he feels as if he is left alone in the wilderness. The *Calcarea* state is no longer going to help him even if he compensates. He goes into the *Stramonium* state. The *Calcarea* situation is the one that is protected, the *Stramonium* situation is the one that is unprotected.

In *Calcarea* the situation is one of seeking security against risks. The *Stramonium* situation demands resistance against terror and violence, and the compensation is just the opposite, namely in the form of a show of courage. So *Stramonium* operates from the situation of being unprotected and threatened and so wants to cling to somebody. *Stramonium* is like a person out in the dark night, wanting to come home, and *Calcarea* is the one inside the house who does not like to go out. The whole situation, the whole reaction and the whole feelings of the remedies are different. Therefore, one cannot fit in for another.

When you compensate, your actions do change but your state does not change. If the state changes, then your whole feeling changes. We see less and less of *Calcarea* adults. The reason is that though most children are in the secure *Calcarea* situation, as they become adults, this security is lacking and it needs more than the *Calcarea* state of mind to face the new situations. Therefore, his state of mind has to change; what it will change into depends on two things:

- The new situation, and
- The other roots that are present in the person.

A *Calcarea* person whose father dies and whose mother becomes dependent on him, one who has no money, finds that he is confronted with a situation in which he has to achieve in order to survive. There is no room now for the *Calcarea* state with its indolence and seeking of protection. Now, the *Lycopodium* root in him, if it exists, will be stimulated, or a *Bryonia* root or even an *Aurum metallicum* one, depending on which roots exist in him. This is probably why we do not see many *Calcarea* adults, especially men.

In the case of a married couple, if both are irresolute, then one will have to compensate for the other's irresolution. Sometimes, when this compensation becomes totally inadequate to face the needs of day to day life, then the state has to change so that a new (and in some way opposite) state comes in. For example, if two insecure people get married, then the one who has a more intense insecure state will become dependent on the other who has to compensate too much. When this is insufficient, he has to become a "naturally" responsible and dominating person. An insecure person with a more insecure spouse (*Calcarea*) could become dominating (*Lycopodium*) or responsible (*Aurum metallicum*) or caring (*Causticum*), depending on the root within him.

Forming a balance

Now, if a couple have two different states, then each of them will compensate for some symptoms and will remain uncompensated in the other symptoms. Thus they will form a balance.

For example, if the husband is responsible (*Aurum metallicum*) and the wife insecure (*Calcarea*), then the symptoms which need to be compensated for by the wife are fear of darkness and fear of being alone (her husband may be travelling, often leaving her alone). The sensitivity to cruelty needs to be in the uncompensated form, since it encourages dependence. This is what keep them together and ensures survival and comfort. Mildness and timidity need to remain uncompensated. In the husband, the symptoms which need to be in an uncompensated form are a sense of responsibility and industriousness, and praying and religiosity. Violence and intolerance of contradiction need to be compensated for. They will not be helpful to him in this situation. You may think that if a person is in a situation exactly complementary to his state, then he has no need to become ill, but we must be clear that in Homoeopathy the state itself is disease; whether it is compensated or uncompensated, it is capable of producing the pathology the person is predisposed to.

Compensation is like a wound up spring to be released

The more we compensate, the more time we need to uncompensate. The more we are not living according to our basic nature, the more we require time to relax, unwind, be ourselves and to feel "at home". The need for various forms of entertainment, relaxation, holidays and weekends comes from our compensation in various aspects of life. That is the reason why physical activities like jogging, swimming and other exercises are popular; that is why sex magazines and films attract; that is why boxing and other such violent movies are enjoyed, or why wars occur. The busy American executive chooses India for a vacation to unwind himself.

People choose that form of relaxation in which they have to compensate least.

Each country's entertainment and relaxation programmes are usually connected with compensatory behaviour. People feel more relaxed when they travel to another country with a totally different life style. Foreign travel thus becomes a common type of relaxation.

Sharing is a common compensatory behaviour. We share our house, places of work, the roads and our friends. Very few things really belong to us exclusively, even if we so desire. That is the reason why collecting things and owning them exclusively becomes a major pastime or hobby. In fact many hobbies represent an effort to uncompensate. That is perhaps the reason one does not observe small children and animals to have hobbies. When compensation starts, hobbies begin.

In our day to day work, we have to heavily compensate in terms of developing personal relationships or during personal communication. The need for parties and social gatherings is an attempt to uncompensate. In the East (for example India), where work and personal communication do not clash with each other, the need for such gathering and parties becomes limited.

Most of us have to compensate for our speed, which is usually slower than we would like it to be. No wonder people in the big cities find it most relaxing to go to a very slow and leisurely place and do nothing. It is natural for the workaholic to work at a fast speed: it does not involve compensation on his part. Therefore, he will have no need for relaxing in a quiet place. Hence, one of the signs that a person is compensating is that he will have a periodical need to do the opposite. On the other hand, the person who is not compensating (even though his present way of life may seem stressful) will feel more tense when compelled to do the opposite.

Compensated features can be perceived more prominently in practice if favourable circumstances for the expression of uncompensated/direct components exist. If they are not expressed by the patient even in these favourable circumstances, then the remedy may be ruled out. The question arises, in which instance will the symptoms be found in a direct form in spite of attempts to compensate for them? They will be seen directly if:
- The exciting factor is very strong and has lasted for a long time;
- The life situation is such that there has been a lack of opportunity to compensate for the troublesome features, for example insecure childhood.

The type of compensation a person will manifest has to be in tune with:
- The other components of the remedy;
- The social situation and norms.

In summary, to decide if a feature that is expressed is compensated or is an uncompensated basic feeling, we can apply the following criteria which determine the uncompensated symptoms:

- A symptom that troubles the patient;
- A symptom (feeling or action) that is felt by the patient as beyond his control. He says: "I can't help it. It is the way I feel";
- Any symptom the patient does not want to have but still has;
- Any symptom that goes against socially approved patterns;
- Any symptoms that are manifested during a stressful situation;
- Any symptom that the patient tries to hide from view;
- When a symptom does not have a reason or a satisfactory explanation;
- Situations close to the original situation of the remedy;
- The patient's attitude towards his disease;
- A patient's choice of vocation and pastimes; for example, we have observed so many *Kalium bromatum* patients with restless fingers opting for pastime and occupations such as typing, computers, playing musical instruments, etc.

Conversely, the reverse of the above would be a compensated symptom. We compensate for those symptoms:

- Which are not appreciated by society;
- Which are harmful to us;
- Which hurt our own self-image.

Those which are useful to us will be found in an uncompensated form, for example the industriousness of *Aurum metallicum*.

By reading the components of a remedy in the Materia Medica, we can get hints about which components will probably be compensated or uncompensated in a patient, according to the above three criteria.

Proving and compensation

In proving not all the components of a remedy can be brought out. In a proving the effect is sudden and acute. These symptoms are experienced by the prover almost for the first time and also in a very intense form. The most troublesome uncompensated symptom will be experienced most clearly and thus nearly exclusively recorded. Those symptoms which are experienced as less prominent by the prover will be overshadowed. By the time these troublesome symptoms could be compensated, the proving will most probably be over.

Selection of potency in compensated cases

I have found it difficult to select the potency in compensated cases because potency is determined by the intensity of characteristic symptoms. In compensated cases, the characteristics are not available in a direct form. They are to be found in compensated form and, therefore it is difficult to determine the intensity of such symptoms.

For example, in the *Nitricum acidum* patient, we saw that he tells himself all the time that there is no sense in taking revenge. This is a compensated form of maliciousness. In this case, how do we determine the intensity of the malice that has been compensated? The answer lies in our definition of health and disease. We generally understand health as a state of peace and freedom. *Compensation involves restricted behaviour, it curtails our freedom to be in the here and now.* In trying to cover up his maliciousness, the *Nitricum acidum* person feels restricted, and his responses and actions can no longer be fully in the moment. So, this is the extent to which his peace and freedom are curtailed, to that extent he is diseased, and in proportion to the intensity of his characteristics, will the potency be selected. The same is true for *Anacardium* for example. To the extent that he is compelled to be kind, he is diseased, and the potency will be determined in proportion to the intensity of the disease.

Likewise, a *Sepia* mother with indifference as a basic feature will often try and do much more for her children in order to hide (*sometimes even from herself*) her indifference. The extent to which she has to do it shows the intensity of the state and therefore the potency required.

The restriction of freedom in people is not equal along different parameters. For example, *Ignatia* has restrictions along the parameters of love and duty and *Bryonia* ha restriction along the parameter of money. In the uncompensated form the restriction will be on one side and the compensated form on the opposite side. For example, a compensated *Anacardium* cannot be cruel even when the situation demands it. He cannot even kill an irritating mosquito. Again you can see that compensation restricts his behaviour. The extent to which his reaction is restricted determines the intensity of his state, and therefore the higher potency.

The difference between true and compensated symptoms

How do we differentiate between a true symptom and a compensated symptom? For example, in an *Anacardium* patient, how do you differentiate cruelty which is compensated, from sympathy? Here are few indications:

- In situations of crisis, we will often see the symptoms in an uncompensated form. He does not attempt to hide or cover up his true feelings.
- In childhood, you will find an uncompensated picture. Children are frank because they are innocent.
- Behaviour of the patient in the house with the nearest relatives.
- Uncompensated behaviour is involuntary behaviour. Compensated behaviour is an act of will. Exaggerated compensation may look involuntary.
- Uncompensated behaviour will be found in acceptable situations such as:
  - Narrating symptoms,

- Social causes,
- When he suffers from a sense of injustice.

For example, cruelty and violence are most often found in a compensated form, but they can become uncompensated in two ways; when under extreme stress, he says:

- "This hand hurts so much that I could take a knife and cut it off"; or
- "The politicians are so corrupt they should be executed."

This is coming from a person who is "very kind".

If you find a patient to be too compensated, ask what the things are that do not affect him, that he resists. Even his total avoidance shows compensation. The need for a man to wilfully do or not do certain things is compensation. *The healthy uncompensated man has no need to do things against his will.* The compensated man's defences are weak, and many things affect him easily. People join organizations, groups, religious practices, etc., to give themselves a legitimate channel to compensate for opposite tendencies.

Difference between compensation and expression

An expression goes in the direction of the symptom and is merely a form of it, a direct form of it. But a compensation is exactly the opposite, in order to cover up the symptom. For example, if a person has fear of being alone, one expression will be desire for company, and another will be clinging. A third expression will be that he is always found in groups. So, the desire for company is not a compensation for fear of being alone, but rather an expression of it. The compensation for fear of being alone would be when a person tries to remain alone all the time, telling himself that there is nothing to fear; he tries to prove himself that he can remain alone.

A child of my colleague was behaving in a very odd manner for quite sometime. He was violent and created a lot of trouble for his parents. When I saw the child, I found that all this had begun when he was in a swimming pool and some creature, maybe a small lizard, came up behind him and somehow it got into his mind that it was a crocodile. Incidentally, a little later he saw a movie where a woman was being eaten by a crocodile, and from that time this child wanted to know everything about crocodiles. He read books on crocodiles, wanted to know how many teeth they have, how long their tongues are, what they eat, where they live and so forth. He is probably a world authority on crocodiles!

This kind of fascination is a sign of compensation for the tremendous fear. Some people who go to mountain climbing and trekking across unknown lands are trying to prove a point to themselves, that they are not scared of danger, that they are not scared of being alone, they are not scared of the unknown, or of the dark. There are others who always want peace and are always talking about the need to meditate, the need to be calm, the need to be unexcited, the need to be not bothered about troubles and not scared or angry: much of this "relaxation response" has to do with the excited remedies of which *Stramonium* is the most important.

186

People talk of non-attachment because they have to let go of things, they must not keep holding on. "We should not allow ourselves to cling on, we have to let go, stand on our own." These people are compensating. This is compensation.

So, look at the words that are used and when they are used with a lot of will: "I will, I must, I should not", whatever they are saying, the opposite is their true quality. People who say: "Happiness is within, and I have to find it within me in my own aloneness, otherwise I will not be stable; so I seek always happiness within and I should not depend on others, this is my aim, my goal", may really be feeling the opposite.

Difference between acute and chronic remedies in compensation

Acute and chronic remedies are terms only arbitrarily given, but normally chronic remedies are considered to be ones coming from a chronic situation. So an acute remedy represents survival in an extreme situation. A chronic remedy has within its range components to tackle a minor crisis too, but if the crisis becomes a major one, it needs an acute remedy to complement it. For example, *Baryta carbonica* has "Anxiety about trifles", etc., but when the situation becomes too acute and there is immediate threat of death, the *Baryta carbonica* state with its irresolution and dependence cannot tackle this. He has to become very restless, panicky and disturbed. This is not in *Baryta carbonica* and so it becomes *Arsenicum album*. Therefore, we find that *Arsenicum album* and *Baryta carbonica* are complementary, *Sulphur* and *Aconitum* are complementary, etc.

When you see an *Aconitum* or *Arsenicum album* state, you have to examine whether the patient after the passage of the acute crisis requires a chronic remedy. For example, a woman during cough gets an acute fear of suffocation which occurs at night. When you take the rubric: "Fear of suffocation at night", you get *Arsenicum album* and when you examine her she is *Baryta carbonica*. When you see *Arsenicum album* in the acute, you have to ask what is the chronic.

What we should not forget is that the chronic may be the same remedy, and the whole case may be curable by just that acute remedy which, in an acute crisis, presents in an uncompensated form, and when there is no crisis, presents in a compensated form.

In a patient needing chronic remedy, many symptoms will be found in an uncompensated form because utility of these components is found in everyday life situations, the insecurity of *Calcarea carbonica*, the business mind of *Bryonia* are useful, even approved by society and are survival-oriented. They can remain for a long time in an uncompensated form and even with a minor crisis the compensated can become uncompensated, as in the anticipatory anxiety of *Lycopodium*. When he is faced with a new, challenging situation, it will come up in an uncompensated form. Such small challenges are quite common in the lives of people, so in patients needing chronic remedies you may find uncompensated symptoms quite often.

The difficulty is in the so-called acute remedies because they come from extreme stress which is not found in everyday life. The components have to be compensated for,

187

especially in adults. The abusive and unsocial behaviour of *Chamomilla* comes from a situation of extreme neglect. Such a situation is rare. Hence, a person in a chronic *Chamomilla* state has to heavily compensate or at least show it in approved ways, for example shrieking with pain, or when his foot strikes the stone, he will abuse the stone. But such occasions will be few and often pass unnoticed in everyday life.

A symptom like "Cruelty" will be heavily compensated for, "Lack of confidence" will also be heavily compensated for, on the contrary a person will speak with tremendous confidence and bravado: "Nothing is beyond me, I have no fears", etc. A case where this was clearly expressed was of a radio personality who would come and behave in a very self-confident manner, so much so that I gave him *Lycopodium* and *Sulphur*. Nothing happened until one day he developed a cough and patch in the lung, and the doctor advised bronchoscopy. He phoned at least twelve times that day to find out what a bronchoscopy is and whether he would be able to tolerate it. He almost collapsed that day. Because of this, I could see the uncompensated picture and I gave him *Gelsemium*, with which he improved a lot.

There is a symptom, "Fear, falling, of, child holds onto mother". Child means a person who seeks protection from someone stronger, who feels incapable of protecting himself. Of falling or when put down means when he is going on a downward path, where there is a danger of falling off, a danger of something happening ("Ailments from anticipation"), there is fear of downward motion and of high places. Then he holds on to the nurse, whom is the protector. This means then, that when a person is faced with a risky situation in which there is a danger of losing balance, falling off, of something going wrong or bad happening, he will hold on someone who is protecting. This is *Gelsemium*. So, I could see his bravado, his tremendous overconfidence and his big talk was a compensation for his tremendous cowardice.

You will find in the acute remedies, for example *Tarentula*, that the industriousness and restlessness will not be compensated for, but will be put into a proper channel, i.e. expression. These uncompensated components along with the symptoms that are heavily compensated, together will make the picture of the acute remedy. That shows us that every feature of the patient which is individual has to be accounted for, otherwise we will lose the remedy. We have also to look at the situation of stress more often than the situation of near normalcy especially in acute remedies.

You will find the uncompensated features in the form accepted, for example people taking great interest in boxing or racing cars or horses. The other signs as we have seen in uncompensation are the hobbies and interests of the person and also the way they relate their complaints: "Doctor, this pain is killing me." This can be an uncompensated form of delusion of being killed.

The foolish laugh of *Hyoscyamus* will give him away always: "Doctor, I went to your clinic and found it closed, ha, ha, ha!" The person laughs where there is nothing to laugh at, or we see the clenched fist of violence. So, the gestures also show uncompensated features.

Also, there is the history in childhood, because in childhood we get the acute remedies in an uncompensated form. In the childhood history, all the moments of stress that the patient has undergone and how he reacted at these times will show uncompensated symptoms.

This gives you the acute remedy in its uncompensated form and that is why Hahnemann writes in Aphorism 5, that "you have to take the most significant points in the whole history of the chronic case" (and how he reacted to them, because at these times the uncompensated features come out).

Lastly, the uncompensated forms come out best in dreams, which is the subject of one of the next chapters.

POLARITIES WITHIN A REMEDY

In writing about the polarities within a remedy, my idea is to make a clear distinction between what belongs to the remedy state itself and what the compensation is for it. The need to differentiate between these two arises because often it seems that a polarity within a remedy is a compensation since it is in some way opposite to one of the features of the remedy. On the other hand, a compensated feature of the remedy may itself seem to be a polarity. We shall look at what polarity means, why it exists, how we can identify it and how we can differentiate it from compensated behaviour.

To take a simple example of a polarity, let me talk about an incident. I was once invited to inaugurate the homoeopathic clinic of one of my students. I agreed and planned to do so on the way to attending a seminar. In my car was a friend to whom I was giving a lift to the seminar. I asked her to come up with me to the clinic rather than wait in the car. She knew my student and she could have come up to greet him on this occasion. She refused to come up saying: "How can I come when I have not been invited?"

To me, this statement represented a little bit of ego. It was like saying: "I am so important that I do not go anywhere unless I am invited." This was how it appeared on the surface. But below that I could see that exact opposite which was: "I am so unimportant that I cannot go anywhere unless I am invited." Both these features were present at that time, together, just like two sides of a coin. It was not that one was the compensation for the other. It meant that she was disturbed along the axis of importance and non-importance and that in some way the feeling of importance has below it the feeling of non-importance, without which it cannot exist. Thus, I could see that importance and non-importance are two polarities which coexist in her at the same time. The expression of it: "How can I come when I am not invited?" is an expression of disturbance on this axis and is included within both polarities.

I am not referring to any particular remedy in this case. In fact, most of time, we cannot determine the remedy based on just one pole of the axis. A remedy is the combination of a specific quantum of disturbance along specific axes, not one but several axes. In each axis there will be polarities. In this friend of mine, ego was just one axis on which there was disturbance and it manifested on both poles. In order to find a remedy we have to examine the other axes on which she is disturbed, and we shall see that on each axis both the poles coexist in a particular expression.

When a person compensates, he compensates for the whole axis and not just one pole. For example, if a person is disturbed along the axis of importance/non-importance, the compensation would be a statement like: "I don't feel the need to be important. I feel quite OK, even if I am an ordinary person, I don't need to become famous or rich." This statement is repeatedly made. So, we can see that a polarity within a remedy represents two poles of disturbance along one particular axis (parameter). Both poles coexist in the same expression, both are uncompensated, involuntary and are usually feelings. Therefore, the provings usually brings out both the polarities of the remedies.

Compensation is the attempt to deny the whole disturbance along an axis. It is always a voluntary act of will and involves an action rather than a feeling.

We shall take as examples the polarities and compensations within some remedies.

Magnesium muriaticum :

The disturbance in *Magnesium muriaticum* is strongest along the axis of friendship. On one side of the axis is the pole of the delusion of being friendless. In direct contrast to this, on the other side, is the pole of unfriendly humor; therefore, we have symptoms like "Sulky", "Repulsive mood", "Forsaken feeling" and "Sadness, mental depression". So, while on one pole of the axis there is a feeling of having no friends, on the other pole we find that he behaves as if he needs no friends.

The compensation for this disturbance is to say: "I have plenty of friends. I am a very friendly person. I feel that one should be very friendly to everybody. I think it is good to have plenty of friends. I never lose an opportunity to make a friend." The need to make such statements constantly to oneself indicates that there is a disturbance along the axis of friendship, but the person is trying to heavily compensate for such disturbance. This example again demonstrates the difference between the polarity within a remedy and the compensation for the disturbance along this particular axis. It also shows how compensations are mainly actions and polarities mainly feelings. Most of the delusions and feelings that we see in a remedy represent its polarities. That is why we usually see opposite feelings in the same remedy.

Sulphur :
— Delusion disgraced, she is;
— Delusion, body, about, as if it were black;
— Delusion, thin, he is getting;
— Ailments from embarrassment;
— Discontented with himself;
— Looked at, cannot bear to be.

This is one pole along the axis of ego or importance, and exactly on the other side, we have:
— Delusion, great person, he is;
— Egotism;
— Indifference to personal appearance;

192

— Delusion, old rags are as fine as silk.

On one side he feels unimportant and disgraced and on the other he feels too important and almost disgraces other people.

The compensation for *Sulphur* would be to tell himself: "It does not matter whether I am important or not, and I should not shun other people."

Stramonium :
Some of the obvious polarities in *Stramonium* are:

– Desire for light;	– Light, aversion to;
– Delusion, divine, he is;	– Delusion, devil, he is;
– Company, desire for;	– Company, aversion to;
– Loquacity;	– Talk, indisposed to;
– Mildness;	– Violence.

The idea of polarity is very useful in many ways. One of them is that when we find in the provings or Repertory a disturbance along one axis, no matter which pole is represented in the Repertory, we can assume that the other pole automatically exists in that particular remedy. Therefore, one can sometimes choose the exact opposite feeling as a rubric. It is not surprising, therefore, if we look in the Synthetic Repertory to find *Tarentula* listed under the rubrics: "Colours, aversion to" and "Colours, charmed by". Similarly, in the rubrics: "Riding, aversion to" and "Riding, desire for", the same remedy, *Psorinum*, is listed. These are merely two examples, but the Repertory abounds with such instances where the remedy has the exact opposite feelings and often modalities. Therefore, sometimes I do not hesitate to use the exact opposite symptom if it is found in the Repertory. However, the basic principle about polarities has to be grasped.

One can see that polarities within a remedy are uncompensated which means that in the original situation of the remedy both the poles (aspects) are needed to coexist for survival. For example, *Stramonium* must have both courage and fear together. A compensation is not needed in the original situation of the remedy and therefore a compensated act does not belong to that state at all, but rather represents man's wilful suppression or denial of that feeling. The compensated form of the symptoms usually will not be found in provings or the Repertory, neither will they be found in dreams. The polarities will be found in dreams, in children and in the childhood history, and in other situations where we can expect symptoms in their uncompensated form.

28

DREAMS

I do not know exactly how I stumbled upon dreams. It was not from any specific case, but at some point I remember asking myself what the difference is between a dream and the waking state. There is the story of a Mulla who woke up and started crying; when asked why, he said: "I had a horrible dream that I am a butterfly." They said: "What is so horrible about it?" And he said: "I am confused whether it is I who had the dream of being a butterfly, or am I a butterfly who is now dreaming of being me!" He did not know the difference between a dream and the state of waking because in dreams often the very same things take place almost as they do in the waking state.

Dreams reveal uncompensated feelings

After prolonged thought, I reached one conclusion which was that in a dream most of our feelings and actions are uncompensated. In our waking state, most of our feelings and actions are compensated. This was the main difference as far as I could see. The reason is simple. Compensation involves an act of will. In the waking state, our feelings are also censored by the barrier between the conscious and the subconscious. We do not allow our feelings any expression many times, even to ourselves, but in the state of sleep, when our will is not so active, the barrier is lowered and our feelings and actions find expression in an uncompensated way.

This much understanding led me to utilize the dreams, since one of our biggest problems in Homoeopathy is to demarcate the difference between compensated and uncompensated symptoms. It can be really difficult to know which is the compensated feeling since the form of compensation depends on various factors like social structure, beliefs and rules, and methods of upbringing and training.

I think dreaming is somewhat like going on a holiday, since, in the dream, things appear exactly as we like to see or feel them in the waking state, whereas in the waking state, we do not allow ourselves to experience and react in the manner we would like to. The disease (false perception about our situation) exists in the dream as well. Disease is not only in the waking state or in dreams, it exists throughout. But what we see in dreams are reflections of the feelings we experience towards various things as well as our uncompensated reactions to them.

Dreams come closest to delusions

Since there is little or no compensation in a dream, it will show you a situation for which the feelings and actions would be appropriate. The situation in the dream comes

195

close to the original situation from which the state comes (delusion), but the dream will never show you the original situation itself. If we had the knowledge of that situation (even subconsciously), then we would be cured, but the dream shows us something very close to the situation, and it reveals our naked feelings and reactions. So, when we see in the dream that our father is a devil, having horns, large teeth and blood flowing from his mouth, we react with terror. We cannot say that this was the original situation. Of course not. But our feelings towards our father in an uncompensated form and our reaction to these feelings in an uncompensated form can be seen in the dream, and we can come close to the situation from which this whole reaction and feeling must have arisen.

The father must have been viewed/perceived the way we saw him in the dream; not exactly that, but something like that, which occasioned our feelings towards him in this manner. The situation which causes the feeling is not known, but the feeling is clear and the reaction is clear. So, the dream comes closest to our deep, but hidden, feelings. Therefore, from the dream, we are able to glean the pure, naked feelings and reactions. When we use these in the repertorial way, and look into the remedy that has these deep feelings and pure reactions, we are very likely to come close to the remedy. You can often hit on the remedy solely from the dreams.

Case

I recently had a patient for whom I could not decide what the remedy was, since nothing significant could be elicited; everything was compensated. He was sitting there, a busy executive, polished and well groomed. He said he had no problems: "Everything is well, doctor", he said. What was the dream he was having? He dreamt that he was lying down with several cobras (snakes) surrounding and protecting him with their raised hoods; he felt a sense of security. This recurs again and again. How will you interpret this dream into rubrics? We can take: "Dreams of snakes" or "Delusion of snakes around her". This is a simple way, but I never use it because it does not represent the feelings, in this case the feeling of fear and the need for protection.

Dreams are concerned with how we feel about the situation as it is, and some dreams reflect the situation as we would like it to be (fantasy). This is the ideal, since how we would like it to be is exactly the opposite of how we think it is. So, when we get a dream that gives pleasure, the opposite of it is our real feeling. Only a beggar needs to dream that he is a king; the king has no such need. When somebody dreams he is a king, it means he really feels he is a beggar.

Similarly, when the man is feeling that snakes are protecting him, he has a feeling of threat associated with snakes. So, the fantasy is that the very snakes that threaten are protecting him. This is how he would like it to be – the opposite. So, I asked him what is the significance of the snake in his life and he said that he was born under a specific star which has something to do with the snake. Somebody once told him that he should perform some rituals in order to protect himself from the influence of the snake. "But, doctor, I don't believe in all this, I have no faith, I did not do anything except that once I bought a little silver snake and put it in the temple. But generally, I don't perform any of these rituals." Now, he bought a snake made of silver and put it into the temple, yet he says: "But, doctor, I don't believe." He compensates: "Doctor, I don't believe in all that." The need to say the opposite of his real nature, to say: "I have no fear, I have no anxiety", this is compensation. That means "Fear" and "Anxiety" are basic symptoms, "Superstition" also is a basic symptom.

Thus, basic symptoms come out in the dream in a completely naked form. The superstition expresses itself as a fear that the snake is harmful to him because he was born under that particular star, and he needs protection from it. So, I took the rubric "Fear, superstitious", and gave him *Rhus toxicodendron*. This remedy has nothing to do with snakes, nothing to do with protection, but it has the theme of the dream.

So, the dream is an uncompensated picture of a man's feelings and reactions towards those feelings, and it is also the picture of the situation which is close to the original situation from which his state comes, or it could also be the opposite, i.e. the picture of the situation in which he would like to be, which is the exact opposite of the situation in which he imagines he is.

Basic dream and situational dream

I started using dreams and I must say that it has rewarded me much more than I ever expected. Here I would like to differentiate between what I call a *basic dream* and what I call a *situational dream*. The situational dream is one which occurs only as a reaction to a particular situation in one's life. So, you had an experience today and the way you felt about that experience occurs in your dream; that is a situational dream. For example, you had to appear for an examination and you felt very shaky about it; and then you had a dream that you are on a mountain and you are trying to come down. It is a bit dangerous and you are trying to keep your balance; at last you come down and you are safe. The theme of that dream is:

- Fear of high places;
- Fear of going downwards;
- Fear of falling;
- Fear of losing control;
- Ailments from anticipation.

All these are symbolized by the mountain and the need to come to a safe place and cross the danger. Fear of high places is fear of dangerous places; going downwards towards a safe place is fear of downwards motion. This is how exams seem to the dreamer and it is the theme of *Gelsemium*. But, just as we saw that a delusion can be a basic delusion or a situational delusion, in the same way a dream can also reveal the elements which are basic to a person and the elements which express the basic nature in a particular situation. For example, we have "Fear of failure" shown in the dream but it is not necessary that the remedy is *Gelsemium*. We have to examine more deeply. Why is this person having such a fear of failure? Underlying this fear may be anxiety about one's image, or fear about

197

achievement, or a great sensitivity to reprimand, or even a fear of poverty. So, dreams that come up as a response to a particular situation, even though they are uncompensated feelings in that particular situation, may not represent the basic nature of the person; they may represent only the expression in a particular situation.

Basic dreams are:

- Those dreams that are repetitive;
- Those dreams that come without any situation on that particular day; or
- Those dreams which can in no way be connected to the existing current situation.

When we ask the patient about his dreams, we must try to see if they are basic dreams. Only through repeated unexplainable dreams can we infer their significance and understand the feelings behind them. These feelings have to be confirmed as part of the patient's basic state, and not merely something that appears in one or two situations; they should be found in the patient as a part of his personality in a chronic case, even if in a heavily compensated form. The dream will give you the hint to look for this symptom, whether in compensated or uncompensated form, and to examine various situations in his life, especially situations of stress; and also to examine his sociocultural background, so that you can get some idea of the compensated aspects of his life.

Symbolic dreams

As I have already indicated, I do not open the "Dream" chapter of the Repertory to look for a specific type of dream. However, there is one exception to this and these are dreams that I see as highly symbolic. In such dreams, absolutely no feelings are involved but one symbol appears again and again, for example water. There is no feeling, there is no fear. They may see snakes, but there are no feeling. In the earlier dream there was the theme of protection. This is not there now – just snakes. The dreams may be of houses, fruit, dead bodies, of funeral or of weddings. When we find these symbolic dreams, especially the ones where there are no associated feelings and this symbol is repeated again and again, then they are a part of the universal symbols. We may not fully understand them and there may be many theories about them. However, these symbols are available directly in the "Dream" chapter and can be used without theorizing. Unless the dreams are of this type – symbolic dreams – I do not use the "Dream" chapter much.

Dreams as delusions

The other section of the Repertory we can use for the dreams is the one on delusions. For example, "Dreams of snakes" can be taken as synonymous with the "Delusion of seeing snakes", because they are similar. Delusion is seeing what does not exist. Dreaming too is to see what does not exist. A delusion is to see things in a different way and a dream also is to see things in a different way. Yet, to take delusion instead of dream is also not good enough. What is important is to get the reaction whether it be a delusion, a fear or an anxiety.

Case

As an example here is a dream of a thirty-five year old male patient who came with tingling and numbness in his arms, which was diagnosed as frozen shoulder. I did not believe this and sent him for neurological opinion which revealed a malignant tumour in his spinal cord. He was operated on and then resumed treatment with us. I was trying to get his history. He came with his father who did most of the talking. In this way, he seemed to be childish, dependent, and except for this I did not get much information. I asked about his dreams, and he said he had absolutely no dreams. I tried to find out the situation in his life when the trouble started. The situation was that he got married and there was a conflict between his mother and his wife, and he did not know what to do. "I was always dependent on my mother right from my childhood and I was always with her. Then my wife came in and my mother and wife did not get along with each other. I could not separate from my mother and, at the same time, I could not see my wife suffering. Ultimately, we (my wife and I) did separate from my parents and this affected me a lot; at this stage my trouble started." I tried to find out what the feeling was at this time. Was it anger, sadness, or something else? He could not say what. I kept on asking for more than half an hour in many ways what the feeling was, but it was not possible to get any clue. Finally, I had a thought: "Tell me, did you have any dream at that time?" "Yes, doctor, there is one dream I remember that came again and again. I used to dream that I am in the sea, there is nobody around me, there is a storm and I am feeling very frightened." I asked: "Are you in a boat or swimming or holding on to something?" "I don't know. I couldn't see that, I could only see myself in the sea, with the storm around me." The beauty was that in the dream he was doing absolutely nothing to get out of this. He was just there like a babe lost in the woods. Therefore, I took the rubrics:

— Delusion, alone, in a wilderness;

— Forsaken feeling;

— Delusion, danger, impression of.

I also took: "Fear, water, of" and "Helplessness, feeling of", because he was making no attempt to help himself, just sitting helpless, with danger from all sides. He is terrorized, feels alone and lost, but does nothing. This was his feeling in that situation. His house was in storm, he was alone, lost like a baby in the woods, and why? Because of his tendency to cling to his mother, so I took the rubric: "Clinging". The child was pulled away from the mother and felt lost. So I took: "Clinging to persons". From this, I came to *Stramonium*, which helped him.

His first reaction after taking *Stramonium* 200 was that he had a dream that he is flying and he has no wings; for a time he feels scared, but then suddenly he realizes that he has the power to fly and makes a very beautiful landing and feels happy about it. This shows a change of feeling, like a baby who was clinging to his mother, now tries out its wings and knows it can fly and it can land safely.

The dreams identified the exact feelings. He was thirty-five years old and was an officer in a bank. So, you can imagine with what great difficulty I got the feeling of his having clung to his mother and feeling forsaken like a baby. He would never consciously

199

admit to such a feeling. As a sidelight, what would the remedy of the mother be? First of all, you can see she is a strong woman, dictatorial, who does not allow her children to be independent and allows them to cling to her. She has kept him clinging for thirty years and then, when his wife comes and wants to share a little bit of him, she gets wild, she would not allow it and that causes quarrels. I have thought of *Lachesis* for the mother on this basis.

Case

I have heard many wonderful dream stories from patients. Here are some examples.

A woman of around fifty years, repeatedly has dreams that there is a fireplace in her house from which all kinds of beautiful, cuddly, strange animals come out. She described it thus: "Oh, the animals are so beautiful, so nice, so cuddly, having white hair, fluffy, with their tails wagging and in all strange forms, but all nice, very beautiful and they all come towards me and I hug them and play with them. There are small rabbits, small puppies, and a cuddly little mangoose, among other creatures. This place is like a garden with all kinds of beautiful plants, flowers and grass and other little things." Very vividly she describes them. "Then, out of this fireplace comes a snake-like monster and I get frightened – the snake-monster is coming out. I don't want it to come out. Then, a big black dog also comes out of the fireplace, but this one is not the fluffy little thing, it is a watchdog. It stands there and it does not allow the snake-monster to come out. It pushes it back inside and that monster is trying to come out and bite all of them."

What is the theme of this dream? We first see innocence and beauty coming out of the fireplace. The fireplace is her own mind, her own subconscious and from this is coming a lot of innocence, beauty, affection and sympathy. From that same fireplace of her subconscious comes ugliness and venom, and she does not want this to come out. She only wants innocence. The monster of the fireplace has to be kept inside and so, the black dog, the guard between her conscious and her subconscious, stops this monster from coming out and pushes it back inside. She knows that if the monster comes out and bites, it will poison all the beauty around. She is anxious about it. I took the rubrics:

— Delusion, sees beautiful landscape;
— Sympathetic;
— Affectionate;
— Communicative;

on one side and on the other side, I took:

— Cruelty;
— Malicious, Deceitful;
— Hatred, Ugliness.

From these, I came to the remedy *Lachesis* and got a wonderful result.

We may have less subtle and more direct dreams, and of these I will give two.

Case

Here is the dream of a man who by occupation is a trainer of stuntmen on motor-cycles. The situation in his life is that these students of his are not obeying him, they are not following his instructions and therefore they are getting harmed. They do not do it the way he suggests, they do it their way and when he tries to warn them, they get angry with him.

The dream: He is riding his motorcycle and is coming to a dead end of the street. He stops, and from behind, a military vehicle (jeep) is going up flying, taking two somer-saults and coming back to the same street. When this is happening, a motorcycle rider is coming from behind him and our patient tells him: "Stop! There is danger." The man does not listen to him, he goes on and the jeep comes and cuts his body into two. The body lying on the floor is cut into two parts and a horsecart comes from behind. The horse frees itself from the cart and grips the hair of the dead body, so that the upper half of the body is in its mouth; it is trying to drag the body away, when our patient tries to grab the head and get it separated from the horse. Suddenly, the head comes to life, attacks him and tries to kill him. The patient wakes up with a fright.

I do not know all the meanings of the dream but I interpreted it in a simple way. First you see something horrible in the dream, so I took: "Horrible things, sad stories, affect him profoundly", and what does he do when he faces this horrible scene? He tries to help. There is a sympathetic attitude. He wants the other people not to suffer but they do not listen to him. How does he feel? He feels helpless, he cannot do anything. So, I took: "Sympathetic" and "Helplessness, feeling of"

He tries to tell the person to stop, there is danger ahead, yet that fellow later tries to kill him; so, also taking "Fear, murdered, of being", I came to *Phosphorus*.

Case

One more case is of a woman of around forty-five. A very successful woman, an assistant manager of a big company in Bombay. She came with a very bad eczema on both her legs, oozing and painful for 2-3 months before she came to me. She was completely disabled, she could not go anywhere, she had to be at home. The interview lasted for only around fifteen minutes. It began with:

— Tell me what is your problem.

She said it is the eczema and it is so bad. I asked:

— Can you tell me the reason for it?

— It could be psychological.

— And what is this psychological thing?

— Oh, some problem, I don't know, some family problem.

— What kind of family problem?

— Some tension, nothing to do with my husband; some tension.

She could not talk about it. So, I said:

— OK, tell me about your dream.

— I get the recurrent dream of stools, passing stool, or stools lying around.

When she was saying this, she never looked straight at me. She was looking from side to side; her eyes were moving quite rapidiy. Then, I said:

— Tell me about the dream of stool.

— OK, doctor, I will tell you the problem. You see I have a son who is mentally retarded and he gets convulsions. Every time before he gets convulsions, I get the dream of stools. During pregnancy I had a dream that there were a lot of stools and the head of a child was coming out of it, and somebody, God knows who, was pushing it back. At that time, I knew that the child would not be OK.

When she was saying this, her eyes were moving very fast. She added in a quiet way, almost in a whisper:

— I feel I could have avoided it. I could have done something.

Nobody in her office knows that she has this son, even though she has been working there for fifteen years. She avoids all social contacts. She is very efficient in her work, but she does not attend any parties, or go out on holiday trips even though she is entitled to do so. Her husband is helpful, but she feels very responsible for the child, as if she alone were responsible. The rubrics:

— Grief, undemonstrative;
— Anxiety of conscience, as if guilty of a crime;
— Anxiety about future;
— Company, aversion to;
— Delusion, she has done wrong;
— Delusion, she is a criminal;
— Indisposed to talk;
— Delusion, she has neglected her duty;
— Going out of home, aversion to.

The remedy I found for her was *Cyclamen*. Phatak's Materia Medica sums it up in three words: *terror of conscience*. Now, we come to the point of the case, which is the dream.

Dream of stool is not found in *Cyclamen*. It is given for five remedies, namely, *Aloe, Castanea vesca, Psorinum, Sarsaparilla* and *Zincum metallicum. Cyclamen* is absent. So, what is the meaning of this dream of stool? Now, we can see the real theme, or feeling, or meaning behind the dream. In symbolic language, the child is now suffering because it was drowning in her own shit, and therefore she is the guilty party, the criminal who has to keep quiet and atone for her crime. She is completely alone because it is her own fault, that the child was suffering. This comes very close to the situation of *Cyclamen*.

The situation of the state :

The actual situation of *Cyclamen* is that of the woman who has done something wrong and out of that wrong act something bad has happened, and so she cannot open her mouth. She has to keep it all inside and just try to rectify it as much as possible. She has to avoid all social contacts, she feels totally alone. That is the original situation of *Cyclamen*. The dream comes closest to this situation. The *Cyclamen* situation is the situation of a man who has messed it up and nobody knows that he has done it. Hence the movement of the eyeballs like a criminal, the unwillingness to reveal the "crime", and the feeling of being solely responsible like a criminal; not a professional criminal but a man who has inadvertently committed a crime. The dream of the woman put the final seal of confirmation on the prescription of *Cyclamen*, which soon cleared up her skin problem.

Which dreams do we remember?

There is evidence that all of us dream. This means that in some way, dreams are useful, since nothing occurs that is not useful. We remember some dreams and cannot remember the rest. Both these types of dreams must have their own utility. One thing to be noted is that people who do remember their dreams usually wake up with a particular mood of the dream, like happiness, fear, etc. Those who do not remember the dreams wake up in quite a normal mood even though they might have gone to sleep on the previous day with anxious thoughts or anger or sadness. We can assume that, in some way, sleep and unremembered dreams restore balance to a troubled mind. In this sense, the unremembered dream completes the day's business and puts man at peace with himself and the world. This happens especially when the situation is not so intense. I am even tempted to say that the unremembered dream is the body's way of healing itself of minor disturbances, especially psychological ones.

However, when the situation (real or perceived) requires some strong specific feelings in order that the person should adopt the proper posture to combat it, the dreams then force themselves into the waking state also and are remembered along with their specific feelings. The more we consciously do not adopt the posture required by the real or perceived situation, the stronger and more vividly remembered the dreams will be.

As a simple example, we may take the case of a student whose survival depends upon his preparing well for the examination, but who tells himself that he has nothing to fear and that he need not study so hard. This student is very likely to get the dream of facing the examination and not knowing the answers. The dream will be remembered and could be useful to him.

We know that disease is delusion, the actual situation may not exist, but the patient perceives the situation to be so. The delusion may be that he is a student whose survival depends on his success in the examination, though here, this is not exactly the case. If this patient tries to tell himself that he has no such anxiety, he too will get similar dreams.

Thus, the person who will have the most vivid dreams which will be remembered with their specific feelings is the one who needs to have those feelings or fears the most.

In other words, he is the only one whose actions are not intense enough for the real or perceived situation. This could be due to his trying to compensate very heavily for his feelings. Therefore, the more compensated the man is, the more his dreams will be remembered. The more out of touch with his feelings he is, the more his dreams will be remembered. The more intense the situation is, the more his dreams will be remembered.

Conversely, the person who does not remember his dreams will be the one whose behaviour is totally uncompensated, who is in touch with his feelings and does not suppress or deny them to himself.

We may conclude that the person who does not remember his dreams at all is the one whose actions and feelings are in tune with (suitable to) his basic perception of reality (basic delusion).

29

MIND AND BODY

Let us talk about the physical symptoms first. We saw that mental components can be connected together if we can understand the situation in which the whole state occurs. In the same manner, we can connect the physical general symptoms. By physical general symptoms we mean the nervous, endocrine and immunological alterations.

Take for example the state of remedy *China*. The *China* state is called for as an adjustment in a person with loss of vital fluids. In such a case, a doctor will advise rest, less intake of solids, with plenty of fluids, especially glucose and saline. *China*'s weakness has just such characteristics: desire for rest, decreased appetite, increased thirst with desire for sour, sweets and juices. The whole physical state of *China*, therefore, is an adaptation to the situation which has arisen from lack of vital fluids.

Let us take this example one step further. With lack of vital fluids and weakness of the organism, the *China* patient also needs to eliminate the bacteria that are causing infection and the loss of vital fluids. So, two things result. Firstly, there is diarrhoea in an attempt to throw out the organism and secondly the temperature increases in order to fight the organism better. Now the fever of *China* occurs in a person with weakened vitality. Such a person cannot afford prolonged intense fever, because that would cause further loss of fluids and a further decrease of vitality. Therefore, the most that this person can afford to do is to produce intermittent fever. Here, there is a sudden high temperature with shaking chills which last for some time, and then the fever comes down with a crash and there are drenching sweats; then the body is allowed to recover its vitality until another bout of fever comes.

This is much more suited to the weak person than is continuous fever. A very robust person, for example *Aconitum*, can afford to produce one big shot of fever which lasts for few days and totally finishes off the offending organism. But a *China* person cannot afford this and, therefore, has periodical aggravation and periodical rise of temperature. What I am trying to put forth is that all the physical generals symptoms of *China*, its sensations, weakness, periodicity, cravings and aversions, etc., can be explained as a response to loss of vital fluids. Now, when we have explained most of the physical components of *China* as an adaptation response to a physical cause, then we can ask what the connection is between this physical state of *China* and the remedy's mental state. Can it be that a particular state of mind is connected to a particular state of body for no reason whatsoever?

Connection between body and mind

The *China* state of mind is characterized by indolence, with feelings of persecution, theorizing and planning. In some way, this mental state must be connected with the state of the body. To my mind, the connection between these two states is that they are most suited to help each other, which means that the state of weakness of the body with inability or unwillingness to move is going to be most helped if there is indolence in the mind. Likewise, indolence in the mind will be most helped if there is weakness in the body. When you examine a remedy's physical and mental states, you will find the connection so strong that it is difficult to deny. Let us take some more examples. One of the best I can give is of *Chamomilla*.

In *Chamomilla*, the physical state comes from a situation in which the person has to scream for help. If you want to imagine a *Chamomilla* state in the simplest way, think of a baby in whose body the diaper pin has been poked by mistake. The baby will then be in a *Chamomilla* state: very irritable, shouting, shrieking, demanding attention, violent and so on. The physical pains will be severe – cutting and violent – and they are so intense and sharp that they extort cries. So, you can see in *Chamomilla* that it is a situation which brings forth violent pains in the body which leads to a mental sate of violence, shrieking and extreme crossness. Of course, it is obvious that if a pin has pierced the child, you have to remove the pin. Giving *Chamomilla* will not help as there is a cause for this condition. But, if you find a person who, without a cause, in this *Chamomilla* state, then the remedy will help. I was examining a lady with small boils on her skin: they were so painful that she was shrieking, shouting, abusive and crying, and demanding: "Cut off this leg." Here you can see the *Chamomilla* state with its sharp intolerable physical pain and the corresponding violence of mind. This is a good example of how the physical state of violent pain goes hand in hand with the violence of mind.

Body and mind help each other

It seems as if the organism feels the need to produce a violent state of mind to combat the stressor (in this case a physical stressor). Initially, it produces a violent pain. But, if this is insufficient to produce violence of enough intensity in the state of being, the mind too is made violent to further intensify the state.

Conversely, the body's intense suffering too goes to help the mind produce the requisite state – cross and snappish. For example, the *Calcarea* person is one who requires a mind that is indolent, who always likes the protective shelter of his home, and is unwilling to move out; so physically he develops aggravation from movement, aggravation from exertion and he also develops a bulky body which prevents active movement. The insecure state of mind is aggravated by this kind of body state, and this kind of body state encourages a timid, fearful, indolent state of mind.

In *Phosphoricum acidum*, the mental state is one of sleepiness, brooding, aversion to business, indifference, hopelessness and despair, and correspondingly in the body there is weakness, lack of energy and disposition to lie down.

It is also interesting to note the physical constitution of our various remedies. If you examine the constitution of *Phosphorus*, you often find that he is lean and fair, with long, curved eyelashes and a graceful walk. In short, a very attractive person physically; and mentally, he is one who tries to attract other people in an affectionate and intimate way. So, it seems to be a body that is made for that state of mind. Similarly, *Sepia* has a mind which is averse to coition and averse to company. No wonder she tends to develop black patches on the face, and can look dragged down and unattractive. *Baryta carbonica* mentally feels inferior, that people are laughing at him and that he is incapable; and his body is underdeveloped and slow.

When we understand these broad concepts, it is easy to go into more detail, like the type of pain the patient has. In some patients we are surprised that their condition, which is normally painful, is actually painless. For example, we may see a boy with inflamed yet painless tonsils. The mental symptom, associated with such a condition, is very likely to be one of "Indifference, does not complain" (for example *Opium*). Similarly, when we find tremendous sensitivity of nerves, especially to injuries and cuts, then in the mind too we find this tremendous sensitivity to hurt, rudeness and especially to insults (*Staphysagria*).

It seems that whenever a person meets with a situation in which the vitality has to cope in an adaptive way, and the mind alone cannot cope, it will take the help of the body; and when the body cannot cope, it will take the help of the mind. If the causation is emotional then the symptoms will begin with the mind, and the body will be called in later, but if the causation is physical, then you will have the physical effect first and then the mental concomitants later. When a person has the physical state of *Arnica*, then his mental state is *Arnica* too, even if the symptoms are not obvious. If the causation is mainly physical, for example he has an injury or has overexerted, then he will develop the physical complaints first and mental concomitants later. But, in the meantime, whatever earlier mental state he had will be suppressed, and no prominent mental symptoms will be seen: only in such a situation are we justified in giving a prescription of *Arnica*.

When needed, the mind calls the body for help and vice-versa. To take another example, when there is loss of vital fluids, then you will not see the persecuted feeling of *China* immediately, but we will see that the whole state has now symptoms of physical adaptation – that is what is required at this time. The adaptation is mainly physical at first, since the causation is physical; but when the physical state remains for some time or it needs more help, then it will drag in the mental state to which it is naturally connected. So later on, you will observe the mental state also of that same remedy. For example, the *Gelsemium* situation comes from two areas, either the mind or the body. From the mind it can arise after bad news when the person feels frightened and shocked; he is almost paralyzed and trembles from fear. Or the situation can come from influenza, and in order to fight the influenza virus, the body reacts with weakness, fever and tremulousness. In this case, the fright and shock will not be so prominent, but they may come up later, in order to help this state of immobility.

Likewise, in the *Gelsemium* state of fright, shock and tremulousness, he may not be totally bedridden and paralyzed if the mental causation is not intense or prolonged.

207

The whole state will be of *Gelsemium* but in bad news, mental adaptation will be more prominent and in influenza physical adaptation will be more so. But certainly you will not see in the *Gelsemium* state (of body or mind) any symptom of any other remedy.

This connection between body state and mental state is nowadays used in some forms of psychotherapy where, for example, the person who feels he is under stress is made to adopt the posture of a very tense person. When he adopts that physical posture, then, similar feelings are excited in the mind. By the excitement of similar feelings, the person gets better due to a kind of unconscious application of the homoeopathic principle.

Practical utility of these ideas

In presenting these ideas I am trying to draw attention to their practical value and utility. So, when you see in the physical state a type of pain, you should ask yourself what kind of mental state can be produced and encouraged by this kind of pain and you will usually find the same mental state in that person. For example, where there is tearing pain, then it usually means "violence" in the mind. Tearing pains in the body can be helped by violence in the mind. And violence in the mind can be helped by tearing pains in the body. Similarly, if you find burning pains in the body, they will produce anxiety and restlessness in the mind, as in *Arsenicum album*, or in *Phosphorus* or *Sulphur*.

I am not only talking about remedy selection. It is simple logic that when you see tremors in the body, it usually means an excited mind. So, however much the person tries to convince you that he is very calm, the tremulousness of his body shows you that is mind is excited. Numbness in the body could mean apathy; a ball-like sensation in any part of the body usually means a hysterical state of mind.

So, from the physical symptom of the person if you can see what state of mind can be encouraged by that pain, or what mental state can produce that kind of physical problem, then you will get very good clues as to the mind and the remedy.

Of course, I need not tell you that the pains we are talking about are non-pathognomonic pains, which means characteristic pains. They are the ones that are not common to the pathology. If a peptic ulcer or acidity in the stomach is producing burning then this is not going to be a characteristic of the person – anyone with acidity will have burning pain. Or if in case of diabetic peripheral neuritis you have burning of the soles, formication or numbness, then this will not help you to find the nature of the P-N-E-I disturbance. But suppose that in a case of a skin ulcer or one of boils you have intense burning, then you can take it for granted that this will be associated with a lot of anxiety in the mind. So, from the nature of the physical complaints one can make a very good guess as to what kind of mental state the person is in. We must understand the principle that the physical and the mental states have to help each other, because they are part of the same P-N-E-I response to a particular causative stress factor. The hint is that from the way the patient is describing his complaints, you easily make out his mental state without even asking about it.

Physical and mental states help each other

As explained above, the physical and mental states help each other. Whenever a person comes with a physical complaint, our mind gets diverted to the complaint itself, for example if it is throat pain we are more interested to find out whether it is better by hot or cold drinks, or worse during the day or night. No doubt we will be successful if we are able to identify the characteristics, i.e. symptoms of the state rather than disease. This holds true of the physical concomitants as well. Yet a far more useful but less used technique is to use the mental state in such case. In such case the mental state comes out very obviously, often without the patient (and unfortunately sometimes the physician too) noticing it. There is no sense in asking the patient to tell you about his mental state. He may not possibly understand your question, but if we understand one thing: that the physical and mental states are in unity, then whatever mental state is being caused, or at that time exists, must be in tune with the physical state. It is much easier to identify the state of mind rather than the physical symptoms. Whatever the physical state is, we must ask in what way does the complaint or state make the patient react or feel mentally. The sum total of the feelings and reactions in the mind will fit into a pattern which is the existing mental state. The selection of the remedy can be much more easily approached from this angle.

Take the case of a five year old child who was vomiting. His vomiting becomes severe and he becomes very uneasy, so much so that he knocks his head against the wall. He wants someone to be with him all the time, and he is holding on to his mother. He is quite restless and rolls about in the bed. He must have a physical state which is in tune with his mental state – restless, fear, anxiety when alone. The remedy *Arsenicum album* is clear from these references. The same rule can be applied in other cases. So, the question always is – what does this (physical) illness make you do (action) and feel mentally?

Mind and body – *Sepia*

Sepia is a person who, through prolonged stress and strain of life (long suffering), feels dragged down, weary, miserable and apathetic, but at the same time retains her sensitivity and reacts with irritability, resulting occasionally in a violent outburst of temper – discarding or throwing away things. Even the things that she used to like before, now produce an aversion.

The *Sepia* woman seems to have no strength to get out of that situation. The best mode of survival for her is to linger on in this sad, miserable state and react violently sometimes. She becomes cold and withdrawn and likes to keep herself busy.

When you examine the physique – out of long suffering and too many deliveries, the body is weakened – she reacts feebly. Her complaints linger on and when exposed to noise, odours, etc., she reacts violently even with vomiting. Such a pleasant thing of life like milk is rejected violently. She develops aversion to her loved ones – husband, family members. *Sepia* likes to be occupied mentally and physically, likes brisk movements as if this helps her to forget her miseries.

The mind reacts to a stressor in the same way as the body. How the body sees the situation, the mind will also see it the same way.

Physical and mental analogy in some other remedies

In my experience, the main action of *Silicea* in the body is usually localized to a particular organ and here it produces the stubborn, hardened lesion, while the rest of the body emaciates. In this local part there is overreaction, a show of strength, of defence, hypersensibility. For example, we see its action in:

- Tuberculous glands;
- Arthritic joints;
- Proud flesh in wounds/ulcers;
- Exostosis in bones;
- Migraine.

We find this weak emaciated patient overreacting in a stubborn hardened way in a particular sphere, especially in the presence of a foreign body, vaccination or infection.

By analogy it seems that the whole body has to concentrate on this spot ("Mono-mania"), and has to show itself as strong and stubborn ("Egotism", "Obstinate"), has to react excessively ("Irritability") with an inner feeling of weakness ("Timidity", "Cowar-dice") – and all this, when exposed to something foreign ("Timidity when appearing in public"). This analogy may seem a bit farfetched but we have many such known examples.

For example *Arnica* in the mind: "Ailments from mental shock" and "Fear of being approached".

Moschus: (in Kent's Lectures) "Mind is hysterical" and so too the tissues are.

Lycopodium: The body reacts to a problem with increased activity, struggle, trying to cope with it. You see the body is struggling to cope; sometimes it is losing, sometimes it is coming up again. It does not have enough strength to produce something violent and fight it out. It is too scared that it will not stand that strain unlike *Nux vomica* which will produce violent reaction and fight it out. But in *Lycopodium* the body is struggling to cope. There is a generalized reaction and not local hardening like *Silicea*.

Beyond mind and body

The essence of the above discussion is to show that both mind and body express the same disturbance. The disturbance neither originates nor is localized to the mind nor the body alone, but it is at a level which is deeper than both. The level of disturbance is the life force itself, the consciousness that pervades the whole being. Health, disease and cure occur at this level. The mind articulates the state best, just like the parliament articulates the state of the nation. In reality, intelligence, awareness and consciousness is a property of the life force itself and is present throughout the being.

The wise man is one who is able to perceive the underlying unity of the body and the mind, and will choose symptoms that come closest to representing the underlying disturbance. If we find those symptoms that represent the underlying state, features that are common to mind and body, our perception will be much more accurate. The underlying disturbance will express itself in the mind and body, but we should be able to see beyond this difference.

For example, when we spoke of the *Lyssinum* case in the chapter "Unsuitable reactions", we could see that itching was violent and coming into paroxysms, the skin was extremely sensitive. In the mind too we saw the same sensitivity and violence in paroxysms. Now, when we look at the two main symptoms of that child:

– Violence in paroxysms;
– Abnormal sensitivity;

we are not referring merely to body or mind but to the underlying disturbance which is the one we have to treat.

30

THE APPLICATION OF THE REPERTORY

Imaginative use of rubrics

As you will see in the various chapters, I have used the Repertory in almost every single case. The Repertory has been a most useful tool in understanding remedies and patients. I feel this tool has been neglected by the profession. There are standard books on the construction and use of the Repertory such as the ones by Bidwell, Margaret Tyler, Kanjilal, Ramanlal Patel, Docykx and Kokelenberg, P. Sankaran and others, and I do not wish to go into this aspect. What I shall discuss in this chapter is the imaginative use of rubrics especially from the "Mind" chapter of the Synthetic Repertory which I use frequently. Before I go into the example I shall give a few hints from practice.

- In the Synthetic Repertory you can trust all inclusions from Kent's Repertory.
- The inclusions and gradations of Pierre Schmidt (ref. no. 7), you can bet your life on.
- Use great caution in the use of rubrics from Gallavardin (no. 5).
- Try to get all the possible cross references from each rubric.
- Use other Repertories as well, such as Phatak's and also cross-check from the original sources. There are mistakes and omissions.
- Remember the Repertory is incomplete; so do not rely on any rubric implicitly.
- Make sure that the remedy you are choosing fits the whole idea of the case and not merely one or two rubrics.
- Read the rubrics one by one; use a standard dictionary to get the exact meaning.
- Use your imagination to guess where you can apply that rubric to patients.
- If you get a rubric with only one remedy, try to understand from the Materia Medica why only that remedy occurs in that rubric.
- Whatever remedy you get, confirm it from the Materia Medica.

Now, I will give merely a sample of the way we can broaden our understanding of the rubrics and how we can apply these rubrics in practice. In the first thirteen rubrics, I have used a style similar to the one used by Dr. M.L. Sehgal of Delhi and I am indebted to him for showing this way. I hope this sample will stimulate the reader to go on to the Repertory on his own and work at other rubrics.

All meanings given here are from Chambers 20th Century Dictionary, 1960 edition.

A. Religious

Meaning	:	Scrupulous, devoted to, bound to a monastic life, strict.
Interpretation	:	One who follows the rules of any Order very strictly and scrupulously.
Expression	:	1. Patient says: "Doctor, just tell me what I have to do. I am going to follow homoeopathic treatment very strictly. I will do exactly as you say." 2. Patient says: "In my profession I am very ethical. I believe that one must strictly follow the rules."

You can see how the rubric "Religious", which one might narrow down to "practice of religion", has now become much broader.

B. Jealousy

Meaning	:	Suspicious or incensed at rival. Incensed – incited. Rival – one pursuing an object in competition with another.
Interpretation	:	Suspicious and incited by one who is you competitor for a particular position or object.
Expression	:	Talking about the patient, her husband says: "Doctor, whenever I have work on a weekend, she gets angry and tries to hold my attention, complaining that I care more for my work than for her."

C. Indifference to personal appearance

Meaning	:	Indifference – without importance. Appearance – show; outward look.
Interpretation	:	Does not give importance to how he appears in other people's eyes.
Expression	:	Patient says: "Doctor, I do as I please, I am least bothered by what other people make of my actions."

D. Throws things away

Meaning	:	Throw – to hurl or to fling. To fling – to send suddenly.
Interpretation	:	To send away suddenly, to cast off something suddenly.
Expression	:	1. Patient says: "My boss said something rudely to me, which I could not bear, so I just resigned on the spot and walked off." 2. "For a long time I wanted to give up smoking and I couldn't and this annoyed me. So, one day, I just flung away the cigarette and from that time I never touched it again."

E. Monomania

Meaning	:	Unreasonable interest in only one particular thing.

Expression : A child of four, with a severe chronic cough, had the peculiar symptom that he was crazy after the colour green. He wanted everything green. Another symptom was that he was very particular that men and women should sit separately, never together. I used the rubrics "Monomania" for his obsession with green and "Fixed ideas" for the latter symptom and prescribed *Thuja*, which worked wonders.

F. Magnetized, desires to be

Meaning : Magnetize – to hypnotize.
Hypnotize – the state in which the mind responds to external suggestions.

Interpretation : The person wishes to do as suggested to him by somebody else.

Expression : "Doctor, I am completely in your hands. I shall do as you suggest. Please do not ask me what I want. I leave it all to you. You know best what is good for me." (This applies especially to *Calcarea* and *Silicea*.)

G. Desires ideal woman

Meaning : Ideal – highest and best conceivable, perfect, imaginary, existing only in idea.
Woman – what man needs to be complete or as partner alongside him (my meaning).

Interpretation : Desires that his surroundings, company, especially his partner, be perfect, which only exists in his ideas or imagination.

Expression : "Doctor, I wish my country had absolutely no crime or corruption and that everybody lived in a harmonious brotherly relationship like one big family."

H. Kill, desire to

Meaning : Kill – to destroy, to overcome, to deprive of life.

Interpretation : To want to finish something completely so that it can never raise its head again.

Expression : "I don't want temporary measures anymore, at whatever cost. I want to finish this problem once and for all."

I. Delusion, snakes in and around her

Meaning : Delusion – false belief.
Snake – venomous creature, ungrateful or treacherous person, anything snakelike in form or movement.

Interpretation : Whatever he sees within and around him, he has a false belief that it is a venomous, treacherous creature.

Expression : "My mother-in-law is a very dangerous woman. She talks sweetly and she knows how to cleverly poison other people's mind against me. So, I wait for my chance and pay her back in the same way."

J. Escape, attempts to, the window, from

Meaning : Escape – to free oneself.
Window – an opening for air and light.

Interpretation : The person feels trapped in a place since the way through which he walked in is now blocked. So, he has to get out from an opening meant for some other purpose.

Expression : "Doctor, I know that Homoeopathy is the best way out of this problem but it is taking too long and probably we are not finding the right medicine. I am just not able to suffer this any longer, so I want to take some allopathic drugs and get out of this acute situation first. After I am out of this, then we can resume homoeopathic treatment."

K. Clinging to person or furniture, etc.

Meaning : Clinging – to stick close by, clasp.
Clasp – grasp, to hold.

Interpretation : Person feels tremendous need to hold on to something either human or non-human.

Expression : 1. "As long as my Guru is with me, I have nothing to fear. I just hold on to him and feel safe."
2. "Wherever I go, I always carry his photograph, I cannot remain a single moment without it."
3. "Hold on to the values in the Bible, it is the only thing that can save us in this evil time."
4. "Doctor, wherever you go, please come back quickly, I just don't know how I am going to carry on without you."

L. Bargaining

Meaning : To take allowance, to get a favourable contract.

Expression : "Doctor, you insist I should stop all allopathic medicines immediately. I am afraid I will have much pain if I do that. Would it be OK with you if we reduce the dose a little at a time." (Patient sounds as if she is making a deal with the doctor.)

M. Hatred, persons who had offended him, of, unmoved by apologies

Meaning : Hatred – intense dislike.
Person – bodily presence.
Offend – displease, harm.
Unmoved – not touched by emotion, firm.
Apology – justification, explanation with expression of regret.

Interpretation : Intense dislike for the bodily presence of anyone or anything which has caused harm, remaining firm despite explanations or regrets.

Expression : "Ever since my diabetes, I have developed an intense dislike for sweets. Though everyone tells me that a little sweet now and then will not do any harm, I just will not go near it."

In the above examples, I am just giving one or two expressions. In fact, there may be several expressions besides the one I have mentioned. My idea is to show you how to look at the rubrics and how to use your imagination in applying them, so that you are scientific, yet you can use the rubrics in a very broad way. This will also help you to interpret into rubrics the various expressions of patients.

I give below some hints to enable you to use almost all the rubrics of the Repertory.

N. Ailments from

This rubric is one of the most frequently used sections of the Synthetic Repertory. However, I use it a little differently from others. For example, "Ailments from disappointment"; new: *Ignatia*, old: *Natrum muriaticum*.

When is the disappointment new and at what point does it become old? It is new as long as it is fresh in the mind, even though several years might have passed. It is old when it has become a scar, to be provoked only when touched or prodded, even though it might be just a few days after the incident. It is not necessary to have the specific causative factor in the life of the patient in order to use the rubric. If from whatever cause (or even without any apparent cause) the patient's whole state (expression) resembles that of a person who has been freshly disappointed, I use the rubric "Ailments from new disappointment". This could have occurred after a failure in examination or loss of a relative or even without any obvious cause. In such a person who shows an expression of fresh disappointment, if we do not find any such incident, it becomes doubly important. Similarly, I use other "Ailments from" rubrics almost as much as I use "Delusions". For example, if the father of the patient dies of cancer and he reacts to it by visiting several doctors, the rubric is not "Ailments from grief" but "Ailments from fright". So, the "Ailments from" is not to be taken from the actual incident but from the expression. The more the expression is uncommon for the incident, the more peculiar it becomes.

O. Fear, children, in

I interpret this as "Fear, like that of children". It is possible to use several "children" rubrics in adults. For example, "Obstinate children", "Restless children", "Weeping children", "Spoilt children", "Desires to be carried". The patient is a child in that aspect. For example, his stubbornness may resemble the stubbornness of a child. In adults who have "Fear of ghosts", "Fear of being alone in the darkness" and other fears which are mentioned in a childlike way, you can take the rubric "Fear in children". Rubrics that belong to old people, puberty and women can also be used in this way.

P. Quarrelsomeness alternating with singing

Interpretation : At one time the person is quarrelsome and at other times the same person is singing. The rubrics with alternating symptoms are very useful, since they show us the two phases that can coexist in the same person at different times. So, when at one time the person is cheerful and at another time (from a slight cause) he can get very quarrelsome, then you can take this as "Cheerfulness alternating with quarrel", provided they are quite intense and marked.

Q. The rubrics under "Insanity"

Insanity does not refer merely to mad people. Insanity means loss of one's sense or wisdom or reasoning power.

For example, insane jealousy is a jealousy which is not reasonable. Another rubric I use is "Insanity, drunkards, in"; a drunkard is a person who is excited and exalted, has lost some control. It does not necessary have to be used only in people who have consumed alcohol. If a person has lost his reserve and is excited, in other words acts like a drunkard gone mad, we can use this rubric. One patient I had just would not let anyone touch her, for no reason whatsoever. In her case, I used the rubric "Insanity, touched, will not be".

R. Delirium

One could also use this rubric for people who do not fall into the category of the scientific definition of delirium. It has to be used more in a dictionary sense, i.e. light-headed, excited, wandering in mind. If you observe carefully, you will see some of your patients talking deliriously.

S. Impatient with children

The rubric "Impatient with her children" would be interpreted as "Impatient only with her children". Similarly, whenever you get such modalities or qualification then you have to understand that it applies particularly to the thing that is qualified. For example, "Violent, to his friends" means "Violence particularly or only to friends"; "Talks of business" would mean "Talks particularly or only about business" or "Talks about most things in a businesslike way".

T. Theorizing, evening

When you get a time modality or other physical modalities, you have to see what it means in terms of the mind. In the above rubric, evening denotes the time when a person is idle after finishing the day's work. So, "Theorizing in evening" means he fantasizes when he is idle (like Walter Mitty). Similarly, the rubric "Anxiety, sitting, while, bent" denotes "Anxiety when a person is sitting relaxed".

U. Weeping, goes off alone and weeps as if she had no friends

There are many rubrics in which there are words like "friend", "family", etc. These relationships have to be understood broadly. A friend is a person in whom you can confide, is one with whom you have a mutual understanding and is one from whom you can expect care and affection. You can have a friendly relation with anybody including your parent, spouse, child or even pet dog. Similarly, family is a group that is interdependent on each other, with different roles assigned to different members. Your "family" could be your play group, professional group, doctor-patient relation, etc. So, it very much depends on what you consider your family. You can belong to more than one family.

Another word that occurs is "home". I had a child who pined away after his parents went abroad even though the boy continued to remain in the same house with his uncles and aunts. I used the rubric "Homesickness" because the boy was missing home. Home is the residence of one's family with its emotional associations. For the boy, home is the place where his parents are.

V. Fear, high places, of

The section on "Fears" also has to be understood as "Fear of reaching a position where there is danger of a person losing his balance or control, falling down and getting badly hurt or even killed". This could refer to any situation in one's life. For example, a person is promoted to a very high position in his company and he gets frightened that he may not be able to keep his balance, he may make a mistake or fail, and then he will fall down from his position and hurt himself badly. Similarly, other fears are to be considered broadly.

When interpreting an expression into a rubric, it is not the words alone that are important but the way they are spoken, the gestures used, the tone of the voice, the expression on the face, etc. These will tell us which kind of rubric we need to choose. The other thing that requires emphasis is that one should confirm the interpretation from other sources, namely from other aspects of the person's life. Once such a confirmation is made, we can rely on our interpretation.

W. Convulsions

Meaning   :   (Dictionary) Involuntary violent disturbance, spasm, fit, violent agitation.

The rubric on convulsions gives us those factors to which a person reacts violently or involuntarily. So, when a person gets convulsions from being wrongly accused (*Staphysagria*), this is one factor which can cause a violent, involuntary reaction.

X. Vaccination, after

The remedies listed in this rubric are the one clinically found useful in troubles aggravated after vaccination, i.e. these are the remedies that are most susceptible or sensitive to vaccine. Vaccines being a foreign protein, it shows us that these remedies are most sensitive to foreign proteins and therefore have a very high tendency to allergic reaction. These remedies are therefore going to be very useful in all allergic, atopic and hypersensitive reactions, and even autoimmune disorders. So, the rubric "Vaccination, after" can be interpreted as increased allergic response.

Y. Case example

Here is a case from my practice with the interpretation of the patient's expression into rubrics.

The patient comes into the consulting room and gives his name. When asked his age he says: "Forty-nine years and six months" ("Conscientious, trifles, about"). When asked about his brothers and sisters, he mentions each of them precisely by age and gives exact detail ("Fastidious"). While talking, he nods his head back and forth ("Head, motion, constant, hitter and thither, rolling"). He sits tensed and leaning forward ("Anxiety"). He speaks of a severe accident which he had. He immediately says: "They didn't pay me any compensation" ("Avarice"). In the hospital he met a man and they became business partners but the partner betrayed him and he was quite angry ("Ailments from anger, anxiety, with"). "Yet, I continued the partnership because I was dependent on the business ("Anxiety, alone, when", "Fear alone, of being", "Business, talks of"). My partner was taking care of the business ("Fear, friend has met with accident, that a"), and I felt that left to myself, I may damage the business ("Injure himself, fears to be left alone, lest he should").

"I am sick now and can't do much, and this man may cheat me further ("Suspicious", "Delusion, thieves, sees, house, in", "Fear, robbers, of"). I don't know what to do ("Irre-solution", "Confusion of mind"). I am losing sleep over this ("Anxiety, night"). Then I had angina pectoris, even though I was very careful with my health. I used to go for a checkup regularly ("Carefulness", "Anxiety, health, about"). I think the angina could be due to the financial crisis I had ("Fear, financial loss, of" – Phatak's Repertory). But today the crisis is over."

"I married late and my wife comes from a middle-class family. I particularly wanted someone from a middle-class family because she won't spend much ("Avarice", "Cautious"). But I find she is very money-minded ("Censorious", "Reproaches others"). I give her money for expenses and she wants more ("Anxiety, expected of him, when anything is"). She saved some of this money and I put in some money too and we bought a garage. Now she says half the garage belongs to her, since half the money is from her ("Estranged, wife, from his"). She says her uncle had given her some money as wedding gift. I know this is not true. It is actually the money I gave her ("Delusion, thieves, sees, house, in" and "Space under bed is full of thieves"). I don't want to fight with her since I have to live with her ("Delusion, offended people, he has", "Fear, alone, of being"). I am anxious as if someone will take away the money behind my back ("Delusion, thieves, house, in"). When there is any noise in the house, I feel uneasy ("Sensitive, noise, to", "Sensitive, voices, to", "Senses, acute"). I close all the doors properly ("Rest, cannot, till things are in proper place"), and I see if there is anybody around ("Searching, thieves, at night, for"). I find there is not a single reliable person. I can't trust my own people ("Sus-picious; plotting against his wife, people in the house, are", "Delusion, injury, they are about to receive", "Delusion, conspiracies against him").

"I have been advised to be careful with my health, to go regularly for walks and drink plenty of water. I do it much more than the doctor advises ("Drinks more than she should", "Walks more than is good for her")."

On being asked to stop all the allopathic drugs immediately, he became very fearful ("Fear, death, of", "Fear, happen, something will", "Fear, alone, of being, lest he dies"). One day he phoned the clinic six times ("Restlessness, anxious", "Carried, desires to be"). Once we started the treatment, however, his anxiety subsided ("Anxiety, railroad, when about to journey by, ameliorated while in train"). He takes his medicines quite strictly ("Religious affections").

One of the impressions I got was of the way he looked at his partner and wife, as though they are people who are slowly eating away at his wealth, like a leech drawing blood, and he has to be very careful not to let them do this. If he relaxes even for a moment, they will start eating away at his property. They appear to him like insects ("Delusion, see insects, rats, vermin") – which usually are active at night and which stealthily eat all the food at night. One has to be very careful, lock all windows, put on the mosquito net, spray insecticide, keep a mouse trap and not leave anything lying about. So, it is because of these creatures that one has to be suspicious, cautious, careful and anxious at night.

Follow-up note

This patient (whose case has been video-recorded) has done well on *Arsenicum album* 200 and later 1M. Not only did we see a clinical improvement in the angina but also his level of anxiety has come down significantly and he has been able to tackle his business problems with much more confidence.

Z. Remedy example

Let us now study a remedy through its rubrics, understanding their broader applications. We shall look at some symptoms of *Stramonium*, and their expressions.

"Clinging":

One prominent symptom of *Stramonium* is "Clinging". The dictionary meaning of clinging is to hold by clasping. The full rubric of *Stramonium* is:

— Clinging, child awakens terrified, knows no one, screams, clings to those near.

Another rubric is:

— Clinging to persons or furniture, etc.

Meaning : Every word in the rubric is important. We shall look at the meaning of each word and find its significance. "Awaken" means to get up from sleep. When he wakes up, he looks around, gets terrified. In this state of terror, he cannot distinguish who is who, cannot identify anyone and clings to the nearest thing or person. A "child" is a person who is not capable of defending himself, one who is dependent upon adults to protect him, so it could mean even a sixty year old, if he has feeling of being dependent for his protection on people with more strength, and he does not have the resources to protect himself. He is like a child. "Asleep" means absorbed with himself, eyes shut, not observing things around,

221

busy in himself, lost in himself. When such a person wakes up suddenly from sleep, he looks around and finds the situation terrifying, so terrifying that his brain refuses to work and he cannot recognize who is who. He cannot wait to find out the best person for protection, he just screams and clings to whoever is nearby.

A woman is sitting and reading a book, relaxed, when she notices a tingling on her arm, something crawling. She does not notice it immediately, but when she does, she screams, runs and grabs a nearby person. This is one picture. She awakens, i.e. becomes conscious of reality, which terrifies her, she does not recognize anyone but just holds the person next to her. This is one more expression of the application of this rubric from children into any adult, away from sleep into waking, but not conscious of reality.

It could also be applied to a person who develops a small, hard swelling in the stomach. Until he feels it, he is relaxed. The moment he feels it, he wakes up to and becomes conscious of it, and this terrifies him. Out of this terror, he just rushes to the nearest doctor and screams out of terror: "Look, what's happened." Now, we go one step further, he says: "Something is happening, I don't know what it is, I must find out what it is. Find out, investigate, take an X-ray, but find out what it is." This takes us to the rubrics:

— Fear, dark, of;

— Light, desire for.

The way he rushes to a doctor reminds you of a child who cannot fend for himself, but when even a minor trouble occurs goes to his protector. Therefore, the rubric:

— Delirium, crying for help.

"Delirium" means when the mind is not fully in its senses, when it is light-headed, wandering, not thinking straight. This is a delirious condition. "Help" means assistance, when you cannot do it on your own, you need someone to assist. How do you ask for help? By crying. "Crying" means to utter a shrill, loud sound. Not like, "Please help me", but, "HELP ME!"

Interpretation : "Knowing no one" takes us to the difference between knowing and not knowing the difference between light and darkness. Darkness is the situation when you do not know what is there and light is when you know what is there. Darkness means also hopelessness, and light is hopefulness, knowledge. A situation with even a slight lack of knowledge or uncertainty is enough to make a *Stramonium* lose his peace of mind. He wants to be clear. He says: "Please find out what is there inside, it's all dark, please throw some light on it. Take an X-ray if you want." He will remove his clothes. "Cloth" is something which covers, keeps parts hidden. There are rubric: "Destructiveness, clothes, of"; "Naked, wants to be". This means to remove the covering and bring it out in open. Nothing should be hidden under clothes.

222

So, we have examined the rubrics "Fear of darkness", "Desires for light", "Delirium, crying for help", "Clinging", etc., but the main symptoms of *Stramonium* are:

— Delusion, she is alone in the wilderness.

— Forsaken feeling.

There is a sensation of danger ("Delusion, danger, impression of") and the sensation that he is alone to face a danger which he is unable to do because it is too terrifying. Everything is in chaos around him. His parents have left him and gone away. He is abandoned, forsaken, left alone in a terrifying place.

Then there is a rubric:

— Anxiety about salvation.

"Salvation" means he has committed a crime and therefore has lost the support of the person who is providing it, i.e. God for man, man for his child. This feeling can be expressed by our patients when they say: "Doctor, wherever you go, please don't stay for more than a week, otherwise I will be lost. I don't know how to manage without you, if something happens, where shall I go?" "Don't leave me and go away" is the main thing for them. Anxiety about salvation as if they would lose your support. The person on whom they are dependent will leave them and they will be left alone, in the wilderness, forsaken. "Doctor, I don't know why, but when you go away, we just cannot manage, we just pray for the day you will come back." In this there is *praying*: "Please, doctor, come back soon." One step further is *begging*. If praying does not work, you beg. This is the way they behave towards you but you can see this behaviour extended to others.

Why do they behave this way? Because, when they become conscious, the world around them is terrifying and they want to cling to someone. If you are not available, they will get really panicky. The rubric: "Delirium, hands are joined" is again a sign of prayer. He feels he is without any protection, like the protective covering of clothes ("Delusion, naked, he is"). The rubric: "Praying" means requesting the person in authority to grant a wish like: "Please, help me."

Interpretation : Night is darkness, the unknown, the scary time. At such time he will pray. One important aspect of our remedies is that they have the opposite state too, at times. If you stay in one extreme you will die very soon, you have to go to the other at times. So, in the daytime, *Stramonium* is laughing. When there is no danger, darkness or gloominess, *Stramonium* is talking, laughing, singing, full of life, dancing. There is longing for sunshine, light and society.

Other rubrics are:

— Weeps all night, laughs all day;

— Delusion, tall, he is;

— Delusion, distinguished, he is;

— Delusion, divine, he is.

He talks a lot about himself ("Affectation"). He boasts that he is bold, not afraid of anything, but when the night comes, he goes and clings. *Stramonium* has bravado when things go well, but when things are not going so well, he can get very scared.

Let us take some more rubrics.
— Delirium, foreign language, talks in a;
— Speech, foreign tongue, in.

What is a foreign language? "Foreign" means something which is not common to the country of residence, something that belongs to another place. "Talks" means speech, "language" means a medium of communication. In his speech he uses a medium of communication that is uncommon to the place in which he resides. It means he is talking French in India for example, or using Greek phrases or an American accent. He is alternating between one language and another language. Using a lot of foreign expressions and different accents. It also means he uses phrases from another discipline. For example, in a meeting of homoeopathic physicians, he might use a lot of psychoanalytic terms, terms which may be foreign to homoeopaths. In everyday language, he may use terms that the other person is unfamiliar with. This too is speaking in a foreign language; you will not understand anything though he speaks the same language as you because the words he uses are uncommon for the place he is in. He can talk of highly spiritual things, like nirvana, samadhi and kundalini shakti. All this can be taken as foreign language, things that the person to whom he is talking cannot understand.

Another rubric of *Stramonium* is:
— Delusion, poor, he is.

"Poor" means lacking in that which is necessary to keep one surviving. You can have poor health, poor fortune, poor intelligence, poor strength. "Thinks he is poor" not only refers to money but also a feeling of lacking something which is necessary for survival. "Doctor, when my fever goes to 102-103 °F, I don't know whether I will be able to bear such a high temperature, whether I have the energy left in me to bear it", says the patient with a terrified voice. "I don't know ("Fear of darkness"), whether I have the energy left in me to bear this ("Delusion, poor, he is")". "Bear this assault of temperature on my body" brings us to the rubric: "Delusion, injured, is being". "The temperature is causing injury to my body, I am scared, I don't know whether I have the strength to bear this injury. Doctor, you do something ("Delirium, crying for help") because, unaided, I will be finished." There is still hope ("Desire for light") with all this terror.

— Delusion, injured, is being.

I have used this rubric in several cases. It means as if things are harming him, causing him injury. In *Thuja*, we saw there is a feeling that the body is brittle, made of glass ("Frail, sensation of being"), as if it can be easily injured. For example, when they shake hands, they are very careful that their bones do not break. This feeling is different from the *Stramonium* feeling. In *Thuja*, the feeling that things are injuring them is absent, for them the surrounding things are innocent, others are innocent, but it is them who are brittle. "Nobody is injuring me, things that are totally harmless can injure me because I am very brittle, I have to be very cautious. If I am cautious, I will not be injured." But in *Stramonium*, there is: "Delusion of being injured", and not the delusion that his body is brittle and extrasensitive to injury. *Stramonium* says: "Doctor, I took your medicine last week and since then, my stomach has got so badly upset, I cannot tell you how much." There is "being injured": "Ever since I started your treatment, I noticed that my hair is falling a lot", and all you have given is placebo. This is the feeling that he is being harmed. "Doctor, the weather is so bad nowadays that I catch cold very often, so you give me some medicine to build my resistance against it." The rubrics are: "Delusion, being injured", "Clinging", "Crying for help".

— Sees dog attacking him, biting his chest.

Why does he see a dog? What is the significance of "dog"? When you are alone in a dark street, it is not a rat, cat or snake that scares you. A snake can bite even in the daytime. When it is dark and you do not know the way ahead and there are no houses around, if at this time you hear the barking of a dog or if a dog is pursuing, you cannot run because of the darkness, whereas the dog can see very well and come and make mincemeat out of you. This is the time when you experience the terror of *Stramonium*. When there is light, and you can see around, see which stone to pick up and throw, see which house to enter for protection, the dog becomes less scary. Dogs are animals which attack when you are helpless; there is the rubric: "Helplessness, feeling of".

— Delusion, sees dogs.

What is meant by "Delusion, sees dogs"? For me, it means he sees people as dogs, sees events and situations as dogs. If he sees an income tax officer, it reminds him of a dog. With great fear, he says: "Doctor, I know they are after me, I don't know when they are going to attack, I don't know what to do. I am so helpless, I run here and there, trying to balance some accounts, I know they are after me" ("Delusion sees dogs, biting him, attacking him, biting his chest", "Delusion, animals jump out of the ground"). They are all the time around you. You can feel their presence near you, they are troublesome, injurious things. It could be your own business competitor trying to harm you.

He gets most scared when things are dark, gloomy and sombre ("Black and sombre, aversion to"). With all this helplessness, terror and fright, you have a choice either to grasp at the nearest thing or person around in order to feel safe and if you do not find anybody to hit out wildly ("Wildness", "Destructiveness", "Violent", "Striking") – "Delusion that he is devil", "Devil, sees people as"; we have a common expression in English: "He brings out the devil in me."

— Kill, desire to.

"Kill" means to finish off so completely that it cannot raise its head again, to eradicate, to destroy not just a bit but to go all the way, exterminate. One of the expressions in the patients is that he does not want his disease to merely subside for the time being, but to go away completely so that it will never recur. The ailment frightens him so much that he does not want it to come up ever again, he is too afraid of it coming to life. "I was so frightened, on taking homoeopathic medicines, that the whole experience would come back again. I think I have killed it, so I don't want to experiment again."

225

He approaches other problems like that also. If there is a leaky tap, he will try to shut it tight and when not successful, he may take the hammer and break off the connection altogether so that it does not leak again. His action is always total. This is how he approaches his problems because problems trouble and scare him. So much that he wants to kill them. Some surgeons are *Stramonium*. Seeing a small wart which has bled a little, he will say: "Oh, it is so terrible, it has started bleeding, we must get it out at once so that it never recurs again." So, we can see the rubrics: "Child awakens, terrified, screams, knows no one, clings to those near" and "Kill, desire to".

Another example, in a throat trouble with a mild infection, the patient wants to take the strongest antibiotics so that it never comes again, he is so terrified of the bacteria. The rubrics being: "Fear, murdered, of being", "Delusion, injured, is being", "Kill, desire to". Also, there is "Threatening": "Doctor, I am troubled too much. I am going to try your medicine for one more week. If within that time I don't see any result, then I will be forced to take some other treatment." It is like: "If you don't give the results, then beware."

The idea of this is to show how each word is important and how all these expressions and rubrics give the picture of *Stramonium*. In short, it is the picture of the child who is abandoned in the wilderness. These expressions are not out fantasy, but from what I have seen in patients.

One of the best *Stramonium* cases I saw was of a man in London. He showed me the poem he had written after he had got better with *Stramonium*. The theme of the poem was about going to an allopath – a neurologist. The poem was something like this: "He poked me here and there, looked at me and told something to his students, he gave me no hope ("Slander, disposition to"). Then I went to Homoeopathy with which I could see light and joy, and I saw myself coming to life." The poem showed a beautiful expressive picture of *Stramonium*. People can get you when it is dark and you are helpless. At this time you react with violence or clinging. I had a case of a child with fever who was holding her ear all the time; the rubric was "Clinging". *Stramonium* wants to be held, some part of his body has to be held, so they hold themselves. I had a case of a man who dreamt of eating glass. He knew it was glass because of the crunch sound it made in his mouth. He spat it out and found that it was really glass and he would have eaten it if it had not made the crunching sound. I took the rubric: "Painless of complaints usually painful". One of Jayesh's patients, a lady, said: "Doctor, I will tell you frankly I have no problem, no fear, no anger, no hatred, nor jealousy, nothing hurts me" ("Indifference, complain, does not", "Indifferent, suffering, to", "Clinging", "Delusion, God, communication with, he is, in"). They believe they have contact with a guru ("Clairvoyance") who will protect them from this terrible world. If separated, even for a minute, they feel abandoned like a child in the wilderness. In this way, *Stramonium* can apply to addictions in a wider sense, not only to drug addicts but to people who need something all the time to cling to; for example, the followers of groups, religious or scientific, etc., who always need the group, master or guru. If that is taken away, they cling to the next thing.

Associated with this is the rubric:
— Religious affections, Bible, wants to read, all day, the (Synthetic Repertory).

"The Bible" signifies any authoritative book. Reading the Bible the whole day would mean that the person needs a book of authority in which he trusts and constantly clings to in order to avoid the uncertainty and darkness he feels around him. The rubric can be used even in scientifics who cling to one particular authority all the time. For example, sometimes we come across a homoeopath who keeps quoting from Hahnemann's 'Organon", as if it were scripture. He is so obsessed with it that he has several copies, he carries it wherever he goes and must read it every single day. Other homoeopaths use Allen's "Keynotes" like this and still others read the Repertory everyday as if it were the Bible. Similar examples can be found in other disciplines. The need for an authority and a constant referral to it, whether it be a book, person or dogma, reflects the person's inner uncertainty and insecurity. This is the deeper meaning of the rubric: "Wants to read the Bible all the day". Incidently, the Bible begins with darkness and this is followed by those famous words: "The Lord said, 'Let there be Light', and there was light", the typical words for *Stramonium*!

As an interesting sidelight, once Jayesh had a case of a child with dog bite. It was a pet dog of a friend. Whenever a new person approached the dog, it became ferocious and bit, so he prescribed *Stramonium* to the dog! "Fear of approach of strangers" is another marked feature of *Stramonium*.

There is also a rubric:

— Delusion, animals, persons are, rats, mice, insects, etc.

This is the only place where it is given very clearly, otherwise it appears as "Delusion, sees dogs, swarm about him"; this means "whatever is swarming about him are dogs". This is how we should interpret. For example, if you see "Delusion, faces, sees, diabolical", it means "Delusion, that the faces he sees are diabolical".

The idea of this is not only to highlight the *Stramonium* picture, but more importantly to show the way we can imaginatively expand the rubrics.

— Delusion that wife is faithless.

This is another rubric which can have a wide variety of expressions. For example, when the patient says: "Doctor, please come back soon, don't abandon us and settle down in a foreign country", this is: "Delusion that wife is faithless". "Wife" means partner whom one trusts and this trustful relationship is the secure basis of one's life. Such a person may become untrustworthy, may break the contract, go away with someone else, leaving this person insecure, abandoned in the dark not knowing what to do, helpless. This can happen in a trustworthy relationship he has with anyone. What must a guru's disciples have felt when he abruptly shifted from place to place?

To expand the meaning of the rubrics in this way is fascinating. What the prover has expressed is the direct experience, but we have to understand what the experience means in term of varied life situations. The prover gave one expression but what is the feeling behind this expressions and how can we see it in the clinic? By using our imagination and looking at rubrics in this new light we will then be able to apply them in a wider context. For this, all we require is the dictionary to understand the exact meaning of the words in the rubrics, imagination and careful observation of our patients.

I want to describe the only *Stramonium* experience I had as a child, when with fever I had this feeling that there was a cotton ball which was slowly expanding and getting huge, occupying all the space in the room and the room was getting too narrow for it. The ball was rolling and I was helplessly stuck to it. I was shrieking loudly with fear, calling for help. I was helped by *Stramonium*. This dream I like because it illustrates the way a *Stramonium* person looks at his problems. He sees the problem and he sees fear and he sees it getting bigger and bigger so that it can suffocate him, destroy him and all he can do is helplessly watch.

There is also desire for black in *Stramonium* along with aversion to black. I have observed most *Stramonium* people wear black clothes just like many *Stramonium* people like dogs very much. It is like making friends with the things that threaten you. It is like the woman who has a fear of snakes and who keeps a boa constrictor as a pet.

One more rubric of *Stramonium* is:

— Insanity, drunkards, in.

This rubric can also be used in a broader sense. A drunkard is a person who is under the influence of alcohol, and at this time becomes excited, exalted and loses his reserve. A *Stramonium* person will talk in an uncompensated way almost as if he is drunk. When there is further stress he can lose his reason. In addition to this, he also behaves like one mad. So, "Insanity, drunkards, in" can be used in a person who is not drunk or insane but who behaves like one who is drunk and insane.

Part III

Case taking and finding the remedy

31

THE HEART OF CASE TAKING

Case taking involves an application of the principles of Homoeopathy. Our firm grasp of the principles alone can guide us in proper case taking. My purpose here is to explain some of the principles and show how in case taking we should be guided by them.

The purpose and the method

Aphorism 83 of the "Organon" reads:

"The individualizing examination of a case of disease... demands of the healing artist nothing but freedom from prejudice and sound senses, attention in observing and faithfulness in tracing the picture of the disease."

See the beauty of this aphorism. In a single aphorism Hahnemann has given the purpose, requisites and method of case taking. He has shown us where to go, how to reach there and what we need to take with us.

The purpose of case taking is "tracing the picture of the disease". The idea is not to try and fit the patient into some remedy or idea, but to trace out the true picture of the disease. The way to do so this is to bring out the individuality of the patient. In this aphorism, Hahnemann is stating the cardinal principles of Homoeopathy which is that disease is an individual affection, and that each patient is an individual, suffering from his own unique disease. When we want to draw someone's picture, we first note his individualizing features. Similarly, "tracing the picture of the disease" requires us to clearly bring out the individualizing features of the case. Only when you bring out the individuality of the patient, can you really claim to have taken the case. Now, we have both the aim of case taking, which is to trace the picture of disease, and the method of case taking, which is to *individualize* the patient.

What are the requirements for case taking? The only requirements are an unprejudiced mind, an observing mind and a mind that draws a very accurate picture. We must not fit people into slots; instead we have to just let the picture come out, without imposing our own ideas on what we see. We must try to bring out and understand the true feelings of the patient not in terms of remedies, but in terms of human understanding.

There are two ways we can take the case. The first is to try out various remedies, like a salesman trying to fit shirts on a customer. I heard of a homoeopath who used this method of interview. For example, in dysentery he knew three remedies: *Ipecac*, *Colchicum* and *Mercurius*. To a patient with dysentery he would ask: "Do you have nausea with a clean tongue and thirstlessness?" If the patient said, "Yes", he would get *Ipecac*. If he said: "No", he would ask: "Then do you have nausea at the smell of food? No? Does your urging persist even after stool? No? Then Homoeopathy has no medicine for you!" This kind of fitting of our limited knowledge of Materia Medica onto a patient is a very deleterious practice. Alternatively we can take all the relevant symptoms of the patient carefully, and then look into the Repertory and Materia Medica for a suitable remedy. This method is much safer and smoother. When the great homoeopath Dr. Pierre Schmidt was asked by a patient if he had treated similar cases before, he remarked: "I hope not!" He meant that each case has to be considered individually, unprejudiced by similar cases we might have seen earlier.

Case taking is the process of perceiving and recording the inner experience of the patient. It is not merely writing down whatever the patient says. This does not mean that we have to theorize or symbolize what we see, but just trace the picture as we see it.

There is a story that once there was a robbery in the house of the great master Picasso. The police said to him: "Master Picasso, you have seen the thieves and you are one of the greatest artists of the world. Why don't you paint a picture of the thieves, so that we can easily apprehend them?" Picasso complied, and on the basis of his sketches they arrested a horse, an umbrella and a television set. We should not be Picassos and theorize or symbolize, but let the pure picture emerge as it is, so that the correct remedy can be apprehended.

What is to be cured in disease?

Aphorism 3 of the "Organon" begins with: "If the physician clearly perceives what is to be cured in disease... " Before we talk about how a case is to be taken, we have to be very clear, exactly what is that we are looking for. We have said that we have to trace the picture of the disease. What exactly does disease comprise of?

One of the easiest ways to find this out is to study our drug provings. After all, drug effects are nothing but artificial diseases. So, when we study our drug provings, we get a good idea about disease. If we study for example the proving of *Bryonia*, we find that in different provers different organs are affected, but most provers have great aggravation from the slightest motion. Similarly, in the proving of *Aconitum*, no matter who the prover is, or no matter which of his organs are involved, there is a very prominent fear of death. General modalities and specific mental states seem to be common to most provers of a particular remedy. This common mental and general state, produced by that remedy can be called its central disturbance.

Each remedy produces a specific central disturbance

Every remedy produced a specific central disturbance, though different provers will have different organs involvement depending upon their susceptibility. The central disturbance supports or causes these peripheral organ effects. The central disturbance is like a stick which is constant but on which different creepers grow, depending on where it is situated. The stick is responsible for the growth of the creeper, but the same creeper can grow on different sticks. In the same way the central disturbance is responsible for organ pathology but the same organ pathology can occur under different central disturbances. For example, diabetes with its common symptoms can occur under so many remedies that it almost seems to be like a creeper which can hook on to any stick.

Our job is not to cut the creepers but to remove the stick that support them. If you cut only the creeper and leave the stick intact, some other creeper can grow on that stick.

Central disturbance is P-N-E-I disturbance

The central disturbance that is produced by a remedy consists of those features of a remedy that are constant, no matter who the prover is. These features are identified as: Mental symptoms, and functional symptoms of Nervous, Endocrine and Immunological systems. Together they form one axis which we can call the Psycho-Neuro-Endocrino-Immunological system (P-N-E-I).

The P-N-E-I symptoms of a remedy remain more or less constant in different provers; but the organ involvement keeps varying and so, one can say that organ involvement comes secondary to the central disturbance, just as the stick comes first and the creeper grows on it later.

Remedies produce artificial diseases. We have seen how, in such a disease, the central disturbance comes first and the peripheral pathology comes later. Similarly, in natural diseases, there is a central disturbance which support all the peripheral pathology. It is this central disturbance that has to be treated and *it is this central disturbance that has to match the central disturbance of the remedy*.

In practice, we find patients whose central disturbance indicates the same remedy but they have different pathologies. In Homoeopathy, when we talk of diagnosis of disease, we do not talk in terms of whether a person has diabetes or schizophrenia. But we say a person now has a *Kalium carbonicum* state or a *Sepia* state. What will be common for all cases having the *Kalium carbonicum* state is that their mental and general symptoms will be of *Kalium carbonicum*. These represent the central disturbance of the patient and they give a clue to his individuality.

Local peculiarities also indicate central disturbance

Even though pathology depends on individual susceptibility, the peculiarities of the local symptoms depend on the nature of he central disturbance. Just as the nature of the creeper does not depend on the stick that supports it, but the way it takes shape depends on the shape of the stick; so, we say that characteristics of the particular symptoms are also an expression of the central disturbance along with the mental and general symptoms.

Thus, local symptoms can help us only if we discriminate between what is common to the pathology from what is peculiar. *That which is peculiar is an expression of the central disturbance.* For example, in a case of peptic ulcer, the patient gets pain when hungry. This is common to ulcer patients. But if he says the pain is relieved by rapid movement, this feature is not in the nature of the ulcer, so it must represent the central disturbance.

Discovering the central disturbance of a case

In case taking, our job is to find out this central disturbance which is often hidden by features of peripheral pathology. It is like identifying the stick which is hidden by the creepers. We can easily understand that, as time passes, more creepers get added, the stick gets further hidden from view, and recognizing it becomes more and more difficult.

In an acute case or one of recent origin, or in the case of a child, the central disturbance is less obscured from view and symptoms are spontaneously forthcoming without much effort on the part of the physician.

In a chronic case, where much time has elapsed, the central disturbance is more obscure and the physician has to make a conscious effort to determine the original symptoms. Two factors contribute to obscure the central disturbance:
– Symptoms of the situation of the patient;
– Symptoms of the pathology.

Hahnemann used the word "striking" symptoms to indicate symptoms that immediately catch our attention. Naturally, these symptoms have to stand out against the background of the patient's situation.

Mental state has to be judged against the situation

Aphorism 211 of the "Organon" reads:

"... The state of disposition of the patient often chiefly determines the selection of the homoeopathic remedy, as being a decidedly characteristic symptom which can least of all remain concealed from the accurately observing physician."

Hahnemann asserts that of all the characteristics of the patient, his mental state is easiest to elicit. What could make this process difficult is that often some part of the mental state is due to the situation itself. Each patient has to be judged keeping his situation in mind. It is only then that one can see what is individual to him.

In India, for example, if a person is half an hour late for a dinner party, he may find that not only is he the first one to arrive, but that his host and hostess have not arrived, and the cook has gone to buy vegetables! His friends will advise him not to be so neurotic about time. I am trying to indicate that there is a certain normalcy for each group. It is said of Indian trains that they have never run on time. One day a train did arrive at the exact time, and some people fainted from shock and were only consoled when they were informed that it was actually the train that was supposed to have arrived the previous day! We Indians work at our own pace. Now, if you find that a person who comes from this background insists on punctuality, it is highly characteristic. But, in Europe, where people seem to worship and get commands from their watches, and where they behave as if the earth will stop moving if there is a delay of more than one minute, in these circumstances insistence on punctuality would no be uncommon or striking unless it is extreme even by European standards. (If Darwin's law of evolution holds true, I suspect that after a few generations, Germans will be born with in-built Swiss watches!)

Different sociocultural traits are like disguises which mask the real person. Our job is to discover in the person before us those features that persist no matter which disguise he wears.

Person's characteristics versus characteristics of situation

A person's age, sex, occupation, educational background, nationality, religion, parentage, etc., each leave a mark on, and produce in the person certain specific features. From the symptoms we uncover, we have to remove those that are explainable by the patient's situation.

A person's occupation, for example, will leave its own mark on his nature. A top executive may be expected to be anxious and irritable or a military commander may be expected to be a strict disciplinarian. But if you get symptoms which cannot be fully explained by his occupation, these are characteristic of the disturbance within. Find those symptoms in the executive or commander that would still have persisted even if he were a priest or a cobbler.

For example, a busy executive complains of feeling very tense. This is common. But he says that whenever he is tense, he leaves his office and takes a very long walk. He keeps walking fast until he sweats; only then does he feel mentally relieved. This modality which cannot be explained, and would have been the same even if he were a cobbler or a housewife, reveals the dynamic disturbance within.

Eliminating situational features

In other words, we have to disregard in the patient's mental make-up those features which are due to his sociocultural environment. We have to remove from the picture all symptoms which are common to the group he belongs to, and which can be explained by his background. What is left is the pure picture upon which you can base a very sure prescription. Sociocultural traits are like clothes on a person. They represent his position, not his individuality. Deprived of his clothes, the man is without any marks of his group or position. This unchanging form, which would remain the same whatever clothes he wears and however much he tries to change his appearance, is the true man.

The question I put to myself when taking a case is: What symptoms would have been found even if he were from a totally different background? These symptoms are of maximum value. For example, if I meet a middle-aged Swiss housewife, mother of three children, well-to-do and well educated, I ask myself after taking her case which of her symptoms would persist even if she were a young, male Tibetan monk, totally unexposed to Western culture, educated in Buddhist scriptures, a celibate whose father had been a shepherd. The symptoms which remain even if she were this kind of monk, are her real symptoms and these would indicate her remedy.

Remedies are fixed totalities; they are the same in any country, culture, or situation. If this were not so, we would have to have a different Materia Medica for different subgroups. We would need one for Swiss females and one for Tibetan males. A remedy is the same anywhere although the expressions may be different. For example, if the symptom of a remedy is conscientiousness, the conscientiousness of the Swiss lady may manifest itself in a high sense of responsibility for her children even if they are quite grown up, while in the Tibetan monk, it may manifest itself as extreme industriousness in learning the Scriptures; but conscientiousness as a trait is common.

Same feature, differing expressions

We can see from the above example that *the same trait can have different expressions in different types of people.* To take another example: if increased activity at night is the trait, the child will be playful at night, the artist will paint at night, the mill worker will always opt for a night shift, the woman will insist on doing the household chores at night after everyone has slept, and the dog will bark the whole night. So, we can see that playing, barking, etc., are the normal activities of the type, but on substracting this, the basic trait can be seen: "Increased activity at night", which is the same for all types. Basic traits are those which do not belong to any particular group of people.

So, when we see an expression in a patient, we have to analyze and reduce this expression to its basic feeling or feelings. For example, if a person is very industrious, working even after office hours and during holidays, then we have to question what is making him like this. It could be due to his conscientiousness or due to his anxiety if a time is set, or it could be that he feels better from occupation or that he is very business-minded and ambitious or that he just wants to avoid the company of people, particularly his family. Maybe, it is a combination of two or more of the above feelings. We have to confirm these feelings in other situations. For example, if we think that his industriousness is due to conscientiousness, then we ask how conscientious he is towards his religion, his family, etc. If conscientiousness is his strong basic trait, it should manifest itself in other areas as well. In this way, we have to reduce expressions to the basic feelings that cause them.

Eliminate features of pathology

The second point to look into is, which symptoms are due to pathology, or, in other words, which symptoms are common to all patients having that particular pathology.

Since pathology is like a creeper that grows on the central disturbance, we have to cut off symptoms of pathology in order to get a clear picture of the central disturbance.

I am not trying to say here that the central disturbance has no role in creating or sustaining pathology. I assert that it does have a very active role, but pathology itself is often not characteristic of any particular central disturbance. At best we may come to a group of remedies which are known to have cured this pathological condition. But since this frequently comes from clinical experience and not from the provings, the list is far from complete. It is always possible that a drug which is not known for a particular pathological condition could produce that pathology if it was proved in a susceptible person. So, pathology is as much a part of the disease as the mental and general state, but it is not its identifying feature. Arms and legs in a man are very much a part of him, in fact they may be the most prominent parts, but often they do not characterize the man as much as a crooked nose or a mole on the chin. In this way pathology, being common to several central disturbances, loses its value as an identifying feature of the disease. The symptoms that can be explained by pathology, therefore become common symptoms.

The question we have to ask ourselves is: Which are those symptoms in the patient which would have persisted even if they had a totally different pathology? If you want to find out the identifying features of a person, find out those features he would have, even if he wore totally different clothes.

The pathology on a central disturbance is like clothes on a person. There can be no pathology without central disturbance, just as shirt cannot stand up without a person being there. Therefore, find out in a case of diabetes those symptoms which would have existed even if the patient had not come with diabetes, but he came with a wart on his nose. In a schizophrenic, find out those symptoms which he would have had even if he did not suffer from schizophrenia but from anxiety, neurosis or asthma. The mental symptoms that do not depend on schizophrenia, and which would have persisted even if he did not have schizophrenia, are the symptoms of the mental state and are part of the central disturbance. The symptoms that are common to schizophrenia, even though they may be mental symptoms, are mental disease symptoms, and therefore do not represent the central disturbance.

How to determine if a feature is situational, pathological or original

If there is a doubt whether the situation or pathology is responsible for a particular symptom, then we can use three criteria to help us determine the true state.

- Has the symptom existed prior to the situation, or prior to the present pathology? If this is so, then it can be taken as a symptom of the central disturbance. For example, if in a policeman we find the symptom "Dictatorial", then the question may arise whether he is dictatorial due to his occupation or he chose the job of the policeman because it was in tune with his dictatorial nature. The best way to determine this is to go back and find out about his nature before he became a policeman. If he was dictatorial even then, it can be taken as part of his nature. To take another example, burning feet is common in diabetes, but if this symptom existed prior to the onset of diabetes, then it assumes some significance.

I often go back in the life of the patient and find out the picture as a child. It is in childhood that the picture is totally clear and unadulterated, and is not covered by layers of culture and pathology.

- The second way to find out the true original nature of the patient is to compare the intensity of his symptoms with their intensity in other persons in the same situation or environment, or with similar pathology. For example, ask if the policeman is as strict as other policemen, or ask whether the aggravation from motion is as intense in this case of joint pain; is it more or less than usual?

- The third way to find out is to ask the patient which aspects if his situation he is comfortable with, and which aspects make him uncomfortable. It is likely that those aspects he is comfortable with are in tune with his nature or disposition. For example, a salesman whose job involves a lot of travel may say: "Travelling is the best part of my job and accounts work is the worst." Another salesman may say: "I have to travel, I have no choice. With accounts, I have no problems at all." One can easily see that the first one likes to travel and the second one is averse to it.

Another question we ask is: "In which position or situation would you be most comfortable?" The situation in which the patient is most comfortable will be in tune with his nature.

The best totality of symptoms would include mainly those symptoms from which one can get no clue about (and which do not depend upon) the patient's age, nationality, occupation or pathology. As the totality gets more and more shorn of the marks of situation and pathology, the clearer will be the indications for the remedy. Therefore, for the purpose of finding the remedy, choose mainly those symptoms from which you can get no idea whether they belong to a Russian grandfather who has cancer or an Australian child who has as cold.

The homoeopath as an archeologist

Many a time the homoeoapth has to do the job of an archeologist, who often finds the original structure covered by the layers of earth, so that its true shape is totally occluded. In a chronic case, what the situation and pathology have added to the central disturbance is like earth accumulated on the monument. Just like the archeologist, the job of the homoeopath is to separate what has accumulated, from what is original so that the true identity of the structure becomes clear.

When he begins this search, he does not know what is going to emerge. He just has to keep separating the false from the true. This has to be done very carefully. One must not remove parts of the original monument itself in the process, nor should one be too cautious and not remove all the earth that has accumulated. In case taking, this would mean that we are not to try and explain away something on the basis of situation and pathology, which may be a part of the original disease. An expert archeologist may be able to make a good guess about the identity of the structure even after uncovering a small part of it. But a scientific and thorough archeologist will uncover the whole structure before he gives his final verdict. Similarly, initial observations or symptoms may give a clue to the remedy, but a good homoeopath will examine all aspects and elicit the whole picture clearly before he decides on his prescription.

All features of a remedy need not be found in every case

There are two very important lessons that we can learn from archeology. The first is that the archeologist will rarely find all pieces of a monument in one excavation. Whatever pieces he does find, he has to discover the type of monument into which they all fit. In terms of case taking, this means that we do not often find all the characteristics of the remedy in any one patient. We have to study all that we do find and see which remedy this fits into.

All the characteristics of the patient must fit into the remedy selected

The second and most important lesson is that although the archeologist does not expect to find all the pieces of a monument in the excavation, he does expect all the pieces he has found to fit into one type of monument. Even if he finds one or two pieces that do not fit, he must seriously suspect his original conclusion. For example, he may find pillars and a dome and so think that the monument could have been a church. Yet, if he finds along with these a butcher's knife, then he has to doubt his original judgement and try to find a type of building in which everything he has uncovered could fit. In terms of case taking this means that we do not expect all the characteristics of a remedy to exist in a patient. For example, we can have a *Calcarea* patient without fear or a desire for eggs. Absence of these symptoms does not rule out this remedy. Yet, whatever characteristic symptoms in the patient we do find must fit. In a case where all other symptoms may fit *Calcarea*, but the patient has a very prominent symptom like audacity or courage, which is not covered by the remedy, this would rule it out. In short, we are not to discard remedies if the symptoms of the remedy are not found in the patient; we have to discard only if the *characteristic* symptoms of the patient are not found in the remedy.

This point is worth stressing again and again because unconsciously we expect some definite symptoms of a remedy to be found in every case of that remedy. For example, if the patient is to be *Pulsatilla*, we expect her to be mild, weeping and thirstless. We also speak of remedies in this manner. For example, we say *Lycopodium* is a coward or *Natrum muriaticum* dwells on past disagreeable occurrences. When we make this kind of statement, it is like saying that we would rule out this remedy if that feature were not present. We must not fall into this trap. Remedies are combinations of several traits; it is not mandatory that all traits be present prominently in all cases. It is not for us to see whether our picture of a remedy will fit or match all the patient's characteristics. If they fit well into one remedy, we have to give that remedy even if our favourite symptoms of that remedy are missing in the patient.

Case uncovering

The plan of case taking that I adopt is one that allows the picture to emerge spontaneously and clearly. Thus, case taking is neither an active nor a passive process. I feel both the terms "case taking" and "case receiving" are not suitable. Actually, it should be called "case uncovering" or "case discovering". Again, Hahnemann surpasses us all when he uses the expression "tracing the picture".

Tracing the background

I therefore usually begin by asking the patient to tell everything concerning his background. When he does so, it is necessary to observe him constantly – his every gesture and movement, his attitude and manner of talking. The initial questions are directed at finding out where he came from, who his parents are, what is occupation is, what the story of his life is. What is the situation regarding education, marriage, money matters, and what are his interests? Against this background, I try to search for the thing which are peculiar to him. At each point it is necessary to carefully discover whether what he is describing is common or uncommon to his background, and how intense and striking it is. This kind of informal talk – even before we have asked about his chief complaints – brings out imperceptibly and unconsciously most of the features of his mind; and slowly details emerge of the way he thinks and feels.

Obtain confirmation of your impressions

The impressions we thus gather have to be confirmed not once but several times, in several situations, before we can rely on them for finding the remedy. If we are climbing a steep, high mountain, our foothold has to very strong and firm, and we have to check it, not once but three or four times before we can put our whole weight on it. If the foothold is not secure and we do not make sure about it before we put our entire weight on it, then one wrong step may take us hurtling down the mountain!

We have, therefore, to be very sure of the symptoms on which we are going to rely. I am emphasizing this because earlier, when I found something which sounded characteristic, I was too scared to get it confirmed as I was afraid I may lose it; and so I defended that symptom with all my life, not allowing even the patient to change or withdraw it.

A symptom which needs to be guarded so heavily is not worth the effort. Let the symptoms be heavily exposed and in fact put them through water and fire before you accept them. Attack the idea yourself, be very sceptical, confirm it in other situations and be very sure before you lean on it for support.

32

SOME HINTS ON CASE TAKING

1. *Ask questions in the opposite direction.*

If you want to confirm that the patient is really mild, you ask him: "Do you get angry?" Often, even a mild patient will say: "Yes." Ask him next: "When did you last get angry?" A mild patient will think a lot and tell you: "Seven months back." Ask him: "When did you get angry before that?" Then he will really have to exert his mind to remember such an incident.

Or, for example, ask a patient who you think is very sad: "When do you remember being very happy?" A sad person will be able to give you only two or three such instances in his whole life. It means that it requires a very, very joyous occasion for him to be happy. Sometimes, even these occasions produce no reaction. If you think a person is a coward, then do not ask him anything about his cowardice. He may straightaway say "No". Ask him to give some instances when he stood up to someone and fought back. These instances will be very rare in the life of a coward.

2. *Always confirm symptoms from relatives and friends.*

Observe the expression on the face of the person accompanying the patient while the patient is narrating his symptoms. You will often find an involuntary affirmative nod of the head or a shake of denial if the person agrees or disagrees with the patient's evaluation of himself.

Sometimes you can turn around and ask the accompanying person if he agrees or disagrees with what the patient has said. This is best done when the patient is out of the room.

3. *Never accept what the patient says at face value.*

4. *Look at the hidden expression behind the symptoms.*

See the way a symptom is expressed. You ask the patient: "Have you any fear of darkness?" He says: "Never, never, never. I have never had any fear in my life. I can walk in the darkest and most deserted streets at night and I have absolutely no fear!" This is to be taken not as absence of fear but as boastful behaviour.

5. *The symptom expressed with spontaneity, clarity and intensity is of highest value.*

So, watch out for symptoms which go beyond the direct response to specific questions. For example, if you ask a patient: "Do you weep easily?", and he answers: "Yes, especially when I see others suffering!", there you can get a hint that the patient is sympathetic or sensitive.

6. *If the patient is markedly irresolute, this symptom will be best elicited when you ask him about cravings and aversions.*

It will take him a long time to answer because he has to come to a decision, and not simply state a fact.

7. *Try to confirm the essential parameters of the person.*

These components will be the same in all situations, only their expression will be different. So, you must use your imagination as to how these essentials could manifest. For example, if you think a person is timid when appearing in public, ask him about all the possible situations where this could become evident, like public speaking, parties, etc.

8. *Try as much as possible to avoid asking the patient directly about his nature.*

Try to lead him through other questions to express it without being conscious of doing so. In South India there is a proverb that we must go in as smoothly and inconspicuously as a needle in a banana.

9. *If you cannot elicit characteristic symptoms in the patient's present state, you have to go back to the time when the last characteristics existed.*

You can look for this in three situations:
– Characteristics after a stressful situation;
– Characteristics of illness before medication;
– If both are not present, then elicit the characteristic features of the patient in childhood.

10. *I give a standard questionnaire form which asks questions about the patient's past history, present complaints with modalities, etc., personal and psychosocial history.*

I have found it very useful for the following reasons:
– The patient gets prepared to answer your kind of questions.
– Sometimes the patient can express some problems more freely in writing.
– It gives you the chance to go directly into homoeopathically relevant questioning rather than losing time in irrelevant details, for example chief complaints, treatments, etc.

11. *The expression of characteristics can often be easily provoked.*

For example by making the patient wait beyond his time of appointment: Is he patient or impatient, mild or rigid, or is he restless or calm?

12. *Beginners in Homoeopathy often feel the need to put question after question; especially if the patient stops talking, they immediately ask the next question. This should be avoided.*

Most patients bring out the best symptoms if you give a pause after the answer. When you ask a question, the patient will give an answer immediately. After this, if you give a pause, he will think about his answer and then may modify or even completely change it. Sometimes, he may say something very spontaneously and this may be most significant. So, a pause means a doctor is telling the patient:

- I am not trying to get answers but I want to understand you.
- Tell me everything.
- I want to know and I am going to give you enough time.

13. *The patient should feel that the doctor is someone who cares, whom he can trust and to whom he can reveal everything: only then will he really open up.*

14. *What the patient asks you is more important than what you ask him.*

Many symptoms like anxiety about health, superstitious fears, fixed ideas, suspiciousness or impatience, can be easily judged from the patient's questions. For example, if you visit a patient with a high temperature who says: "Doctor, how soon will my temperature come down, so that I can get back to my business immediately?" The patient has a high temperature, lack of appetite, tremendous weakness and the whole family feels anxious about his health, and his only question is when he can join his business again. That becomes a highly characteristic feature of him.

15. *If you come to a dead end in case taking and just do not know how to make the patient talk, just ask him to describe one typical day in his life, his routine from morning to night, you will find many leads from this narration.*

33

TECHNIQUES OF CASE TAKING

Case taking is so easy and yet it is a most artistic and skillful procedure. In case taking, the internal state of the person in front of you is gradually revealed. It is a very interesting and fascinating experience, as much as it is fascinating to know yourself. There are really no standard techniques or fixed rules in case taking. It is just an effort to understand the person in front of you and one can use any technique to suit one's temperament. I sometimes joke with students that, if necessary you can even take the patient out for dinner in order to know everything about him! As long as you are able to feel the patient's feelings, whatever technique you use is good enough, but in my practice I have evolved certain techniques that have helped me immensely. These techniques are the practical application of all the ideas that have been mentioned in the various chapters of this book. I have tried to collect them all together here and to illustrate their utility in the clinic. For a fuller understanding the reader is advised to refer to the original chapters themselves. None of these techniques is absolute nor compartmentalized. They are all interlinked. Naturally, they have certain things in common. They are not to be followed like a rule book, one after another, rather you will often need to jump from one to another. You can devise your own techniques. It is not necessary to use all the techniques in every case. As we go through these techniques one by one, I shall give examples and explanations.

Observation

It is the most important and useful technique and the one that needs to be developed the most. In fact, if we train ourselves well, many a time observation alone is enough to know the patient. It begins right from the time the patient makes the appointment, or when you meet him outside the clinic situation. Observation has to be totally unprejudiced, which is why Hahnemann used the expression "unprejudiced observer", and by so doing, he laid down the most difficult condition. In fact, I can even say that if you have learned to be an unprejudiced observer, you have learned how to live and how to relate, because we always judge the present from the view point of the past. This is prejudice. When we see something, we link it to a similar experience in the past and we say this must be like that, and thus we deny ourselves the experience of something totally new. The person in front of us is absolutely unique, and our present experience with him is also for the first time. With this in mind, we have to observe without interpreting his actions hastily into this or that remedy or idea. The day we start fitting people into categories (remedies) and we think we know people before we really observe, that day we have become useless as homoeopaths.

So, what do you observe? Basically you observe what is it in this person that makes him an individual, what is it that makes him different from other people. For example, the way he makes an appointment. One patient will say: "Doctor, I would be so grateful if you could see me", and another will say: "Doctor, I must see you immediately." There is a difference in these two ways of asking, which shows the state of mind at that time. Observe how he conducts himself, how he has filled in the questionnaire, how punctual he is, how he is dressed, how he enters, how he sits – at the edge of the chair or behind, what his hands are doing, what his feet are doing, his facial expressions, his manner of communication and how he reacts to the person he has come with. If he has brought some medical files, how well he has arranged them, how he has brought them, has he brought them at all. Every single thing has to be observed: his movements, his postures, his speech, the way he explains himself and what atmosphere he creates in the room. None of them really indicate the remedy, but the state and frame of the patient's mind. This will be confirmed by other information later, but during this initial observation, looking and feeling are important.

One good way to begin an interview is to put your observation back to the patient and ask him if he is experiencing this. From here you can get straight into the heart of the case. For example, you might say: "You seem to be tense, what is bothering you?", or "You seem to be in a hurry." He is caught unaware and the answer spontaneously jumps out; now, if you attempt to go behind the answers, you will straightaway find something very deep in his personality.

I had an interesting experience in Germany, when I was in the clinic of one of my colleagues there and she was interviewing the patient in German, a language I do not understand. Yet I was able to tell the remedy. This experience I have had several times especially in non-English speaking countries. Even in my clinic there are people who speak languages I do not understand. You just have to develop this kind of observation. In children especially, observation plays an important role.

I will mention one case where observation helped me in prescribing. It was the case of a twenty-four year old unmarried girl who worked as a research scientist in a research institute. She presented with a chronic cough. I observed that her hands were very restless and along with this she would glance from side to side to see if anyone else was in the room. Even though she easily gave a lot of physical complaints, when I came to her mind, she would become silent and again glanced around, saying little and answering "No" to most questions. This whole attitude – secretive, glancing from side to side with restless hands – was noticed by me and gave me the idea that she was behaving like a criminal. The rubrics are:

— Restless hands;

— Answers in monosyllable, "No" to all questions; and

— Delusion, she has committed a crime.

From these I came to the remedy *Kalium bromatum*. There is another rubric "Delusion, thieves, accused of robbing", *Kalium bromatum* too!

246

Then I asked her: "Why are you so scared. What have you done that is making you so worried?" She was taken aback and told me how she was in love with a scientist from the same institution and this was not approved of by their parents and so they had to keep it all a secret. This was surprising because both were independent and could just have announced it and got married. She felt as though she was committing a crime and that others would find out. I gave her *Kalium bromatum*. She did well and ultimately got married to that man. My observation was confirmed when I asked what her interests and hobbies were – she liked to knit and play the sitar, which involves the use of hands. She liked to keep busy mentally and physically, especially with her hands.

In conclusion, observation is aimed at trying to understand the state of mind of the person. The observation has to be accurate. If you see a restless child ask what kind of restlessness is there in the child – does he want to change place or is it the restlessness of touching things or changing occupation, or is it restlessness of a kind in which he wants to be carried about? What feeling could lie behind his restlessness? Such accurate and sensitive observation is the sign of a good homoeopath. That is why Hahnemann wrote in Aphorism 211 about observation:

> "This holds true to such an extent that the state of disposition often chiefly determines the choice of the homoeopathic remedy, being a decidedly characteristic symptom that can least of all remain hidden from the accurately observing physician."

He places so much emphasis on observation.

Mode of narration of complaint

If you develop sensitivity to hearing the patient's manner of narrating his complaint, you will often be able to prescribe on this technique to the exclusion of all others. It will show his state of mind and his attitude towards his illness. Usually this attitude towards his illness is representative of his general attitude and his emotional state. Different people will react to the same illness in different ways and this will be in tune with their mental states. I can even say that most of us use illness to further our mental state. Or in other words, the state that we are furthering represents our true state. If we take a simple example like tonsillitis, a patient having acute pain in the tonsils could react in a number of ways. His attitude can be any of the following; he could say:

– This can lead to cancer.
– I am interrupted at my work by this pain.
– I need support.
– How unlucky I am that this is happening to me.
– How will the task in my hand get completed?
– If I miss work due to this pain, what will the boss say to me?

In most of these attitudes, anxiety about health could be a common feature. But there could be other attitudes like: "This is due to my past karma", or "The pain is so severe that I don't feel like working", or " I need to become extra cautious to avoid this in future." To find out what is the basic attitude, one has to ask further and further non-leading questions. For example, if there is anxiety about health, we have to find out why there is anxiety about health. Sometimes this comes out by itself from the casual remarks of the patient, but most often from the patient's questions and doubts. If we keep this in mind, this idea about the patient's attitude to illness, then we will be very alert for any such incidental remarks. We need to observe the words that he uses to describe his complaint.

Case n. 1

I had the case of a lady who had an intense sciatic pain. I learned that she was a college professor and was being troubled by her senior in some ways, and she had to protest about this. She was very sincere in her work. So, taking the features, namely, sincerity, niceness and the occasional sudden explosion of anger from a feeling of injustice, I gave her *Staphysagria* which did not work.

I saw her again and this time she said: "Doctor, this pain is troubling me so much. It is not allowing me to do my duty." As she felt that she was being troubled by the leg and due to this trouble she was not able to perform her duties for which she felt guilty, I took the rubrics: "Delusion, that he is persecuted", "Delusion, that she has neglected her duty" and "Anxiety of conscience, as if guilty of a crime". Through this process of thought I came to the remedy *Cyclamen* which ameliorated her pain immediately.

Case n. 2

Another case was of a boy who had a stammer and said: "I just don't know how I am going to get out of this stammering habit." I interpreted this to mean: I am now trapped, I am making an effort to get out of this trap alone and I have to help myself out. (He could have said: "Doctor, this habit is so embarrassing and only you can make me well", or "Doctor, how did this start and how long will it take to go away?") I took the rubrics: "Fear of narrow places", "Delusion, succeed, he cannot", "Delusion, deserted, forsaken, he is", "Restlessness, anxious, compelling rapid walking" and I arrived at *Argentum nitricum*. This is how an *Argentum nitricum* patient will usually complain.

Case n. 3

I remember seeing a case with my colleague in his clinic. A lady had a varicose ulcer and she wanted to know whether Homoeopathy could help. My colleague told her that it could but she was not satisfied with the answer. She said she wanted to know if he was sure that it can help. He said that nobody can guarantee but she can try out for a month and see how it works. She was afraid it may bleed in a month because the surgeon had told her so, and hence had advised surgery. My colleague said, if she is so afraid of bleeding, then she can go in for surgery. Then she added that her friend had told her that after surgery the ulcer may reappear again. At this my colleague asked why she was not waiting then. She was about to reply when I saw that my colleague was getting irritated and intervened. I could see that her main state of mind was her inability to trust anyone. I therefore took the rubrics:

— Suspicious, mistrustful;

— Restless, anxious;

— Anxiety about health;

— Fear of death...

Arsenicun album.

What I am trying to illustrate is how the casual remarks and the way the patient approaches us can give us leading indications in prescribing.

Typical of the way a *Bryonia* patient will conduct himself when he comes for consultation is that he will speak to the doctor as if he is talking to his financial or legal adviser, and you will get the impression that his health is a matter involving a business deal. For example, when told he has a bad prognosis, he will typically sit back in the chair with arms folded, stiff and stern, and will ask very unemotionally and dryly: "So, doctor, what options are there open to me now?", as if he is dealing with a business crisis. Here we could take the rubrics:

— Delirium, business, talks of;

— Business, talks of;

— Delusion, business, he is doing;

— Determined (Phatak's Repertory).

Case n. 4

A woman thirty-thirty-five year old came with asthma. She was telling about her complaint in great detail and with many fears, fear of ghosts, dogs, etc. In her case I took the rubric: "Fear in children". Why did I do so? Because her manner of talking and her fears were like those of a child. In this way I have used a lot of rubrics that are to do with children. I have used rubrics in adults like:

— Irritability in children (irritability as of a child);

— Fear in children (fear like a child);

— Obstinate children (obstinate like a child);

— Religious affections in children (religious like a child).

I have also applied the rubric, "Desire to be carried", in adults. This rubric means that he desires to put all his weight on someone else's shoulders and would like that person to bear the whole burden. When I find that a person puts the whole burden on someone, as if his feet are too tired to support him, then I use this rubric even if he is an adult.

Accompaniments to the suffering

The state of mind that is produced during pain or suffering is often the state of mind of the patient in an uncompensated form. For example, a patient with a skin eruption may shriek: "This pain is too severe, please do something or cut off my leg!" We see here violence, shrieking, abusive and want of support. This is a state of *Chamomilla*. These accompaniments are most important in case taking as they enable us to get a good picture of the patient. In the West, I have experienced people talking in terms of depression, or inferiority complex for example, but without really talking of their true, untainted feelings; and so observation and the accompaniments of the sufferings are useful because they cannot make a fool of you.

A villager is able to give mental symptoms more exactly. He will say: "Doctor, I get so angry I feel like stabbing someone with a knife", but the executive from a multi-national company with the same feeling will understate it and say: "I am a little irritable but that is required in this profession, otherwise, I will not be able to get my work done."

Case

I remember a case of asthma which was not responding to treatment because she had hardly any mental state symptoms during the attack-free period, and during the attacks, she would take allopathic bronchodilators and get relieved. I had to admit her to the hospital and observe her during acute episodes. I found that during the episodes, which usually occurred at night, she would develop tremendous anxiety and fear of death by suffocation. We also found that she was not willing to talk and was quite reserved. One of the physical concomitants she developed was very marked hoarseness and loss of voice for no apparent reason. On the whole, we found her very mild, and quite indolent. She was worse lying down, worse during sleep from which she would get up during an attack of breathlessness. She was timid, restless during the paroxysms and wanted open air. Now, if we forget her physical complaint altogether and just consider her mental state, what symptoms do we have? We have:

- Anxiety at night;
- Anxiety, open air ameliorates;
- Anxiety with fear;
- Anxiety during sleep;
- Anxiety on waking;
- Fear at night;
- Fear of suffocation;
- Fear of suffocation at night;
- Frightened at night;
- Mildness;
- Reserved;
- Restlessness at night:

- Starting;
- Starting from sleep;
- Talk, indisposed to;
- Timidity.

When we look at these symptoms, the remedy which emerges is *Spongia* and *Spongia* was confirmed from Phatak's Materia Medica, where he begins his paragraph on respiration with: "Hoarseness with many complaints". Also he gives: "Fear of suffocation". This case gave us a hint that if this girl has cough at night and that produces anxiety and fear of suffocation, then she must have a mental state which has anxiety at night and fear of suffocation.

Interests and hobbies

This includes everything that a patient does in his or her spare time. We are not just referring to things like stamp collecting, but everything that the patient feels good doing (such as music, dance, fiction, painting, knitting, jogging, being with people, gossiping). You need to ask what would give him the biggest thrill or most happiness. What would you enjoy doing the most? Why? What does that interest involve? What appeals to you in that interest? It is important because a profession is often chosen because of skill and talent, but hobbies are chosen according to one's mental framework. Therefore, they bring out uncompensated behaviour. Compensated behaviour is like a wound up spring. When the patient needs to relax he will do exactly the opposite. People enjoy travelling because they feel free and uncompensated at that time. In another land or even when out in other towns or villages, you can do exactly the opposite of what you are bound to do in your own city or accustomed environment.

Different people compensate for different things depending upon the state of mind they are in. In a city the *Rhus toxicodendron* person will have problems because he needs a lot of activity, exercise and space to move, so he likes to go out and have a holiday where there is a lot of space, whereas this is not necessary for a *Calcarea carbonica* person. An activity a person enjoys the most is likely to be one in which he can be free and uncompensated the most. The need for such an interest shows that he is compensating in his routine activity, and the qualities of that interest will show features of that uncompensated state.

Case

A boy of twenty years came for consultation for his asthma. In the second or third consultation he revealed that he was faced with a serious problem. He could not decide whether to talk to a particular girl or not to talk to her. He explained the situation and I could see that he had tremendous irresolution. He wanted me to take the decision for him. Going into his case further, I asked him about his interests and hobbies. He said that he liked to watch movies. When asked what type of movies, he said: "Horror movies." He described to me a movie that was really horrible. It was about ripping open somebody's abdomen by an extraterrestrial creature and vomiting in it and passing on the corpse to someone else to do the same thing. The narration of the whole incident was quite horrifying, but the boy was narrating it in a very calm manner. I asked him whether, after seeing such a movie, he felt frightened or sleepless. He said: "No, Doctor, on the contrary, I get better sleep after such movies." Hence I took the following rubrics:

— Unfeeling, hard-hearted;
— Moral feeling, want of;
— Irresolution;
— Will, contradiction of.

I prescribed *Anarcadium* for him. Of course, two more relevant rubrics were:
— Confidence, want of self;
— Cruelty.

This case shows how interests and hobbies represent one's uncompensated state of mind.

For example, *Kalium bromatum* likes to keep hands busy with activities like knitting, painting, typing which appeal to him because these activities help him uncompensate for the restlessness of hands. The thing that appeals to you the most may also be the one opposite to you, just as opposite people attract each other. This would be a complementary relationship. A coward will like to read and fantasize about courage. Who needs to fantasize? It is a person who cannot do it in real life. The king will read about beggars, and beggars would rather see a movie about kings. You must be careful not to get confused over this.

Patient's nature as a child

We can understand the mind of the patient in an uncompensated form if we know how he was as a child, because in childhood he compensated much less. You may be able to find in him the same nature now as in childhood but in a more compensated way. The remedy is often the same. You can use his nature as a child as a clue to understanding his nature now.

Case

There was a friend of mine, a lean man with a bald head, who was very sociable, diplomatic and got along well with everybody. I guessed that this man would need *Phosphorus*. I took the history and there was craving for ice-cream, chilliness and a helpful nature. When I asked him about his nature as a child, he said he was tense before exams, and shy. My whole perception of him changed and I gave him *Silicea*. This sociability was a heavy compensation for his shyness and self-consciousness. The uncompensated state comes out by asking about one's nature in childhood. Unless there has been a radical change, you can even rely on the childhood picture to prescribe, if the picture right now is not so clear. Childhood symptoms, like being obstinate, mischievous, yielding, going against parents, shy, courageous can be used in the adult if there is still a hint of them.

Typical behaviour

There are certain things which the patient does that will characterize him. If you ask a relative, he will begin by saying: "Just the other day..." These elements show his uncompensated nature. A patient rang up: "Doctor, I want to know the exact time I can meet you because I cannot wait." A relative says he is so restless, he typically gets into the wrong bus since he cannot even wait to see if he is getting into the right bus. He walks very fast. The remedy is *Histaminum* because of: "Restlessness, from waiting", "Hard walking ameliorates mental symptoms" and "Quarrelsome".

Case n. 1

A six year old child was looking down from a window and threw a pebble on another child one floor below. This typified him; to throw, to strike, to destroy and the cunning nature – all fit in *Tarentula*.

Case n. 2

One man said: "When I was riding my motorcycle I was thinking so much of my future that I forgot to turn at the right turning and went four or five kilometers ahead before I realized my mistake." This is *Spigelia*, because of the rubric: "Absorbed, buried in thought, about future". So, out of typical behaviour, we can come to know the state of mind.

Example

Take the example of Mother Theresa. When asked whether she will continue to go to work in spite of fever, she replied in a way typical of her. She said: "Is it not better to burn in this life than in the next?" This one sentence has so many components:
- Delusion, neglected his duty, he has;
- Conscientious about trifles;
- Industrious;
- Religious;
- Answers in questions;
- Contradiction, intolerant of;
- Obstinate.

Her remedy could be *Aurum metallicum.*

Reactions in life situations

How the person has reacted in times of stress and strain in his life. The true nature comes out in times of stress; whether he is bold or timid, whether he wants to escape or

253

stand up and fight, or is suicidal and depressed, or elated and joyous. I believe that the nature of reaction during and after a stressful situation reveals the uncompensated state of the person more than at other times.

Case n. 1

The owner of a soap factory had four daughters and a son. He came with diabetes which started after the death of his son in an accident. I asked him how he reacted and he said he could not even cry as he was in a state of shock. He was now anxious as to "What will happen to my daughters in case I die?" The reaction to that stress was: "Anxiety for others", "Anxiety for his family", "Fear as if something will happen", "Cautious, anxiously". I came to *Causticum*. There was grief and sadness, but anxiety for others was much more intense.

Similarly, after a business loss or disappointment in love, what are the feelings that come up? At that time one's specific not-OK feelings can often be seen more clearly and from this it becomes easier to identify the mental state. Of course, you must make sure that the state you have identified is the basic state of the patient and that it persists, albeit in a compensated form, at all times.

Case n. 2

A man aged around sixty years, a famous radio programme personality, used to come to the clinic. He was very buoyant in his attitude, was quite talkative and made a show of himself as if talking on the stage – quite a confident looking person. This man developed a lung problem. It was suspected to be tuberculosis; so he was advised bronchoscopy. The day before undergoing bronchoscopy, he rang me up, talking as if he was almost collapsing. He rang up seven times that day. Based on the behaviour, I found his remedy to be *Gelsemium*, something that was eluding me in the past, because I had given him *Sulphur* and other remedies.

The symptoms indicating *Gelsemium* were:
- Extreme fear of surgery; so: Ailments from anticipation;
- Anticipation, physician, dentist, before going to;
- Fear, of death;
- Fear, happen, something will;
- Ailments from fright;
- Clinging (seven phone calls);
- Company, desire for;
- Confidence, want of self;
- Cowardice.

Gelsemium not only helped his lung problem but also a joint trouble which he had subsequently developed.

Central feelings of the patient

What are the feelings of the patient that are revealed by his various expressions? The patient says a lot of things, but where do they all come from?

Case n. 1

For example, a girl said: "Doctor, why are you not giving special attention to my case? What have I done?" Here you can see quarrelsomeness and lamenting, but what is the feeling? Her feeling is that she is not being appreciated, in comparison with others, a feeling of being neglected and jealousy. I gave her *Calcarea sulphurica*. For details of this case, the reader is referred to the chapter on "Delusions".

Case n. 2

The next was an interesting case I had treated in my early practice. It was a boy, who, when I was taking his case, said that he was very ambitious. He liked to go on long walk alone, and thirdly he was very lazy. I gathered the impression that he was a very timid person. Therefore, I first put together the four things:

- Timid;
- Lazy;
- Ambitious;
- Takes long walks alone.

Then I began to wonder what does an ambitious but a lazy and timid person do when he takes long walks. Then I got the idea that he must be fantasizing or theorizing. From this situation I concluded that his central feeling is that of a person who only fantasizes but does not do anything to fulfil his dreams. I took then the rubrics:

— Theorizing;
— Indolent;
— Timidity;
— Cowardice.

The remedy that helped him was *China*. Of course, I confirmed those rubrics from him. What I am trying to show here is how the symptoms are not just mere symptoms, how when we put them together, we immediately get the impression through our human understanding of what must be his deep subconscious thoughts.

Case n. 3

A lady developed a problem of pain in the shoulder and inability to move her joints after the death of a neighbour. I could have taken it as "Ailments from grief" but I found that this lady was quite a reserved and shy type, and the neighbour was the only person in the building with whom she was able to communicate because the neighbour spoke the same language as the patient. From this, I got the impression that the death of the neighbour had created an anxiety in this lady as if she had lost a crutch, a support; so, I took the rubrics:

— Delusion, he walks on knees;

— Delusion, legs are cut off;

— Fear of strangers (because she was unable to face new people; she wanted to be in the company of familiar people only).

I also took the rubric: "Delusion, beloved, dying".

Who is the person who will have this delusion? It is the person who is tremendously dependent upon the friend. Of course, in this case the friend was actually dead, but we want to discover the personality of this lady – she is a type of woman who is so dependent on her friend that the smallest trouble to the friend will make her feel: "If my friend dies, what will happen to me?" There is:

— Anxiety, others, for;

— Anxiety, trifles, about;

— Confidence, want of self.

All the feelings represented by these rubrics reveal inferiority, a feeling of dependence. I gave her *Baryta carbonica*, which helped.

Dreams

These represent uncompensated feelings because here one's will and morality are at their weakest, and one's feelings come out through symbols. When dreams are placed alongside other observations about the patient, they can show a sharp contrast and these can be integrated into a "picture of the person". A person who is nice, good and saintly has dreams of violence and bloodshed. The boy who felt trapped had dreams of being in a vast area whose boundary he could not see and he was running helter-skelter trying to get out. These dreams represent his frame of mind – fear of narrow places (even though in the dream it is a vast space), of being trapped in it, anxiety, restlessness and failure to get out; all fit into *Argentum nitricum.*

The state of mind of the mother during pregnancy

In a large number of children and adults too, the state of the mother during pregnancy is duplicated, especially if that state was very intense.

Case n. 1

In a case of *Lyssinum*, the mother, during pregnancy, was furious with the Goddess and she was agitated and violent in her expression, with a very severe toothache. In her son, almost since birth, there was a skin eruption. When he came to me (at the age of ten), he was violent with the Goddess because of his dermatitis. The mother's exact state was duplicated and he did well on *Lyssinum* (for details of this case, see chapter: "Unsuitable Reactions"). Similarly, *the state of the mother and of the father at the time of conception* can give many clues.

Intense, real and extreme situations faced in the life of the patient

These are what I call "epidemic situations", since an epidemic is due to an intense exciting cause that can produce a similar effect in a large majority of the population. Such situations have the same effect on most human beings, no matter what their original nature was. For example, if a bomb is going to blast, most will react in the same way. You must carefully search the childhood history to see if he has gone through such intense situations.

Case

This patient had been brought up in his childhood in his aunt's house. He was treated very badly there, but he could not do anything about it. He passed through this condition for twelve years and felt helpless, unfortunate and tortured. After this he became an Air Force officer for thirty years and then retired. After retirement, at the age of sixty, he did not opt to do anything and spent his time drinking and reading books on communist philosophy. He liked to talk and discuss politics with friends. The only other point in his history was that he was much affected by the death of his mother at a very young age. He still weeps when he thinks of her. He says he was very much attached to her.

We have enough clues for *China*, here, namely:
- Indolence;
- Theorizing;
- Sentimental;
- Dipsomania;
- Timidity (he can only read communist philosophy but has no courage to do anything about it).

But most of these symptoms are in *Sulphur* too. We need some more points for confirmation. Here it is very helpful to know that he passed through a typical *China* situation in his childhood, with the tormented, persecuted feeling, the unfortunate feeling, and with the timidity and indolence too.

What feeling the patient creates in you

There are two things that can happen to you in the presence of the patient. At one level, you can react from your own state and you will find some things are agreeable and some others are disagreeable in the patient. You can understand some things but there are some things which you cannot. All this will depend on your own conditions for feeling OK. If you know these conditions and if you have some understanding of your own state, then you can ask yourself what it is in the patient that makes you react in the way you do. So, if you are getting angry, or you are falling in love, or getting bored or annoyed, then what does it tell you about the patient?

The second level is to remain still and silent inside and observe the feeling that is generated by the presence of the patient. If you can look beyond your own state and its reactions, you will find that you can mirror the patient's state in your own mind, not intellectually but through your sensitivity. You can experience the feeling of the patient, a process that is known as empathy.

It would be interesting to see, also, what kind of patients are attracted to you as a physician, and especially which ones stick to you. Usually you find that they belong to states which are complementary to yours, and you will observe this complementary relationship often in practice.

In this connection, it is interesting to note what you involuntarily tell the patient during or at the conclusion of the interview. This is often a reflection of the patient's own state. For example, if you tell him: "Don't be afraid, nothing will happen", it could mean that the patient has fear of something happening, even though he might not have expressed this feeling in so many words. Similarly, the advice like: "Don't worry, I will help you through", reflects the patient's dependent feeling.

In conclusion, I may say that it is at least as rewarding to look at ourselves during the interview as it is to observe the patient.

What are the qualities in others and in yourself that you cannot tolerate or understand?

These questions will bring out mental symptoms in their uncompensated form. When we ask the patient this question, several of his own features come out clearly and much more easily than when we ask him to talk about himself. Let us find out how to use this information. Normally what we cannot tolerate in other people are their actions which make us unhappy. When somebody says: "I cannot tolerate his indifference to his family", it means, I want him to be caring, and then I will feel OK.

Such an enquiry will lead us to examine the patient's conditions for feeling OK. That is, what he needs to be and what he needs others to be, in order to feel OK. The information about what he needs to be can also come from the question: What is it in others that you cannot understand? Usually, the qualities we cannot understand in others are the opposite of those which are compulsive behaviour for us. For example, if we are fastidious, then we will not be able to understand how someone can be sloppy. A single question that we can ask the patients is: "Describe any person/relative/friend, and the qualities in him that you cannot tolerate or that you detest." The person will then make a list of the various things in others that he cannot tolerate, cannot understand, cannot appreciate, cannot approve of. Usually, these are the very things which he cannot tolerate in himself and he has the compulsive need for the opposite quality. This need is a part of his state and is therefore his uncompensated symptom.

One answer could be: "I cannot tolerate a person who is slow, dull, unambitious and lazy, and who does not do his job well." This shows that the state originally comes from a situation that demands the opposite, namely higher intelligence, ambition, conscientiousness, and industriousness. On the whole, this is a very easy way to get a case because it gives a chance for a person to criticize others (which he does not mind doing) and incidentally reveals his own nature.

Another important question is: "When are you angry with yourself?" The answer represents the conditions he has to fulfil in order to feel OK. Together both these questions will give you all the conditions for his OKness.

All the conditions that we impose on ourselves and others usually come from our own feelings or fears. For example, if we are afraid of being alone, we impose a condition on others that they should be with us all the time and we cannot tolerate if they go away. If we have a fear that we shall misplace something vital, then we shall be overly careful and fastidious. Such feelings (sensations) and compulsions (functions or actions) arise from our perception of the situation (basic delusion).

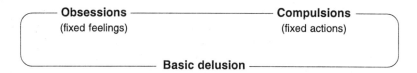

We have to try to understand the case from the above two angles, namely sensations and functions, so that we can perceive what the basic delusion is. It is in the understanding of the conditions or compulsions that the question about what you cannot tolerate or understand in others becomes extremely useful.

To add one incidental point, the qualities which we like and dislike in any person usually come from the same source. For example, we like somebody's achievement but we do not like that he is not caring and affectionate. If we look at it, both are two sides of the same coin but we accept only one side and so have problems in relationships. What we accept or cannot accept is due to our own conditions.

What does the physical state indicate?

The physical and mental state are parts of the same underlying state. In fact, as we observe more, the differences between the physical and the mental lessen and ultimately disappear. If you want to confirm your impression about the mental state, you have to find out what the physical state indicates. If a person is mild, soft, yielding and quiet, and if you find characteristic physical pains which are violent, sharp and darting, and if these pains are indicative of the central state of the person, then you have to reconsider your assessment of that mild, yielding state. In fact, you can even go the other way and ask what quality of mind does the physical characteristics indicate. If you see violence in the

259

body or restlessness or stubbornness or acute outbursts in the body, these are also to be used as symptoms indicating a mental state.

Person's occupation and area of work

It is important to know whether he has selected the occupation himself or circumstances made him choose it. In any case, how does he function in his area of work and what branch has he chosen? For example, if he is a doctor: is he a surgeon or homoeopath, and what kind of Homoeopathy or surgery does he practice? This indicates his nature. Look at the motivation involved. What is individual to a person is the important question we must ask.

Take homoeopaths for example. You can see so many differences among them in the way they do Homoeopathy. Some practice the intuitive way, they feel things almost through extrasensory perception ("Clairvoyance"). Some ridicule them ("Censorious") and do it the mechanical way, taking each and every symptom into account ("Conscientious about trifles", "Fastidious"). Some wants shortcuts ("Indolence"), others want rules ("Irresolution"). Some will keep changing the prescription ("Capriciousness"), others will stubbornly stick to it, insisting they cannot be wrong ("Egotism", "Obstinate"). Some are very careful to select a low potency ("Cautious"), some do not mind giving the high one straightaway ("Rash", "Defiant"). Just the way an individual practices Homoeopathy reveals a lot about his nature. Which books he uses, which teachers he follows, what hours he works, what kind of cases he likes to see, what else does he do in the profession besides practice, which groups he associates with; literally everything has components of his nature. This applies to all professions.

The idea in relationships

A man will form a relationship with a person or a group that is complementary to him by nature. By complementary we mean that it is opposite to his nature and fits him like a key into a lock. The lock and key will have opposite qualities. Man forms a balance in a system and we must see his part in that balance. This balance is subjective and individual. For example, when I do a seminar, a balance is formed between myself and the audience. I want to speak and they to listen, I want to teach and they to learn, I lead and they follow. It is a disease when my need to dominate or to be a speaker is my condition for feeling OK. Mother Teresa is responsible, moral and industrious. She will make a balance by choosing to do something that requires morality and religion and gives her the feeling of doing her duty.

The situations that the patient has created in his life

What kind of script is he writing? Which actors is he choosing to play the other parts? Usually the kind of situation the patient will set up will closely resemble the original situation from which all his feelings arise. In fact, in a chronic case, he will set up a very similar situation in his life to the one in which in his imagination he has already reacted.

This gives him security and confidence that his delusion is absolutely correct. A *Lycopodium* man will marry a *Pulsatilla* woman, and will say: "How can I survive if I don't dominate because she will do nothing by herself. I have to dominate." *One reason why children are more easily curable than adults is because they have not set up situations to encourage or aggravate their state.*

Interview with friends and relatives

It would be useful to confirm our impression of the patient by interviewing the people who have known him for some time. It would be ideal to do this at length but if time is short, or we believe we already have an accurate picture of the patient, then what we can do is to ask the friend or relative to describe the patient's nature by using four words to indicate four important features. When we hear these words, if they fit in with our understanding of the patient, then we can be sure. But if there is the slightest difference in the quality of our understanding from what the relative tells us, then we have to go into much more detail with him.

The best technique

The best technique is not to use any of the above techniques directly, but to watch what happens spontaneously. Indeed, the best case taking is done through silence, not questions. The above eighteen techniques are to be used consciously only if you reach a dead end and do not know how to proceed further.

The way the patient follows up

If we keep our minds open even after making a prescription, we can get a lot of information from the way the patient follows up the treatment. Some of them will come only when there is pain. Such people are likely to say: "Doctor, cure me later, but ease my suffering first" ("Indifference, recovery, to" and "Fear, suffering, of"). Some patients will come and say: "Doctor, I think the medicine was too strong for me, so I stopped it after the first dose" ("Delusion, glass, she is made of", "Frail, sensation of being"). You will get a patient who says: "Doctor, I have written datewise what happened after the remedy" ("Carefulness").

I could give several examples, but the point I wish to make is that the case taking process never ends. It has to continue each time the patient comes to you. Even the way he reports the reaction to the remedy is part of the case taking process.

34

THE ESSENCE OF CASE TAKING

In Aphorism 83, Hahnemann says:

> "The individualizing examination of a case of disease demands of
> the physician nothing but freedom from prejudice and sound senses,
> attention in observing and fidelity in tracing the picture of the disease."

"Freedom from prejudice" are the most important words he has used and this is also probably the most difficult condition he has laid down. A good homoeopath is one who will be the least prejudiced. Prejudice means judging the present on the basis of past experiences, which leads to a fixity and rigidity of thinking. Prejudice arises because of our insecurity and unwillingness to be in the moment; because it feels unsafe to live in the present. Prejudice represents readymade solutions. It also comes from indolence, preventing us from really seeing what exists and observing carefully without any preconceptions. We can experience prejudice at every moment of our life. Whenever we look at something, an object, a person or a situation, we already have some thoughts about it. We look at one aspect of the situation, then we classify it and finally we fix it into a pattern that exists in our mind. We merely have to make one or two observations, look at one or two aspects, and already the assumption is that we know everything about it. This prejudice is bound to be there, but our ability to live in the moment depends on our ability to keep prejudice out.

Prejudice is like darkness, it cannot be pushed away. It can only be removed by bringing in light. Light is the awareness.

The same applies when we look at ourselves. Again we experience preconceived notions about ourselves and these prevent us from knowing who we really are and what is going on within us. In the same way these notions prevent us from really seeing what is going on outside and in other people. To be unprejudiced demands letting things be as they are, and observing without fitting them into any category. Life demands this of us and so does Homoeopathy.

What do we require in order to take a case? Knowledge of Materia Medica and Repertory, of miasms, essences, Psychology and Pathology? In fact we are required to be fools, to know nothing. That is why Hahnemann wrote that disease requires individualization. It actually demands nothingness which is freedom from prejudice and sound senses. This means that all our senses, including our awareness and observation and the inner senses, have to be present at that time in that place totally. We have to be completely

263

focused. We need to focus our senses, attention and observation. To observe means to look without judgement, to witness without analysis. What do you observe? You observe things as they are without prejudice, seeing what is in front of you, what is around you and what is within you. Without preconceived notions, you observe what is going on at that moment. It means that like a sheet of glass, you are allowing everything to come to you exactly as it is, without colouring it, without making it bigger or smaller or removing anything.

Case taking demands that kind of stillness of mind, that kind of openness and space. If you are able to create this, then the case will come to you. The person sitting in front of you is unique, there was never anyone like him before nor will there be any anyone like him in the future. How exactly does he think, what are his exact feelings? We have to understand how he views his life and the space around him. This will come to you, not from intellectualization or analysis, nor from rationalization, but from unprejudiced observation; you can then perceive his exact and true feelings.

It is this perception of the state with its feelings and its expressions, both in the body and the mind, which will be translated into rubrics. Only after this will the remedy start appearing in your mind. If this method is followed, you will be a good case taker and if it is followed in life, you will have learned the secret of living, of relating and of communicating.

Ultimately, the way you take the case reflects the way you live, the way you think, the way you feel and the way you relate.

35

PERCEIVING

Most of the time we are trying to find the symptoms of the patient, and when we do so, our aim is to elicit a group of symptoms giving us a totality of the case. The symptoms we are trying to find are rather discrete; for example, we may have the symptoms: "Sympathetic", "Fastidious", "Desire for music", etc., and we say the remedy is *Carcinosinum*. In this list we may get "Sympathetic" from one incident, "Desire for music" from another and "Fastidious" from the third. We just combine these together and we are able to find a set of symptoms that fit into a particular remedy. This is one way of doing a case or one might say this is the common way of analyzing the case.

The idea of this chapter is to take us beyond this random listing of symptoms or random collection of symptoms into perceiving behind the expression of the patient, perceiving the whole totality of the case. One might say that behind every characteristic expression, there lies the entire totality of symptoms if we learn to perceive it that way. Going a bit further, I might add that the entire totality of symptoms is actually one symptom, i.e. to say it all comes from one single delusion. Let me give some examples.

Example n. 1

The simplest case that we can consider is of a woman who comes into the clinic and says: "Doctor, I phoned you up an hour ago to find out if I could come and you told me to come. I came, but you made me wait so long. Why do you do this to me?" She says this in a very friendly voice, in a kind of friendly quarrelsomeness, all the while sitting quite close to me. Then she carries on: "But where else can I go? I have only you as a support. If you tell me to come and wait, I have to wait."

The idea of this chapter is to show that perceiving begins with the first contact with the patient and those things that come from observation, that come involuntarily from the patient, that come not in response to questions, especially of the mental state, are the most important things. In this lady, we can see the way she speaks has got the kind of familiarity which is assumed with me. It is as if she is talking with a close relative or friend. Added to this, she says she has no choice but to do as I say, and that she will act as I instruct. The combination of symptoms we see in this patient is "Affectionate" and "Desire to be magnetized", which works out to *Phosphorus*. In this way one can see in this expression two important elements of the case being revealed.

When we go on to the next case, we shall find that if we are able to perceive, we will find many, many more expressions and symptoms or components in each expression.

Slowly we shall see that almost the entire totality of symptoms comes out from the characteristic expression of the patient.

Example n. 2

While leaving after the consultation, the patient asks: "Doctor, I have to ask you a very important thing. I plan to buy a machine to make wool in my house and I want to work on it. But, a few days earlier, I heard that somebody developed cancer by working on this type of machine. Doctor, tell me, should I buy the machine or should I not?"

In this expression, we see the entire case. On one side we see that she has been frightened by a story of cancer, so we might consider the rubric: "Horrible things, sad stories affect her profoundly". As a result of this horrible tale that has frightened her, she rushes to a person in authority and instead of just asking the pros and cons of the situation so that she can take the decision herself, she transfers her entire will into the person of authority and lets him take the decision for her. Again we see the "Desire to be magnetized". When we combine these two rubrics we get *Calcarea carbonica*. If we perceive a little bit further, we see that this fear is like the fear of a child. So, we might take the rubric: "Fear in children". And again, as a frightened child turns to somebody in authority, so you have the rubric: "Company, desire for; alone, when, aggravates". Seeking the security of a person in authority, the *Calcarea carbonica* personality likes to feel all the time protected like an oyster within its shell. In one expression of the patient, one can see the entire totality of the remedy.

Example n. 3

Talking about her dream, the patient says that she dreamt that she was going shopping with the most famous actress in the country. Now, behind this one dream lies a lot of significance. How do we interpret or use this dream? See the elements of the dream.

To go out for shopping with somebody means to be seen in public with that person. To be seen with a film actress in public and not only that, but to be seen shopping with her, it speaks of a kind of class. So, in her fantasy, she feels she should be of that class, for whom it would be quite common to go out shopping with such a famous personality.

So, we have the rubric "Egotism" and we have the idea of appearing in public and so "Timidity, appearing in public, when" and this indicates the remedy *Silicea*. This speaks of an image, that she is someone who has class, who goes out, mixes and rubs shoulders with the most famous people. Later on we shall see that the whole idea of *Silicea* is that it is a princess. It is the delusion of being a princess which very much fits into this dream.

The idea of this chapter is to show that we are not dealing with symptoms, but the patient's perception of the situation that lies behind every expression. It is this perception that we have to understand. If we do understand that, we shall see the entire totality in each expression.

Example n. 4

After mentioning several complaints, the patient points to the veins on the back of her hand and says: "Doctor, don't these veins appear more bluish than they should be?"

This is a very simple example. The main rubric would be: "Rest, cannot, until things are in their proper place", but added to this would be "Fastidiousness", "Carefulness" and "Cautious". The idea is that if she let these veins be a bit more bluish and if she did not bother about it, it would slowly increase and would finish her. So, she is very particular of the smallest detail and if anything appears a little bit out of order, she has to take note of it and correct it immediately. So, you have the rubrics: "Suspicious" and "Impatient", "Hurry" and "Restlessness, anxious". Here you see the entire gamut of *Arsenicum* symptomatology in one single expression. *Arsenicum*'s vision of reality is as if there are thieves at night unnoticed by him. You see the perception behind this expression.

Example n. 5

A new patient while entering the consultation room, pauses at the door and asks: "Doctor, should I leave my slippers at the door or can I wear them into the room?"

In my whole career, so far no patient has ever asked me this question before. One naturally assumes that in an office one can wear slippers and nobody even bothers to ask me if they have to be taken out. Therefore, it makes this expression of the patient extremely characteristic of her. It is our job to see what is her perception that made this expression possible. The first thing we can see is that she is careful and cautious, that she tries to find out what is the norm of the clinic before she does anything. Going behind, we see that she is being very careful and cautious because she does not want a reprimand from me, that she does not want to be admonished, that she could not do something that is not correct.

Therefore, behind "Carefulness" and "Cautiousness", we see "Sensitivity to reprimand" and "Sensitivity to be admonished". Now, behind this sensitivity is that if she will follow the rules properly, she will not be admonished. So, there is a desire to be always correct and always fair and following the rules. Behind this, one can perceive the whole of her delusion, which is that as long as she is following rules of the person in authority, she is OK. Her perception of reality is always that she is under somebody whom she has to obey and whom she has to follow. So, instead of looking at me as a doctor, she looks at me as her boss or as a person in authority, whose rules, just or unjust, have to be followed for fear of being admonished or punished. This is the idea of her delusion. The remedy was *Staphysagria.*

Example n. 6

Before I went on a trip to Europe, a patient came and said to me: "Doctor, please come back soon and for heaven's sake don't settle in Europe, since we will be lost without you."

Again, in this case one might be tempted to use the rubrics, but it is better and it is more important to be able to see what is the patient's view of the present situation that is making him say that. It is obvious that he feels frightened of being left alone just like a child lost in the wilderness and that the person who is to protect him or to support him goes away and betrays him. He will not come back and when he does not come back, he is finished and is left to the wild animals to be eaten. It is that idea of being frightened and alone in the dark in the night, in the forest with animals, in the terrorizing world with the only source of support going away, nobody to hold on to, nobody to protect him, that makes him shriek out and ask that I should come back as soon as possible. This might sound theoretical. But one has to observe the expression of the patient's face, the tone of his voice to be able to notice the urgency of his plea and the fear that makes it come out. The rubrics one could use are:

— Clinging;

— Praying;

— Delirium, crying, help, for;

— Fear of being alone at night;

— Delusion, that she is alone in the wilderness;

— Begging;

— Religious;

— Delusion, wife is faithless (wife, a trusted companion, will leave him and go away to somebody else).

In this way, from one expression, one can see the entire gamut of the symptoms that characterize a *Stramonium* state. The idea is not to point to the list of symptoms that one could derive from one expression, but it is to show that all these symptoms come from one single perception of reality and that one should be able to see the same perception behind all the symptoms and expressions and especially be able to see that even from one single expression one can get straightaway to the person's central delusion, to his central perception of reality, which is the heart of case taking.

To explain a bit further, one could say that now we can see that all symptoms of *Stramonium* are in fact one symptom. That there is no difference between the clinging of *Stramonium* and the religiousness of *Stramonium* and no difference between religiousness and praying, praying and begging, between begging and entreating, between entreating and fear of darkness, fear of darkness and desire for light and company. The whole *Stramonium* expression is actually one thing and it is one thing that we are trying to understand both in the patient and in the remedy, and not the conglomeration of symptoms that make the totality.

36

BRINGING OUT THE PATIENT'S PICTURE

How did you learn to bring out the picture? I have no questionnaire so I have to take all the mentals and physicals. I go into a lot of details in mentals. I get a lot of different pictures of many remedies. How do you grasp the picture of one remedy? It so happens that the better I know the patient the more difficult it becomes to prescribe for him. How did you learn to understand man in terms of a remedy, to make this connection?

Human behaviour usually cannot be reduced to one essence. It is too complex to be brought down to one point. It is multifaceted, but despite many facets it forms one picture. If you want to understand an object, for example ice, it has many qualities. It has coldness, hardness, transparency, colourlessness, the ability to melt. Now, if you ask which is the central point of ice – coldness, melting ability, etc. – you will find that there is no central point. There are many qualities that come together to form ice. These qualities come together in a very purposeful way to make something which has a particular utility, or something that fits a particular place or role. Similarly, with human and remedies. Each human or remedy is also made of unrelated qualities, but these qualities come together to make a picture that fits a particular place or role, that fulfills a particular purpose. We have to understand the picture. When the picture is grasped, the essential of the picture will automatically come up and the remedy will be easily seen.

I fully aggree but still I have difficulty. A man has different facets. He might have facets of a remedy, which are unknown to me. You are able to grasp the feeling that comes out clearly from many facets. How do you do this? Probably it is easier in India than in Europe, where I see that several remedies seem indicated in the same person.

The problem is that you are looking for facets. Look for the man and facets will come. In my experience with European patients, I did not have much difficulty.

Even if solely limiting to the mind?

Yes. No difficulty, no big differences, may be a few, but nothing obstructive, the method is the same. We have to stop being symptom collectors. We have to be patient or human understanders. The case does not have to be a conglomeration of symptoms but a trait of the patient. We have to be able to portray the patient and the essentials of him will come up. If we do not get lost in questions, the picture comes out on its own.

37

SELECTION OF THE REMEDY

A group of computers experts in Bombay asked me whether I could make an expert system. I was tempted to do so especially as I wondered whether I could systematize my own method of selecting the remedy. This gave me a chance to think about what I do, step by step. I shall attempt to put these thoughts into this chapter.

Image of the patient

The first thing I do when I see a patient is to observe everything about him. It is not only observation of details such as how he dresses, talks and walks but it is also the impression that he makes. As I go on with the case taking, I note his every gesture or act and every peculiarity of his nature as narrated in his history. Slowly, I build the picture of a person in mind and, in the formation of this image, I try to depend upon his uncompensated features.

Initially, his general appearance, such as whether he is excited or calm, dependent or independent, hurried or slow, strikes me. Later, I start noticing specific things. We have to go from the general to the specific. That he is an anxious person is more important than what his anxiety is about. The rule I use is *what the person is... is more important than what he has.*

If we proceed in this fashion, the mistakes are minimized. We ask: "When do you get angry?" "I get angry after sleep", the patient replies. "Anger after sleep" is the rubric we may select. Here we may make a mistake since the anger might have some reason such as his neighbour making a lot of noise in the morning, and his helplessness about it. In this case, "Suppressed anger" is the more appropriate rubric, since it represents the basic nature of the person rather than merely his one symptom.

I once read a book about Bach flower remedies and though I never used them what I found interesting is that the remedies are not prescribed on symptoms but on the whole state. You are compelled to define the state first and only then the symptoms. What state the person is in has to be understood first and only then the symptoms that he has. No doubt, I listen to his words, but more important is his use of the words, his tone and manner of saying them and the context in which they are said. Gradually, an impression of the person is formed in my mind. Then I go further. For example, in an anxious person, I try to find basically what his anxiety is about. This may happen spontaneously, I need not ask the question as it is quite likely that answers will emerge. I keep them in a corner of my mind and proceed with the history. I see whether anything goes against this idea which I am forming in my mind.

I am very skeptical about my own judgements. That is a key to success. The scientist or physician who is willing to prove himself wrong will be successful. The more certain you are, the harder you need to try to prove yourself wrong. I am not talking about remedies at all. The more I keep remedies out of my mind, the more successful I will be. *The secret in prescribing homoeopathic remedies is to be unprejudiced, to experience every case as a new case, to go into the patient's case as if you have never seen a similar case before.*

From basic components to situation

What is useful is to examine the person's situations in life and how he views them. You will always find a difference between how they are and how he views them. I especially try to understand the conditions that he has set up and try to go into the feelings from which these conditions arise, and find out where in his life he faces restrictions or blocks. These feelings and compulsions give you the basic components of the person, on which the totality of symptoms of the mental state can be erected. Each component has to be confirmed and when put together, these components will give a good picture of the patient's mental state.

From this I make a picture of the situation in which he imagines himself to be and therefore requires all these components. Here we are touching the deepest, hidden feelings of the person. We have to be very cautious not to fit the person into something we already know. The patient himself is not very sure at this point so even he may not be able to confirm or deny what you say. You could push the wrong idea of the patient if you ask leading questions. So, this is an area where you have to be very careful. If you are not very sure, it is better to stick to the components. It can also be an area which is very rewarding if followed carefully. Once I have done this, my understanding of his state is complete. Then I understand physical generals and peculiarities. Most of the time I am able to connect physical generals and peculiarities with the mental state. If however I find that some physical general symptom or local peculiarity is not covered by the remedy I am considering, then I review the whole symptomatology and see if there is a remedy which covers the physical and peculiar symptoms as well, and which has a similar mental state. The idea is that *mind and body are often two expressions of the same basic disturbance and must be equally covered by the remedy.* If this does not occur (which happens rarely) then preference is given to the remedy that covers the mental state. If there is a very strong physical characteristic, then we have a strong reason to carefully consider a remedy which covers this. Put together, these aspects form my totality of the case.

Fit the patient into the remedy

I then go to the Repertory, unless I can see the remedy without an iota of doubt. I have to compare several rubrics and make cross-references in order to find the exact rubrics. I may interpret a rubric imaginatively, yet at the same time I have to be very careful not to fit a symptom into a particular rubric just because the remedy I have chosen is there. I take care to see that the important symptoms of the patient are in the remedy I select. Yet, the important features of the remedy should be found in the patient too. By important I mean the symptoms which are nearest to the basic feelings of the remedy. Some of these symptoms may be found in a compensated or overcompensated form, which may deceive us unless we look at the uncompensated behaviour such as found in dreams. The less important symptoms of the patient need not be found in the remedy. Similarly, the less important symptoms of the remedy (like its particulars) may not be found in the patient. I have made a formula upon two Aphorisms, namely 164 and 211 (I call this formula "375").

> Aphorism 164: The small number of homoeopathic symptoms present in the best selected medicines is no obstacle to the cure in cases where these few medicinal symptoms are chiefly of an uncommon kind and such as are peculiarly distinctive (characteristic) of the disease; the cure takes place under such circumstances without any particular disturbance.

> Aphorism 211: This holds good to such an extent, that the state of the disposition of the patient often chiefly determines the selection of the homoeopathic remedy, as being a decidedly characteristic symptom which can least of all remain concealed from the accurately observing physician.

From these I gather that Hahnemann had the same idea, i.e. we need not try and fit all the symptoms of the patient into the remedy but the symptoms of the mental state (which will be reflected in the physical generals since they come from the same source) must fit the remedy that we select.

The task of selecting the remedy, of which I have given broad and general guidelines, is in fact a very laborious but artistic process. With great circumspection, observation, understanding, empathy and with the use of reference books such as Materia Medica and Repertory, you will make fewer and fewer mistakes. Referring to this process of selection of the remedy, Hahnemann in the footnote of Aphorism 148 says:

> "This laborious search demands a study of the original sources."

Case example

A medical doctor aged twenty-eight came with severe rheumatoid arthritis. She was born in Delhi. During pregnancy her mother had no problems. When she was five-six years old, the family moved to Bombay, and she used to get attacks of sneezing. During her second year of medical college she starting getting trouble in one small joint. She had taken treatment, developed tuberculosis and had been treated for this one year before she met me.

Some features that emerged were that she does not get angry easily but remains depressed. She is always thinking with a negative, pessimistic attitude. She remains tense due to illness, feels helpless and fears she will get crippled. When she is alone, she broods and feels left behind, she weeps when consoled and feels better by weeping. The only cravings I could elicit were for sweets and spices.

Observation

I found that her pace was quite slow and she had no hope. She came to me to see if I could give her some relief from the pain. She could not accept it when I told her that she could improve and get cured. She refused to believe me. She had been to a homoeopath earlier and her condition had worsened. She said that as a medical practitioner she knew that her prognosis was very poor and on the X-ray bony changes were seen which were irreversible and there was no sense in my offering hope. I told her that there was hope and offered to show some cases like hers which had improved and could be confirmed by X-rays. She still refused to believe me. I sent her away without medicine because I thought that unless she was positively motivated to take the treatment, it was useless. I suggested some books on holistic medicine and asked her to see me after a month. She came back after two months. She brought her sister along. This time she began the interview by saying that she had taken gold injections without relief and the rheumatologist had pre-scribed chloroquine (quinine preparation) with steroids and that the chloroquine has helped. She said she was interested in taking up a job in a pharmaceutical company because she was interested in knowing about the recent advances in medicine.

She had several thoughts. One of the thoughts was to make a lot of money and then at the age of thirty-five to retire and buy a nice house in a village. Sometimes she had the thought that she should go and help Mother Teresa or some other social worker. When she had these thoughts she felt quite optimistic about getting well, but the rheumatologist had said: "How can your shoulder get better when the bone is eroded?" When she asked for my opinion I said it was possible. She asked how it could be possible when we know that bony changes are irreversible; how could the medicine bring back the bone?

Since the day her rheumatoid arthritis was confirmed, she became pessimistic. She felt crippled and that her ultimate destiny was a wheelchair and becoming totally dependent on others. She felt what was the use of living, but lacked the courage to commit suicide. Again I tried to motivate her to give up the allopathic drugs gradually and to look for total cure in any system. She refused to take the risk. Again this time I sent her away with more books on holistic medicine though she was repeatedly requesting me to at least give her medicine to alleviate the pain.

On one occasion she even called me senile because I refused to give medicine. I was not giving medicine for two reasons. Firstly, I wanted to be sure of the remedy, and secondly, it was no use to prescribe if she was not motivated. From the sister I got the impression that she was a mild person, who was gullible and could be easily fooled. After the illness, she had become introverted, despairing, pessimistic and resigned to her fate. She was not strong emotionally. "Resigned to one's fate" was coming up again and again. I did not see anxiety in her but only that she had firmly accepted her incurability; she just wanted some relief from the pain.

She was young and here I was offering her not just hope, but strong hope. Not only was I showing her cured cases from my practice to prove that what allopathy considers incurable can be cured, but I was also showing her books written by allopaths themselves that even cancer can be cured, even without medicine.

She was unwilling to listen. She was so completely fixed with her feeling of hopelessness, that she could not accept even slight reassurance. She was a dull, slow, pessimistic person, resigned to her fate. She only felt afraid of the suffering. The disease was troubling her but she could do nothing about it. Even towards me, the reaction was the same. When I made her come three-four times without giving any medicine, she would request a remedy from me each time and when I refused, she would walk away resigned as if I was troubling her and she could do nothing about it. This was the impression I was getting. Somehow, by the fourth interview, I was able to motivate her and she could see I was sincere in my efforts and in my faith to make her well. Then she was able to accept that as my medicine started giving her relief, she could reduce the cortisone and the other drugs. But to make her do this was for me a herculean task. She was a very difficult patient because she could not accept hope. She should have felt fortunate that, in spite of her illness, she had found a person who assured her of help. Resigned to one's faith, unable to accept good fortune was most important in her state, so I took the rubrics:

— Delusion, unfortunate, he is;

— Indolence;

— Timidity;

— Cowardice.

She is slow and lazy and she will not take any step because she feels the situation is so bad that nothing can be done about it. "It is my bad luck I am getting crippled. The disease is troubling me but I cannot fight the disease."

There is only one moment when she is optimistic, i.e. in her thoughts, either making money, building a house or helping society: ideal things. At this time she feels good but reverts back immediately as if she has woken from a happy dream into the reality of misfortune. There is a need in her to build big dreams, fantasies. Her reality was opposite to her fantasy; only a beggar needs to have the fantasy of being a king.

But, does she really feel she can fulfil the dream? No! Only the thoughts gave her pleasure.

— Theorizing;

— Plans, making many;

— Absorbed in thoughts.

"Theorizing in the evening", i.e. after the day's work, when the planning has no practical use. When you plan in the evening, you do not want to do anything about it. It is just fantasy. Her interest is in working in a pharmacy and discovering new medicines, which again is "Theorizing". You see the confirmation of this feeling that she is "Unfortunate", "Timid", "Cowardly", "Indolent, can do nothing"; and in her fantasies she is just the opposite: "Lucky", "Fortunate", "Building houses", "Active", "Courageous".

She has also:

— Suicidal, but lacks courage;

— Discouraged;

— Obstinate.

What is the situation she imagine herself to be in? The situation is that she is being troubled and suppressed by this disease and she can do nothing about it. She cannot fight back, she is totally helpless. She needs to be pessimistic without hope, because hope is harmful. So, the only thing she can do is to sit and fantasize and think nothing can be done to help her. This is the reason she was unwilling to accept hope and unwilling to accept good fortune. When we study these rubrics, we get *China* which is confirmed by the craving for sweets and spices.

An interesting thing was the relief she got from chloroquine, though administered empirically and in the crude form. It was as if she was taking *China* in the mother tincture. I immediately stopped the chloroquine and started her on *China* 200. I have been treating her with *China*, given twice in seven months. She has done wonderfully well. We have brought her cortisone (of which she could not miss a single dose) down from 2 mg twice daily to nil. Not only are her joint pains better, but the mobility of her shoulders is coming back; something she could not have hoped for even in her wildest dreams. Now, she has asked me to suggest some books on Homoeopathy because she is interested in studying it.

Understanding the patient is just like creating a portrait. In a portrait we do not start with the nose or eyes but with the outline, then slowly we fit in all the details. In the same way we have to approach the person in a broad manner, make a general outline first, and then slowly all the details will fall into place beautifully.

I also realized that to make a computer expert system to select the remedy does not sound right. It is we who have to become experts, instead of trying to make an expert of the computer!

38

HOMOEO-PSYCHOTHERAPY

Recently, I conceived the idea of giving the "similar stimulus" through words and images instead of medicines. I put it into practice with very encouraging results. By itself, it is a logical consequence of our understanding of Homoeopathy. But even more, it helps us to sharpen our methods of understanding the core of a case. In order to examine the idea of Homoeo-psychotherapy, we have to ask certain fundamental questions on how exactly a homoeopathic medicine acts. What we know about the action of homoeopathic medicine is that it produces a state of being that is similar to the state in which the patient already is; and such creation of a similar state proves curative. The idea of Homoeo-psychotherapy is that by producing a similar state through words and images it is possible to produce a curative reaction of the Vital Force. We should first know that a state of mind produced through homoeopathic medicine can be produced through other means of communication as well. Similarly, such a state can be created by our talk; can we not use this in lieu of medicine?

To do this we must confront the patient with an image of his own state, which is similar to his central feeling, so that the person sees through his mind's eye the image of his exact feeling. We can do this by taking his case first, and then throwing back his basic feeling to him. We already know that a remedy, which has the basic delusion from which the whole state arises, will act curatively. The very delusion from which all his feelings and actions arise, if brought home to the patient, may achieve the same result. Once a person appreciates his own delusion, this begins to work on him like a homoeopathic remedy.

Homoeo-psychoterapy in practice

Taking the case

Now, I come to the actual process of administering this therapy. As is usual in homoeopathic practice, the case is taken in the maximum possible detail, especially with regard to the mind. We have first to understand the situation of the patient: his background, his occupation, his family life, social relations, his cultural and economic status as well as his childhood environment, etc. At the same time, we also observe how he has reacted to the situations around him. These observations about the patient, in the course of the talk in the clinic itself, are very important. The way he expresses his feelings – whether he is excited or dull, weeping or cheerful, slow to answer or hurried, mild or vehement – should be carefully noted.

With all this information, we have to use our human understanding and ask the following questions to ourselves:

– What are the patient's conditions for feeling OK (at peace with himself and others)?

– What are the basic feelings about himself or his situation that necessitate such conditions?

– What are the other expressions of such a vision of himself in terms of his feelings and actions?

This whole process of finding out the patient's delusion (his perception of reality) need not be a very quick process. Surely, we should try to avoid guess work or putting the patient into a readymade theory or remedy picture. The process should be gone through gradually and each step should be confirmed by the patient (the physician keeping his mind open all the time, knowing that he could be wrong). He may begin with some ideas but there should be great flexibility in his thinking so that he can change those at any stage, based on his observations and the patient's responses.

Step by step, the physician helps the patient advance to find out what are the conditions that he has to fulfil in order to feel OK. What does the patient feel about himself and his situation that makes it necessary to have these conditions, and how has this feeling influenced his whole life and activity including his job, relationships, social activities, etc. At this point, the patient will realize to some extent that the conditions he has created are in response to his perception of reality, and often this perception of reality is far too exaggerated.

For example, he can see that his whole activity resembles a man being chased by a lion, but actually it is only a dog that is chasing him. Exposure to such an image automatically creates the whole mood of that state which is similar to the state he already is in. This experience proves as effective as the homoeopathic remedy for the simple reason that it is in fact the "homoeopathic remedy through word-images."

Case

As an example, we can look at the case of a woman who came with the problem of abnormal behaviour caused by her depression, such as slapping her husband, and other actions which necessitated psychiatric treatment. In this case, I went into the history in detail and discovered that all these complaints started after her marriage. The situation in her home was that she had a sister-in-law who got along much better with other in-laws. The sister-in-law was an extrovert, more beautiful and in fact was a model. Our patient felt inferior and developed severe "not-OK" feelings about herself. I went on step by step to find out her conditions for feeling OK. The prominent thing that emerged was that she wanted to be like her sister-in-law. The statement which was going in her mind was: "I will be liked and cared for, only if I am like my sister-in-law." From this feeling she tried to imitate her sister-in-law, but was unsuccessful, and from this failure she became depressed and developed abnormal behaviour. What is more significant is that in this process she failed to develop her own potentialities. I spoke to her husband and found that he cared for her as she was, and he did not feel the need for her to be like her sister-in-law. So, the patient was now confronted with her own perception/delusion (that she had to be like her sister-in-law to be loved and cared for), while in reality this was not possible nor necessary. It was the delusion (false perception) that left her no choice but to be depressed and hate herself. When exposed to the difference between perception and reality, the patient agreed that she could see to some extent that her feeling was too exaggerated for her situation. This exposure to her delusion acted effectively.

After this, she was advised a simple relaxation technique to be practised for a few minutes every day and was sent away without any medicine or even placebo. The whole process took around two hours. A week later, the patient reported a marked amelioration of her state. She could now shift back from her parents' home to her husband's, and was able to face the situation much better. She could now look at herself more positively and decided to take up some work that suited her talents. This change was significant since we had discontinued all her psychiatric medication. Her husband happily confirmed the improvement.

Incidently, in this case, if I were to prescribe a homoeopathic remedy, I would have chosen *Lac caninum* on the following symptoms:
- Contemptuous for self;
- Anxiety from doubts about success;
- Delusion, she is looked down upon;
- Delusion, she is diminished, short;
- Confidence, want of self;
- Delusion, despised, that she is;
- Sadness, mental depression;
- Undertakes many things, perseveres in nothing.

Case

My second example involves a young man of around twenty years. He was referred to me by a colleague who had treated him with some remedies without much success. His main problem was tremendous depression. He wrote in the questionnaire: "I am an unhappy person, I don't know what is joy." The most of the questions he answered: "I don't know." He was withdrawn, completely pessimistic, and had made some attempts at suicide.

We went through his situation in life, and found that he was the only son of a businessman and had four elder sisters. Being the last child and the only son, he was highly pampered and overprotected. At the age of fifteen his father suffered a heart attack and the boy was suddenly called on to shoulder responsibility, something to which he was not used. The boy who was already timid, became extremely nervous, and felt very lonely. He became chilly, his hands became cold and he had several dreams of his father dying or the business crashing. With these feelings he could do nothing and went into depression.

In this case, we tried to examine his basic feeling, or basic perception of reality behind these feelings. It was a difficult process because the boy could not distinguish between reality and his delusion. *The sicker a person becomes, the less he is able to discriminate between delusion and reality.* In fact, one can say that this is the real measure of sickness.

In spite of this, I tried to expose this boy to his own delusion. The feeling (delusion) was one of incapacity to face the problems and risks involved in business. He felt he was lacking, not equipped to face the big hurdles in business and therefore, his response was to do nothing.

Since he was lacking in confidence and he could not do anything about it, the only way of survival for him was to sit back and do nothing, be depressed and have suicidal thoughts. He was like a lame person who comes in front of a mountain which it is imperative for him to cross, and he knows he is totally unfit and lacking in ability to climb it: he feels that even small stones can topple him and he will fall. So, he sits back, feeling inferior, depressed and scared to death. In reality, the situation was not so severe. The boy was brought to the realization that he was behaving like a lame man in front of a mountain, but he was neither lame nor was there the mountain in front of him. After this discussion, the boy was given placebo and asked to report after a week.

A week later the boy reported an initial aggravation for two days in his whole state with several memories of his past coming back to him and this was followed by relief. This sounded to me like homoeopathic aggravation, almost as if I had given a potency higher than was needed. After another week, he reported that he was not feeling so good but on looking at him, he seemed better and this time he was more open to my words. Also, his watch was missing. Here I must mention his watch which I had observed when I saw him first. It was a funny watch which had on its dial a spider's web and on one hand of the watch was a smaller spider which went round and round. The boy mentioned that he liked this watch and the spider because the spider represents to him a creature that does not give up even if it fails.

The third time he came to me, I reinforced the talk (just as if I were repeating the dose) and sent him away. When I last saw him, he was significantly better despite the situational problems.

For those interested, my prescription for him would have been *Psorinum*, based on the following symptoms:
- Delusion, he is poor (poor means lacking in something which could be money, strength, talent, courage, etc.);
- Fear of poverty (means fear of losing something);
- Fear of failure in business;
- Despair of recovery (recovery means coming back to original sound position whether in business, health or after a loss);
- Suicidal thoughts;
- Forsaken feeling;
- Ailments from anticipation;

- Anxiety with fear;
- Anxiety about future;
- Delusion, he was going to lose his fortune;
- Doubtful about recovery;
- Discouraged;
- Fear of misfortune;
- Fear of disaster;
- Indolence, aversion to work;
- Sadness, mental depression.

Homoeo-psychotherapy and the question of potency

Nowhere is the question of potency more clearly solved than in Homoeo-psycho-therapy. First of all, we should understand what we mean by potency and what are the qualities of high and low potencies. Potency is the power of any substance (or even thought force) to bring about change. The potency of medicine is its inherent ability to bring about a change in the state of health. The power increases with the potency. The higher the potency, the more intense influence it can have; the lower the potency, the less intense is the effect. Now, we should know that the more intense the central disturbance is, the clearer the mental state will be, and the clearer the mental state, the more intense the delusion will be. Therefore, the higher the potency of the drug, the greater its power to produce such an intense state that the prover can distinguish to a lesser and lesser extent the difference between delusion and reality. The lesser the potency, the milder and more vague is the state, and therefore, more the difference between delusion and reality.

Similarly, when we talk about Homoeo-psychotherapy, we can say that we have administered a higher potency of the therapy if the patient got a very specific and intense vision of the delusion. We can say we have administered a low potency of the therapy if the vision is less specific and a more vague description, or only a general idea of the delusion, rather than a specific intense experience. This is obvious since by definition, the higher the potency, the more intense is the change in the state of health it can produce. As we proceed in this process of therapy, we will find that, depending on the intensity of the state in the patient, we will have to modify the potency of our therapy. A person with an intense state is hardly going to be influenced by a low potency of the therapy. We will have to take the potency higher and higher until we reach the level where he shows some reaction. We have to stop at this point and let him go because a more intense experience could cause unnecessary and sometimes unsafe aggravation. In fact, the beauty of the therapy lies in this, that:

- We can modify our potency on the spot and slowly increase it to the desired level;
- The reaction can be seen instantaneously.

Thus, this therapy scores over traditional Homoeopathy in the way that potency selection and remedy reaction can be properly modulated and controlled, and the reaction can also be seen on the spot. Going back to the two examples I gave, we can see that in the first case I did not use a specific image for the delusion of the patient. I merely gave a general idea that she felt she had to be like her sister-in-law to be loved and cared for, which in reality was not correct. This itself was sufficient since her state was not so intense and hence she could at once see the difference between delusion and reality.

In the second case, I had to give a very specific and intense image since the boy was quite deep in his state and would not have responded to a general description as in the previous case.

Advantages of Homoeo-psychotherapy

I should mention here the major advantage of this therapy, viz. that it can be administered even though we may not know the remedy homoeopathically. Secondly, it is possible that a remedy for the exact condition does not exist. For example, we may find that in a patient there are some specific conditions for feeling OK. We may discover the delusion, i.e. his perception of reality that led to these conditions, but we may not know the remedy that has this delusion. Maybe such a remedy is not proven enough for us to know its delusions. Here we can administer the therapy with success.

Of course, this therapy is not so easy; it needs skill and art. If you administer the therapy wrongly, the patient will immediately reject it. Worse still, he may accept it and get the wrong label, which can be very difficult to remove. Circumspection and tact are required. Even though Homoeo-psychotherapy was initially conceived as giving an image to the patient, *I have found it advisable to merely guide the patient into himself, to merely point out his obsessions and compulsions*, to ask just very brief questions at the right points, so that the patient tells you his deepest feelings rather than you telling him. This way, fewer mistakes are made. The physician stands back supporting the patient and leading him to the point of awareness.

In the case of children, we have to devise other techniques like telling fairy tales and stories, and watching their reaction. In much smaller children, pictures and movies could be tried. We will have to develop these techniques.

Every homoeopath will be well advised to try to understand and apply this therapy. Even if he does not apply it in an individual case, the very process of taking the case and reaching the core of the mind will sharpen his skill and enhance his understanding of the mental states of people, an ability which is essential in finding the Similimum.

Part IV

Materia Medica

39

THE SITUATIONAL MATERIA MEDICA:
ITS ORIGIN AND UTILITY

My idea of situational Materia Medica started with the case of the dumb boy (*Veratrum album*) which I presented in the chapter "What is disease". I realized that the state for which I would have given *Veratrum album* was a suitable reaction to a particular situation. I understood then that disease itself is a posture for a particular situation. Drugs are nothing but artificial diseases. Each of them must be a posture suitable for a specific situation. I therefore started studying the symptomatology of the remedies, especially the mental symptoms, and with correlation from my practice I was able to understand from what possible situation that particular remedy state arises. This made me understand the remedies in a new way and allowed me to see the place of various symptoms in a remedy. It made it easier to remember and apply, and also compare one remedy state with another.

I was initially working at a remedy being a characteristic combination of components but later it was made to connect these components through situational Materia Medica. What is important to note is that every single aspect of the patient fits into one state, because the whole posture represents a survival mechanism in a specific situation. So, we must understand that every symptom which exists must fit the pattern. If some symptom does not fit, the selection may be wrong. The ideas of situational Materia Medica is to study a pattern behind the conglomeration. It compels us to perceive the whole state of the patient as a survival mechanism in a particular situation. It is a question of what situation needs such state and then of identifying a remedy whose state originates from a similar situation.

In essence, situational Materia Medica is nothing but the basic delusion of that remedy state. It is the viewpoint from which all the expressions of the state arise, with their obsessions and compulsions.

The situational Materia Medica has been devised to understand the remedy. It is not to try and locate or choose the remedy based on the present situation of the patient. If there is an excitable root inside, any situation may excite it; therefore, the actual situation of the person is not important. For example, if a person has a *Calcarea fluorica* root (with "Fear of poverty"), even if his health is bad, the first thing he will worry about is money and not his health. Though he comes from a situation of bad health, he is reacting as if he is in a situation of poverty. *So, what is important to trace is not what situation the person is in but to what situation he is reacting*. If you find that out, the situational Materia Medica will be useful. The situation to which he is reacting might have occurred earlier in his life, or in his mother during pregnancy or in his parents. That will merely confirm your prescription but will not be the indication for it. The indication will always be the totality of his expressions including his dreams and his delusions from which we get an idea of his perception of the situation. For this you have to ask in which situation should he behave like this. Of course, we have already mentioned that a state will try to create a situation similar to the original situation; so we can also ask which situation he has created. For example, *Aurum metallicum* invites responsibility and *Natrum muriaticum* invites grief.

Using situational Materia Medica, I have been able to compare remedies, which I will illustrate later on. The interesting part is that once I had understood situational Materia Medica, I was able to predict most of the symptoms of the remedy given in the Materia Medica, and I was easily able to understand how these symptoms occurred in the remedy.

The person who understands the situational Materia Medica is one who has thoroughly grasped the concept of disease as a posture, as a state of being, and not as a conglomeration of symptoms or pathology.

In the following pages, I shall describe the situational Materia Medica of some remedies. Through the situational Materia Medica I have been able to come in contact with the state of the remedy. I am often able to recall a similar (though less serious) situation in my own life, and through this recollection can have a direct experience of the remedy state, almost as if I were proving the remedy. I also found that in patients an exposure to the situational Materia Medica of their remedy often acts as the remedy itself. This is similar to Homoeo-psychotherapy.

The examples given in the following pages are meant to be read only after one is familiar with the standard Materia Medica for that remedy. It will be useful to precede the reading of a remedy by reading it in M.L. Agrawal's "Materia Medica of the Human Mind". Then one can see how varied and seemingly unconnected symptoms form a pattern.

Initially, I have given the method I use to discover the situational Materia Medica of a remedy, so that the reader may explore the whole Materia Medica on his own.

I must state that in reality, we do not know the whole situation of any remedy. We know big parts of the situation of some of the remedy-states, but surely not the whole of it. Each time we discover newer and newer aspects of our remedy-situations.

40

DISCOVERING THE SITUATIONAL
MATERIA MEDICA OF REMEDIES

How do you discover the central state of the remedy? What is the method you use to understand the remedy?

This can be best illustrated with a remedy I have never used, because then we will be looking purely at Materia Medica and trying to understand it from the symptoms recorded in the provings alone rather than in terms of what we have seen in clinical practice.

We will take the remedy *Hura brasilientis* of which I have never read any cases. Not only is there no clinical experience from my side, but hardly any clinical experience is available.

I read each remedy in various Materia Medicas, but I have especially been using the book "Materia Medica of the Human Mind" by Dr. M.L. Agrawal. This doctor has rendered a unique service to Homoeopathy by producing an alphabetical list of mental symptoms of each remedy appearing in Kent's Repertory. He has also demarcated the "single remedy" symptoms. *Hura brasilientis* has the following single symptoms:

— Cheerful in the morning at 8.00 am;
— Delusion, thinks she is about to lose her friend;
— Delusion, sees persons hanging three feet from ground, on falling asleep;
— Fear, of fever on going to bed;
— Fear, of misfortune in the afternoon at 2.00 pm;
— Laughing, followed by chill;
— Every paroxysm of pain excites a nervous laugh;
— Weeping when singing.

Among the delusions are:
— Delusion, has lost affection of friends;
— Delusion, alone, world, in the;
— Delusion, his friends have lost all confidence in him;
— Delusion, sees dead persons;
— Delusion, deserted, forsaken;

— Delusion, floating in air;
— Delusion, he is unfortunate;
— Delusion, sees spectres, ghosts, spirits;
— Delusion, despised, that he is;
— Delusion, fancies herself lost;
— Delusion, repudiated by relatives;
— Despair of recovery;
— Despair, religious, of salvation.

Other feelings that the remedy has are:
– Anxiety about salvation;
– Affectionate;
– Thoughts of death and desires death;
– Discontented;
– Fear of misfortune;
– Forsaken feeling;
– Sensation of isolation;
– Indifference to pleasure;
– Sadness;
– Sulky;
– feels unfortunate;
– Reproaches himself.

Among some of the actions are:
– Biting himself;
– Biting his hands;
– Break things, desire to;
– Destructive;
– Impatience;
– Obstinate;
– Restless;
– Causeless weeping.

If we study all these symptoms of *Hura brasilientis*, we find a lot of them have to do with forsaken feelings. There is a specific feeling of forsakenness, which is reflected in the delusions that she is about to lose her friends, that her friends have lost affection for her, people are casting her away, they do not want her. Therefore, she is alone in the world; she is not liked, she is despised and hated. Why has this happened? Because of bad luck, she is unfortunate – this feeling is strong: "It is my bad luck that something has happened to me because of which I have lost my friends and they have started hating me."

Now, when I think about this, I ask myself what is the situation in which these feelings are justified? Here is the situation of a man who has lost the affection of his friends. All his friends and relatives now hate him and do not want him, they have cast him away, and so he feels left out, forsaken, isolated and feels unfortunate.

The rubric "Despair of recovery" means that it is difficult for him to recover from this position. The chances of getting back to the original position are slim; so there is sadness and mental depression. He becomes quite frustrated and bored (ennui). He can get destructive, even destructive of himself. He gets angry with himself, bites himself, feels unfortunate and reproaches himself.

Various possibilities occur – maybe he has committed a big crime. If that was the case, "Anxiety of conscience" and "Delusion, he is a criminal" should have been there, but they are not. What is available is unfortunate feeling, some misfortune has happened. So, what could the misfortune be that has made his relatives hate him? What could the misfortune be from which he cannot recover? When I go into this feeling, I get a strong impression of leprosy. A leper is a man who, through a stroke of bad luck comes into a position where all his friends have deserted him, they hate him, despise him, lose affection for him and, however much he tries, he cannot compensate. The old feeling cannot return; once a leper, always a leper.

All this reminded me of how lepers were treated in the past. Even nowadays, they are isolated, cast away, nobody wants them and nobody cares for them. Forsaken, deserted, repudiated by relatives, lost the affection of friends, despair of recovery, bites himself, etc.; all these fit into that one situation. I am not saying that this is the only situation, but what I am saying is that *Hura brasilientis* feels like a leper. That is the feeling one can get from reading the totality of *Hura brasilientis* mental symptoms. It may be in any situation: he feels like a leper, feels cast away and hated with no chance of coming back. This is the theme of *Hura brasilientis*.

When I got this idea, you can imagine my joy when I went through Clarke's "Dictionary" and found that *Hura brasilientis* has been proved and it has brought out the best symptoms in people who had leprosy in the past, and *Hura brasilientis* is a known remedy for leprosy. I am not saying that *Hura brasilientis* should be used in leprosy, but what I am saying is that leprosy could have been one of the original situations in which the *Hura brasilientis* state must have been produced. There could be other similar situations. So, any person who in normal life has these feelings, though he is not a leper, requires *Hura brasilientis*.

I imagine that Hura brasilientis *could be a remedy for AIDS patients, probably they might have this same feeling.*

It is quite possible for an AIDS patient to have this same feeling, but if you find this feeling in an AIDS patient, it is not important. It does not indicate the remedy unless the feeling is overwhelming. If any of these symptoms come out in a leper or in an AIDS patient or in a person in a similar situation, such a state becomes common. Therefore, we have to search for symptoms that are uncommon, outside of the known, recognized situation. For a leper to feel despised and hated is common. We have to see something else there behind this. From this despised feeling, what feeling is he getting? He is getting the feeling: "Nobody likes me, nobody wants me, what will I do for food?" One leper may feel like this. Another one will feel: "I am not liked, I am not wanted, what will happen to my daughter? May be they will say that she is the daughter of a leper. How will she get married?" This is a strong feeling in the second leper.

The feeling of been unwanted would be common in most lepers; it does not individualize any one of them. It is what is uncommon, what is peculiar, that denotes what is basic and not what is situational. If this feeling comes in a person who is not a leper nor an AIDS patient, then *Hura brasilientis* will be the remedy because that will be his basic state, which is not due to a situation. In a person who is in a similar situation, we have to search for symptoms beyond his situation, look for the symptoms that reflect his individuality. In a person who is not in that situation, these feelings would be highly characteristic and the remedy would be indicated without doubt.

Once we understand the situation of *Hura brasilientis* and its basic feelings and reactions, we have to compare it with other remedies which have similar feelings. *Lac caninum* has got tremendous contempt for self, he feels worthless and has such feelings as:

  − Delusion, that she is looked down upon;
  − Delusion, that she is diminished, short;
  − Delusion, that she is despised;
  − Delusion, that she he is dirty;
  − Want of self-confidence.

So, these two remedies come very close. There will be confusion. What is striking in *Lac caninum* is its marked hatred, maliciousness, desire for company, want of moral feeling, anxiety from doubt of success, undertakes many things but perseveres at nothing, absentminded and antagonism with self.

Now what does all this show? We see that *Lac caninum* has also the feeling of being left out and rejected, a feeling of low self-worth; but she blames somebody else, that means somebody else is responsible for her condition, and therefore she develops hatred and malice. This feeling is: "I am responsible but somebody else is also responsible."

  − In *Hura brasilientis*: "I am not OK, you are OK."
  − In *Lac caninum*: "I am not OK, you are also not OK."
  − In *Anacardium*: Lack of confidence, malice and hatred, cruelty.

The *Anacardium* patient is one who is suppressed very badly so that his confidence is shaken, and he develops hatred and malice. *Lac caninum* is in a similar situation.

One step further from *Anacardium* is where the person has been literally thrown out of the house. Then she develops the feeling, "everything is OK with me, but it is you who are the devil." *Platinum* – "Delusion, devil, everybody is, and that she is great".

In Hura brasilientis, *it is quite obvious that there are delusions. What about remedies like* Calcarea sulphurica *where there are no any delusions?*

Where there are no delusions listed in the remedy, then I study the other symptoms of the drug. One thing is sure, that all symptoms of a remedy are based upon delusions – every single symptom without exception. Because delusion is disease and since symptoms are an expression of disease, they can be expressed as delusions. So, from the expression we to go to the delusion.

In the expression itself, delusion is available if you are able to perceive it. So, what will you do with the remedies in which no marked delusion is available? I study the single symptoms of the remedy. Symptoms against which only one remedy is found in the Repertory are single symptoms. When we study the single symptoms, we are able to get single delusions.

For example, *Calcarea sulphurica* has two single symptoms:
– Lamenting, appreciated, because he is not;
– Hatred of persons who do not agree with him.

Based on these two symptoms we can build up the whole picture of *Calcarea sulphurica.* I have had several confirmations of this remedy in my clinical practice. Let us analyze these one by one.

— *Lamenting, appreciated, because he is not.*
What are the symptoms? First is lamenting, i.e. complaining. What is the difference between complaining and lamenting? Complaint: utterance of grievance. Lament: passionate expression of grief. So, it is much more in degree than a complaint. Complaint is merely to say something, and lament is to say the same thing with a lot of passion or force.

The situation is of a man who is not appreciated, who feels somebody else is appreciated. The situation is of one who is jealous and so laments: "I have to make a passionate complaint of my grief that nobody cares for me, nobody does me good." It shows a situation of dependence. He does not break away and go, but is dependent and afraid of going away, so we see the rubrics:
— Timidity;
— Fear at night;
— Fear of dark.

He is a person who belongs to a family on whom he is dependent. The parents have three children and he is the second or third child. He has not yet learned to struggle on his own, cannot be independent, but the parents appreciate the other children more than him. So, he laments passionately so that they come to know what he is feeling. But they do not always listen as we see in the situation. So, we have sadness, mental depression and at times he does nothing but just sits quiet and meditates. There is discontented feeling, irritability and despair.

There are people who come and tell him: "No, no. You are talking nonsense. Actually, everybody is being treated fairly." But this does not sound true to him, and for such people he develops hatred – "Hatred for the persons who do not agree with him". Therefore, he is called obstinate and quarrelsome, and also malicious. This is the picture of *Calcarea sulphurica*.

You can say *Calcarea sulphurica* is the third daughter, and the second daughter is much more beautiful than her. All the attention of the family is directed towards the beautiful looking one. All the clothes are being given to her. All the jewelry is being given to her. She even gets married first. This girl cannot break away and so she tries to tell everybody that she is not being treated fairly, but nobody listens to her or they say she is just imagining it, so she develops hatred for these people.

In the chapter on "Delusions", I told of the girl who came into my clinic and said: "Doctor, I have come here to quarrel with you. Why are you giving attention to all your patients, but not to me? You must have some bad feelings towards me. You do not like me as much as you like others." Again the same lamenting that she is not appreciated, hatred, malice, obstinate, quarrelsome, offended easily, sadness, depression, timidity and dependence. So, I said to her: "Why should I differentiate between you and the other patients? I am not your father", and everything cooled down; she started laughing. I gave her *Calcarea sulphurica*.

We must study the Materia Medica carefully, symptom after symptom, and try to understand from where the symptoms come, what they mean and what the delusion is. We may not find the delusions explicitly mentioned. For example, I had a patient in whom everything fitted *Baryta carbonica*. She was feeling as if she had no friends. I took the rubric: "Delusion, friendless, he is", but there was no *Baryta carbonica*. Then I looked at "Forsaken feeling": no *Baryta carbonica*.

So, where is it given? You will find: "Goes off alone and weeps as if she had no friends" under "Weeping". That is a delusion, of course, but it is not the basic delusion. Why does she feel friendless? Because she cannot remain without a friend, which shows dependence. This point is given under: "Delusion, beloved friend is sick and dying". "Without that friend how shall I survive?" This is the fear. She feels as if her legs are cut off and she is walking on her knees, this is dependence again, so we see the features:

- Craving for company;
- Irresolution about trifles;
- Anxiety about trifles;
- Cannot do anything on her own;
- Feels people are laughing at him.

This is *Baryta carbonica* – how easy to understand the dependent man! The lame man is *Baryta carbonica*, literally, a man who has his legs cut off, a dwarf, a three and a half foot man. Especially the normal man who feels he is so.

There are many methods to understand remedies. One is through delusions and rubrics. Then there are other methods. I believe one of the best methods to really understand a remedy is to prove it on yourself, and then you will get the exact feeling, and you can almost forget about the rubrics. The only problem is that you will not be able to prove many remedies in your life. So, your Materia Medica will be short if you only depend on that. Jürgen Becker of Germany is doing this. He will prove the remedy on himself and on some volunteers, and then hear them and try to feel the experience of the remedy, the situation of the remedy, especially through dreams. Unfortunately, our "Dreams" chapter in the Repertory is not so good. The reason is they have given the dream but not the sequence of the dream. If they had given the exact sequence of the dream and the feeling of the dreamer, then it would have been more useful. So, Jürgen Becker tries to get the whole sequence, and the feeling behind the dream, and from this he attempts to understand the remedy. He does not use the Repertory so much, or even the Materia Medica. His descriptions of the remedies are very impressive, coming from direct experience.

My method is more analytical, but at a particular level I can also feel the remedy. I am able to feel the differences between remedies and reduce them down to rubrics, and also make them very standard so that it is not just my opinion but how it is recorded in the books. When Becker and I compared notes, we found our ideas to be similar. It was fantastic. He did not know many rubrics and I did not know any of the dreams and both of us were saying very similar things.

For me this way to study a remedy (through situational Materia Medica) is very exciting; otherwise it is just copying of ideas, copying of prescriptions. If we have the idea of how to study a remedy, we can discover a remedy on our own. Can you give us some guidelines?

Some remedies were very difficult to get, some were rather easy. Here are some guidelines. The situations we are talking about should not be very uncommon situations. In fact, they should be as common as the remedy is common. We should not postulate that "*Sulphur* is a king who has lost his kingdom". There are not many kings now, we have to relate to something more common. The most helpful guide is our feeling. If we look at the remedy and study the symptoms of the mind from the source books, we will be able to feel the state within ourselves and there will occur a connection with some situation in our own lives.

The situational Materia Medica of the remedy will be a similar situation, only much more severe. Have we not felt unappreciated in our life? In which situation did we feel like shouting: "Oh, why do they not appreciate me?" In this situation we were dependent on somebody, and they were giving importance to somebody else. They were neglecting us and telling us that this was not so. There must have been such a situation in our own life. So, most of these situations are common. In some way or other we must have experienced all of them.

The delusion itself (as we have said in the chapter on "Delusions") is a symbolic presentation of our own feeling. So, there is hardly any delusion which we have not experienced. We have experienced all the feelings which are symbolized.

One of my colleagues, whom I know well, told me: "Rajan, I want to give up all my homoeopathic activities. Now I just want to retire and not do anything. You had better take charge of all the things I am doing now. I want to give up. I am feeling completely finished. I am totally exhausted." How did this happen? We traced out that he had done a lot of mental work, had overexerted intellectually, and had landed up in this state. I gave him *Picricum acidum*. With that he recovered beautifully. At this time a student was with me and we started studying *Picricum acidum*.

What are the symptoms in *Picricum acidum*? We find mainly:
  - Difficult concentration;
  - Confusion of mind after mental exertion;
  - Dullness;
  - Unable to think long;
  - Aggravation from mental exertion;
  - Indifference;
  - Indolence;
  - Weak memory;
  - Prostration of mind;
  - Inclination to sit down;
  - Lacks the power to undertake anything;
  - Mental work is impossible.

This is more or less the mental picture of *Picricum acidum*. Now, there are two delusions which belong only to *Picricum acidum*:
  — Delusion, arms reach the clouds when going to sleep;
  — Delusion, tongue seems to reach the clouds when going to sleep.

What is the meaning of this? At that time, in some other context, I was mentioning the poetry of Rabindranath Tagore, where in one of the stanzas he describes how he wants his nation to be. He says: "Where tireless striving stretches its arms towards perfection." The student got a hint from this stanza. What is tongue and what is hand? Then she read in the original Materia Medica proving that: "Forehead seems to extend towards the clouds". So, what is tongue, what is hand and what is forehead?

The forehead is for thinking, the hand is for writing and the tongue is for speaking. These are the three organs of intellectual ability, and they feel stretched to the limit; they seem to extend right up to the clouds. That is what the prover in German is trying to convey. "I feel that my intellectual capacity, and the organs used to express it, are stretched beyond the limit, so that now I need to rest and bring them back to health."

This is the idea. This is the situation of *Picricum acidum*, where a man has extended beyond his limit, has used his organs beyond their limit so that they are stretched beyond the clouds, and now he needs to shut up, cut off and take rest. To help him do this, he gets increased sexual thoughts which is the opposite to the intellect.

This is how we slowly figured out some of the meanings of the delusions and started to understand delusion as nothing but an expression of the patient in a symbolic and exaggerated way.

The remedy *Piper methysticum* once interested me. I have never prescribed it for anybody but when I studied it, I found that it could be useful for a large number of people.

The symptoms of *Piper methysticum* are:
- Amusement, desire for (which it shares with *Lachesis* alone);
- Cheerful, gay, happy;
- Dullness, sluggishness;
- Ennui, entertainment ameliorates;
- Excitement ameliorates;
- Exaltation of fancies;
- Fear of suffering (which it shares with very few remedies);
- Hurry while eating;
- Indolence after sleep;
- Industrious;
- Irritability from noise;
- Active memory;
- Mirth in evening;
- Occupation ameliorates;
- Talk, indisposed to;
- Thinking of complaints aggravates.

These are the only symptoms, except "Mirth after emission" (Kent's Repertory), which is a single symptom.

Now, what do we see? We see two things: "Desire for amusement, entertainment and excitement", and "Thinking of complaints aggravates". That means it is the situation in which he should not think about his complaints, i.e. his grievances. He should not think about his complaints because they are too painful and nothing can be done about them. Therefore, he avoids thinking about them and he keeps busy the whole day:
- Industrious;
- Occupation ameliorates.

In the evening he gets bored, and seeks entertainment and excitement. There is a sense of boredom associated with suffering:
- Fear of suffering;
- Thinking of complaints aggravates.

There is pain – problems that cannot be solved, either health, financial, emotional or spiritual problems, and it is better not to think about them, but escape through

295

entertainment and amusement, or remain occupied and industrious. Work in the day and, in the evening, without a single minute wasted, jump into some form of entertainment until sleep ("Mirth in the evening"). So we can understand that there is a desire for:

- Amusement in the evening, industrious in the day;
- Mirth in the evening, occupation in the day.

So, he can work a lot without fatigue and is quite lively and cheerful, but inside is the fear of pain, fear of suffering, and out of this fear he keeps seeking occupation or entertainment, and probably he does not want to talk. There are vivid fancies, dreams which are vivid and adventurous which is exactly the opposite to the boring routine of life, with no relief and no possibility of easing it.

Take a man who is financially poor. He has nothing good in life. He works hard the whole day and needs television and some entertainment at night – some radio, some dance, some music – that's all, he does not want to think about anything else. In the West, however, there is emotional and spiritual poverty, not material, but again it is the same thing. In the East it is material poverty, so all the people rush to the movies. Movies are the most popular thing in India. Why? People want to avoid the pain and suffering that would be caused if they thought about they own situation.

At some stage every human is in this state and we may get the impression that half the human race is in it. But we should be careful not to overuse it. It should be prescribed only when we find such a state to be very intense, or to exist in a person who is not in this situation at all, whose life is neither painful nor unexciting, but who behaves as if it were so.

Whether the problem is mental or physical, when a person feels the need to avoid thinking about the pain and keeps his mind off it for fear of feeling it and suffering from it, then we find the occasion for *Piper methysticum*.

41

SITUATIONAL MATERIA MEDICA
OF SOME REMEDIES

ANACARDIUM

Anacardium has two feelings which are its main components. These are "Cruelty" and "Lack of confidence". Both are extreme as is the situation from which the *Anacardium* state arises. It is a situation in which a person is dominated and suppressed. *Anacardium* could be the son of a very intense *Lycopodium* person who habitually dominates and suppresses the people around him. One who has undergone this suppression develops a "Lack of moral feeling" and "Cruelty"; he becomes "Malicious" towards the person in authority and disobedient. A lack of moral feeling is necessitated in a situation of very severe suppression. To give a crude example, severe suppression by religious authority may give rise to it; when a person's desires and natural feelings are crushed, he becomes indifferent to morality and takes on antisocial attitudes.

As I understand it, it is a situation of child abuse. When parents are too strict with children, when they impose all their desires forcibly on their children and do not allow them either to think or do anything on their own. This creates a state of child abuse such as seen in *Anacardium*. In such a case, the child's desires are never fulfilled, he cannot take any decisions, to the extent that he cannot wear the clothes he wants to wear because that also would be decided by his parents. It is a situation of overstrict, overdominating and overimposing parents (or any authority figure).

Now, if this child (or later adult) starts taking decisions, then he will be punished. The parent or the person in authority will be hard on him. So he becomes nervous. It serves him to be irresolute, because to him decisiveness will cause suffering. Indecisiveness will save him. So he develops lack of confidence and irresolution.

But at the same time, if he keeps putting up with this domination, he will suffer again. So he reacts against this by cruelty, malice, want of moral feeling and antisocial behaviour. *Anacardium* can become very hard and cruel, and at the same time have lack of confidence.

This combination will be found in *Anacardium* patients where it will resemble a situation as if the patient is being dominated too much and as if he is being persecuted.

Anacardium could be the wife of a selfish tyrant, who rules with an iron fist and does not allow her any freedom to take even small decisions. Whatever she decides is wrong, and so her survival lies in deciding nothing. Therefore, there is tremendous "Irresolution", "Always two wills", "Lack of self-confidence", "Weak memory", "Dull-ness" and "Confusion". Her self-confidence is completely shattered from fear of people and so she may seem childish, idiotic and timid. Such timidity and fear can paralyze her thinking, as may be seen when appearing for an examination.

These are people who are tormented, hurt by criticism, punishment and abuse. Inside they harden up and become "Violent" with a "Suicidal" or "Homicidal tendency". They become "Abusive" and "Stubborn" and avoid company. On the one hand, there is fear of punishment, telling him to do good, and on the other, hardness and cruelty, telling him to do bad. This gives us an important feature, namely the feeling as if an angel and a devil are on either shoulder. The angel creates feelings of guilt, and the devil creates feelings of cruelty and want of religious and moral feeling. The angel gives rise to orderliness ("Fastidious", "Cannot rest until things are in proper place") and the devil to breaking things.

In one case I found the two symptoms together in a very peculiar way. A lady with paralysis gave the symptoms that after the death of her husband she felt nothing. In fact, when the funeral had left, she cleaned the whole house. The cruelty of *Anacardium* will more commonly be found in a less obvious form: usually, it will be hidden or compensated for.

ARGENTUM NITRICUM

A patient whose case was taken by a student had so many symptoms that I could not make any sense of it. The patient then narrated a dream which he used to get repeatedly.

He was in a large empty area. Everything looked old and broken, and he was alone. The trees looked burnt and there were dead animals around, giving the place a haunted look. Nothing was alive. It was a large open space and it looked as if the animals were dead, and had suffered something; there were skeletons all around. He wanted to escape from this wide open space but it was endless. He felt trapped, trapped by the space. He could not see beyond this large open space. He wanted to get out, tried to, but could not. It was beyond his capacity. No one had survived these ruins.

Another dream: He was pushed from behind off a height. Before he reached the ground, he woke up. He was then chased by men who wanted to kill him, they were throwing spears and he was running fast.

The patient was a boy, eighteen years, stammering (especially in front of people), timidity appearing in public, stammered quite a lot, very nervous.

Main themes:
- Sensation of isolation;

- Situation of disaster and danger
- Trapped and unable to get out;
- Unsuccessful efforts.

Rubrics:

— Forsaken feeling, sensation of isolation;

— Delusion, fail, everything will;

— Delusion, succeed, he cannot; does everything wrong;

— Fear, narrow places, in;

— Ailments from fear and fright;

— Stammering;

— Anticipation, stage fright;

— Anxiety, walking in open air.

"This stammering is something I'm trying to get out of, but can't", said the boy. The situational Materia Medica of *Argentum nitricum* is a situation from which he himself has to struggle and nobody is going to help him; he is trying but not succeeding. When the situation reaches the level where he can do nothing about it, he goes into the state of *Gelsemium*. So, *Argentum nitricum* and *Gelsemium* are complementary. In *Argentum nitricum* there is restlessness, activity, hurry, impulsive actions. *Gelsemium* is slow, sluggish, dull, paralytic, and does not want to be disturbed.

That is why closed places, high places, any situation can aggravate *Argentum nitricum* patients, and they can act in an impulsive manner in order to get out of this trap. Whichever situation in life reminds him of a trap aggravates an *Argentum nitricum* person. Such situations could be:

- Crowds;
- Closed spaces;
- Bridges;
- Tunnels;
- High places – for example buildings on fire;
- Aeroplanes;
- Any place where the exit is blocked.

The expression they like to use very often is: "There is no way out", or "I don't see the way out." The compensation is to see the way out all the times. So, they will never enter into a situation unless they can see the way out. They will never go on a journey unless they have the return ticket booked, i.e. the way out is not a problem. When they go to the cinema or theatre, they sit next to the door. In their own life, whenever they make a plan, they will see the way out of it. They cannot bear uncertainty: Phatak – "Suspense aggravates". When a time is set, again there is the feeling of something being limited, that the exit is blocked. It creates great anxiety because they are trapped in the time frame.

They are always trapped in an isolated way, always alone. They do not know how to get out of it. Another situation is the stage. They are anxious to go on stage, but when persuaded, feel isolated and trapped. They are alone and the exit is blocked. When the time is set, it creates suspense and they have the feeling: "I want to get it over because the time is passing too slowly" ("Hurry for the appointed time to arrive"). Always hurried and impatient. So you see this restless walking about: "Must walk" (Phatak's Repertory), "Restlessness, anxious, compelling rapid walking", "Walking quite hurriedly".

They avoid doing things, do not undertake anything because of this fear of being trapped. When they feel trapped they do almost suicidal, impulsive things. In physical terms, it is like throwing yourself out of the window, but in psychological terms, it means they will impulsively get out of the situations in which they feel trapped. For example, in their business, if they feel anxious or tense about it, they could suddenly impulsively drop the whole thing and leave even though they may lose a lot. So, you have the rubric: "Indifferent to business affairs". They have the look of a trapped animal. Even when talking about their health, they feel there is no way out and they are in danger, as if about to die. Then suddenly, they take an impulsive decision to drop the treatment they are taking and jump into some other form of medication/therapy. All this is worse when *Argentum nitricum* is alone because his feeling of isolation is aggravated.

In every expression, in every gesture, in every sentence, in every act of a man is his disease expressed. It is up to us to be able to see it. For example, the *Argentum nitricum* fellow said: "I am trying very hard to get out of this stammering and I am not succeeding." "I am trying very hard" – I have to try alone (sense of isolation); "To get out this stammering habit" – he is trapped in it; "And I am not succeeding" – feeling that he will not succeed.

It is important that the stammering is something that is bothering him. Stammering has to do with stage fright and appearing before people and this bothers him also. So, it is the picture of a claustrophobic/trapped man who cannot get out: that is the state of *Argentum nitricum*.

CALCAREA SILICATA

This is a very useful remedy. Some of the main mental symptoms:
- Anxiety regarding health;
- Anxiety regarding money matters;
- Fear of poverty;
- Sensitive to reprimands;
- Yielding disposition;
- Talks to dead people;
- Anxious restlessness;
- Frightened easily;
- Anxiety;

- Seeking support, i.e. Desire to be magnetized;
- Cowardly;
- Confusion of mind after mental exertion;
- Thinks his disease is going to be incurable;
- Sadness, causeless;
- Bashful timidity;
- Hurried, impatient;
- Irritable from consolation.

The closest remedies are:

- *Arsenicum, Staphysagria, Calcarea, Silicea, Gelsemium, Stramonium, Baryta carbonica.*

Physical symptoms I have observed:

- Tremors;
- Cold sweating palms;
- Blue line on edges of gums;
- Cold moist finger tips.

Anxiety regarding money and fear of poverty show that the person is coming from a poor family (situational). *Silicea* does not have this but instead has an air of egotism. *Calcarea silicata* does not have egotism but rather bashfulness. Poverty is like a primary disadvantage.

Silicea behaves like a princess, *Calcarea silicata* rather like a pauper. He has to be careful in spending money, being poor puts him at a disadvantage. Therefore, he has to become yielding, he cannot at any time assert himself, he would rather escape than stand up for himself. *Calcarea silicata* is not as obstinate as *Silicea*. *Silicea* has rigidity along with conscientiousness, which is absent in *Calcarea silicata*. Therefore, *Calcarea silicata* compares with *Staphysagria*. Both have high sensitivity.

Sensitivity to reprimands is an advantage. When you are starting at a disadvantage, then sensitivity keeps you safe. For example, if you are working under an irate boss, if you are sensitive to his reprimands, you will avoid any arguments and so prevent getting fired. *Calcarea silicata* therefore is a man who is poor and at a disadvantage. He becomes sensitive to reprimands and yielding, and also timid and bashful since these will help him.

It is a situation where supports are available, unlike that of *Psorinum*, where there is fear of poverty but no support, so he becomes despairing. In *Calcarea silicata*, support is available, so he turns to people form support, puts his trust in other people, goes to get psychotherapy, i.e. "Desire to be magnetized" (*Silicea, Calcarea*).

The divergence from other remedies comes with "Anxiety about health". It is not an ordinary anxiety but a severe one. It is seen in teenage boys who ought to be out enjoying life but who come to the clinic, spending hours there, worrying about some sneezing, a cold or the delusion of heart problem. The fear is of having an incurable disease. It is not a simple fear. It is a fear that paralyzes them and prevents them from going ahead in life. The only advantage of the fear is that it makes them non-achievers, more dependent. It gives them an excuse for non-achievement and dependence, and this is where it differs from *Staphysagria* and *Silicea*.

Staphysagria	:	is the competitor.
Calcarea silicata :		is the defeatist, loser.
Silicea	:	is a person who will try to reach high ideals.
Calcarea silicata :		is one who gives excuses not to reach.

It seems that they come to the doctor with the hope that they have a serious disease, as if they would like it to be so. They appear frightened; you see fear of disease on the face, but subconsciously they use these fears to do nothing. At this stage, when you contradict him saying that he does not have anything, he can get irritated ("Consolation aggravates"). Total lack of confidence exists in this remedy. *Silicea* also has "Irritability from consolation" and "Desire to be magnetized".

This appears to be contradictory. *Calcarea silicata* wants support, but would not like it to be said, that they do not have anything. This great dependability on people, especially financially and socially, brings it close to *Baryta carbonica*. When such a person dies (supporter), *Calcarea silicata* can be devastated. He can go into a shocked state – automatic conduct. He will sit still and do nothing or as a survival mechanism he may imagine that these people are not dead, "Talks to dead people" (Kent). She imagines that her husband is in the next room. They are wives who are emotionally and financially dependent on others.

Calcarea silicata is a person who is financially and emotionally dependent on somebody else, and due to some disadvantage (real or unreal) is not able to face the world of competition, and so avoids the world. *Calcarea silicata* acts as if he were a disabled son of a not-so-rich father.

The original situation comes from disabled state, i.e. not so well-to-do family. *Baryta carbonica* is very similar. *Baryta carbonica* is disabled in another way. *Calcarea silicata* is disabled in a way that he is not able to achieve what his parents want him to. Therefore, he needs an excuse for this. The really disabled man does not need an excuse, but *Calcarea silicata* consciously looks for an excuse not to achieve. The very fact that he has to produce these excuses shows that he knows he has to achieve. What the family wants him to achieve is usually money. Poor class parents expect their son to reach a high status but the boy finds that he is unable to fulfill their expectations. As it is, there is the relative disadvantage of being poor. He finds the goals set by his parents too high. So he has to be financially dependent, and in order to be so, he becomes mild and yielding.

Calcarea silicata is the boy whose not-so-rich parents expect him to achieve things beyond his capacity. This is the situation of *Calcarea silicata*. It explains three things:

- Why are most of the *Calcarea silicata* patients male? Because in India the male is expected to achieve.
- Why are most *Calcarea silicata* patients teenagers or just over this age? Because this is the age when the demands of the parents are maximum.
- Why are most *Calcarea silicata* patients really non-achievers? Because they come from demanding yet supportive families.

Baryta carbonica situation: the person is really disabled and so feel incapable. *Calcarea silicata* consciously feels the need to achieve which *Baryta carbonica* does not feel. In *Staphygrasia* survival depends upon achieving, as also in *Silicea* and *Lycopodium*, whereas in *Calcarea silicata* the patient has almost given up efforts at achieving, and his survival depends upon finding excuses not to achieve. *Calcarea silicata* are not total failures (non-achievers). They do achieve but much less than what was projected for them.

In short, *Calcarea silicata* has to do with money (relative poverty), expectations and neurosis. No wonder it is one of the most frequently indicated remedies in India, which has to do with poverty and expectations.

CARCINOSINUM

Carcinosinum is prepared from cancerous breast tissue. It was first used by D.M. Foubister on the main clinical indication to "Sleeplessness". It was initially used only clinically on the basis of a past history of cancer and later provings were made.

Situational Materia Medica: The situation of *Carcinosinum* is one of a child with a strict upbringing. The parents insist that the child should be perfect. Therefore, he shows "Sensitivity to reprimands". He becomes more "Fastidious" and there is suppression of desires. He has an artistic disposition with a love of music. "Dancing" is the way he can express himself and so this becomes his survival mechanism.

Out of this control, *Carcinosinum* patients feel they must be perfect and from this arises "Anticipatory anxiety". If they organize a party, they are not so much concerned that the party should get going as that everything should be perfect. Sometimes this can be so extreme that they become "Suicidal".

Staphysagria is the closest complementary remedy but the situation of *Staphysagria* is caused by being insulted by the person on whom he depends, whereas in *Carcinosinum* the situation is that of being heavily controlled by him. *Carcinosinum* patients are often the children or the partner of either *Lycopodium*, *Aurum metallicum* or *Nux vomica*.

Carcinosinum are controlled children who have good manners; they sit and behave themselves and are not mischievous. One of the most striking features of *Carcinosinum* is: "Fastidiousness". They are very well dressed people with good taste, unlike *Lachesis* who dress very gaudily. This *Lachesis* feature is seen in women approaching menopause in an attempt to maintain their charm. *Carcinosinum*, then, are conscious of good taste and desire perfection in everything. They may become neurotic about perfection. Neatness and cleanliness are not enough for them, they must be perfect; furniture must blend with the surroundings, with everything matching. *Arsenicum* patients want order, *Nux vomica* patients want everything in its place, but *Carcinosinum* craves "Perfection".

Carcinosinum people can be very "Mild" and "Sensitive", like *Pulsatilla* and *Ignatia*. They are very "Affectionate", "Warm" and "Sympathetic". This is similar to *Phosphorus*, but *Phosphorus* craves consolation and affection, while *Carcinosinum* is "Averse to consolation" and is "Offended easily" ("Ailments from reproaches"). They are caring and concerned for others; they are friendly, sociable and cheerful people who always come to you smiling. They will tell the doctor they are feeling better even though they are worse (unlike *Kalium carbonicum* and *Arsenicum*), as they feel sympathy for the doctor and do not want to offend him (*Staphysagria*).

Though they are sensitive and get easily hurt ("Sensitive to reprimands", "Easily offended"), they do not show it. Like *Ignatia*, there is a tendency to suppression, but hysterical weeping and involuntary sighing is absent in *Carcinosinum*. They accept every-thing with a kind of resignation and it all accumulates inside without any expression to the outside world. They have a lot of grief stored inside them, but are very yielding. So even though disappointed and dominated, they live without any expression of their sensitivity. They have a tendency to "Suppress" everything. They have tremendous "Anxiety about health" with a great "Fear and dread of disease", especially cancer. Another side of *Carcinosinum* is their very artistic nature. They are lovers of music, dance, painting, literature and poetry (*Staphysagria, Phosphorus, Lachesis*; opposite to *Bryonia, Arsenicum, Calcarea fluorica* who are materialistic). They are "Ameliorated by dancing" (*Tarentula*). They are nature-lovers and are "Ameliorated at the seashore" and þy thunderstorm and lightning (opposite of *Phosphorus*). So, in spite of an internal grief and many disappointments, they can still enjoy nature, the sea and thunderstorms.

Six striking elements of *Carcinosinum* blended together:

Fastidious	:	Desire perfection.
Sensitive	:	To hurt, reprimands and offence.
Yielding	:	Tendency to suppression and bearing all emotions without any protest.
Artistic traits	:	Sensitive to nature, music, dance.
Anxious nature	:	Anticipating always, since obsessed with the idea of perfection; not worried about success or failure. Anxiety about health, fear of disease, especially cancer.
Affectionate	:	Warm and sympathetic.

Physical elements:

– Blue sclerotics;

– Position in sleep – lying on abdomen;

- Desires eggs, fats, chocolates, milk;
- Moles on skin;
- Past/family history of infectious diseases, viz.:
  - Tuberculosis,
  - Measles,
  - Mumps,
  - Chicken pox,
  - Malaria,
  - Typhoid;
- Past/family history of cancer.

CAUSTICUM

The situational Materia Medica of *Causticum* is of a person who is facing a threat from outside and, in order to face this threat, he requires that the whole group should fight together. Being the strongest member of that group, the one who is the most capable of putting up a fight, he regards a threat to any one member of that group as a threat to himself. If he does not forestall the threat, it would affect the whole group and he will be weakened.

It is the situation of a man who is the only educated member in a group of illiterate workers on whom the management is pressurizing unfairly. The whole group has to fight back and if any of the workers is threatened, this man takes his side, fights for him, because if he does not and something happens to the worker, the group as a whole is threatened next. He, being the strongest member of that group, has to take care of the rest of the group, and he becomes very much concerned if anyone is troubled. His strength lies in the strength of the group and he is the one who looks after it. This can happen in a family too. One of the partners, the husband or the wife, realizes that the rest of the family is very weak, unable to face external threat and he/she has to take care of the family, to keep it united and safe. The survival of the family depends on it. If anybody who has gone out is a little late in coming back, he/she will get very much perturbed and feels tremendously anxious for his safety ("Anxiety about others"). This is the "Sympathetic" side of *Causticum*.

Nitricum acidum is very sympathetic too. In the Repertory, both *Nitricum acidum* and *Causticum* are listed in two marks; they are equally "Sympathetic", because *Nitricum acidum* comes from a very similar situation. The only difference is that *Nitricum acidum* is actually fighting a very hard battle with an enemy. It is not merely fighting unfairness like *Causticum*, but it is fighting with a person who has harmed him, and *Nitricum acidum* fights a long and unforgiving battle with him. For this battle he requires the support from all his friends. So, *Nitricum acidum* is very sympathetic to all his supporters. He cares a lot for them. He can do anything for them. Towards his enemy he can be just as hard and cruel as he is sympathetic/caring for his supporters. So *Nitricum acidum* is a man who is fighting the battle, he is very "Sympathetic" to his friends and has "Hatred" towards his enemies. This hardness of *Nitricum acidum*, its cruelty, is combined with its sympathy. So he says: "If I am a friend, I am the best friend and if I am the enemy, I am the worst enemy." So the rubric of *Nitricum acidum* is: "Delusion, as if engaged in a law suit", which explains "Malicious", "Obstinate", "Unforgiving", "Hatred" and others qualities.

The third remedy which is listed as "Sympathetic" is *Phosphorus*. *Phosphorus* is the only remedy which is listed with three marks. While there is a kind of selfishness behind the sympathy of *Causticum* and *Nitricum acidum*, in that they stand to gain by their sympathy, *Phophorus* is a genuinely sympathetic remedy. *Causticum* will be sympathetic, meaning he will be anxious for others, but *Phosphorus* feels the anxiety of others. So, there is genuine sympathy in *Phophorus*.

In *Causticum* the child goes out and comes a little late, the child is enjoying itself, but *Causticum* is worried. With *Phosphorus* this is not so. *Phosphorus* feels the anxiety of the other person. When the other person is anxious, *Phosphorus* feels it. *Nitricum acidum* is sympathetic conditionally. "As long as you are my friend, I am sympathetic; once you offend me, I shall kill you." So, this is not genuine sympathy – it is conditional sympathy. In *Causticum* too, there is conditional sympathy; but in *Phosphorus* there is unconditional sympathy. He really feels the suffering of others. It is very genuine and he "Desires company", "Desires sympathy from others". It is not so much the case in *Nitricum acidum* or *Causticum*. They do not desire company or sympathy as *Phosphorus* does. *Phosphorus* has got a genuine give and take relationship like the one who can make friends the quickest. You can communicate with a *Phosphorus* very easily; not so easily with *Nitricum acidum* or *Causticum*. Both will take care of you. But you cannot have a good communication with them.

CHINA

China is the man who had an ambition to do something, to make a fortune, to make a living like *Sulphur* or *Lachesis*. But people did not allow him to get on with his work, they troubled and hindered him all the time ("Delusion, work, hindered at") and so he did not achieve. He feels very frustrated, angry and persecuted ("Delusion persecuted") and develops a "Contemptuous" attitude towards everybody. He will not leave others in peace. He has no courage to break away and is "Indifferent" and "Hopeless". He feels "Suicidal" but without the courage to do it. He is frustrated in his ambition, and fantasizes about it in his spare time. He builds castles in his thoughts, becomes the King or Emperor. He plans step by step just how he will advance in his career. In his fantasy, he does what he would have done if he had not been hindered, but he knows that both theorizing and planning are useless.

China is within all of us. We all have plans and goals and somehow people come in the way and hinder us. We are frustrated but we know nothing can be done. We fantasize about what would have happened if the circumstances had been favourable, if we had good luck. We feel so unfortunate. Just our bad luck. *China* is probably the remedy for

China itself: the students have been so frustrated by the government and are left to fantasize what would have happened if their luck had been good.

FLUORICUM ACIDUM

The components of *Fluoricum acidum* are as follows:
– Immorality;
– Aversion to responsibility;
– Sexual desire increased;
– Aversion to his wife;
– Indifference to loved ones;
– Animated (attractive) to strangers;
– Increased energy;
– He requires little sleep.

Now, how can we connect these together? When does immorality become necessary? When does a person need to be immoral, irresponsible and sexually minded?

It would be a situation where, if he is moral, then he will suffer. It would be a situation where, if he is responsible and has too much anxiety for his family, then he will suffer. So, what is the situation where he will suffer from morality, responsibility and care?

As I understand, it is a situation where there is an incompatibility in marriage which is causing him suffering. He needs to break away from this marriage. Therefore, he needs to become irresponsible, he needs to become immoral, he needs to increase his sexual drive. He needs to talk pleasantly to strangers and at the same time becomes indifferent to his family. This state will enable him to break away from this incompatible marriage or relationship.

Therefore, if we read the rubrics in the Synthetic Repertory: "Delusion, marriage, must dissolve" and "Delusion, bethrotal must be broken", we find *Fluoricum acidum* under them.

So, a *Fluoricum acidum* situation is one of an incompatible relationship. Now, an important factor to remember is: please, do not look for a cause in a patient. If you see a *Fluoricum acidum* patient, do not think that he should necessarily have an incompatible relationship. Or if anyone has an incompatible relationship, please do not prescribe *Fluoricum acidum*. You have to only bear in mind that a remedy could be understood better if we try to understand the causative factor and the picture which develops from it. It only helps us to understand the Materia Medica of different remedies in a much better and easier way by trying to logically connect the components of each remedy.

Like for instance, in a *Veratrum album* case, we saw a patient behaving as if he was a king, though he had become a pauper; as a king who had lost his social position. He is a person who actually has not lost anything and he has no need to behave in this way. He required *Veratrum album* since he reacted unsuitably and out of proportion to the existing situation.

When the cause does not exist, the state becomes even more characteristic. But the seed of the situation which causes the state of the remedy originally has been created somewhere in the earlier generations. This is then transmitted as "roots" into the subsequent generations. For instance, in the *Veratrum album* case we can understand that somebody in his earlier generations must have lost his social position and created the *Veratrum album* state. This state has subsequently been transmitted as a root into this patient. Often such a history can be traced out.

Every remedy originally comes from such a state created by earlier generations. Such a cause need not necessary be found in the patient. But the totality of the patient's symptoms indicate that he behaves as if he is reacting to a particular cause or for survival in a particular situation. If we understand the particular situation, the whole picture of the remedy becomes very clear, and we can also very easily differentiate remedies.

This idea I have called "the situational Materia Medica" – understanding a remedy through the original situation in which the state could have been caused.

GRAPHITES

There are two very striking features in *Graphites* which blend together. Let me describe them one after the other and then we will see both blending.

The first feature is that the *Graphites* patient is very excitable. He becomes excited from the smallest possible thing. Excited would mean anxious, sentimental, despairing, irritated, sad. The slightest cause is sufficient to create a turmoil within him. Rubrics from the Synthetic Repertory are:

— Anxiety about trifles;
— Conscientious about trifles;
— Despair about trifles;
— Irritability about trifles;
— Laughing about trifles (this laughing about trifles demonstrates that *Graphites* can become happy quite easily too);
— Sadness about trifles;
— Trifles seem important;
— Weeping, anxious;
— Weeping after anxiety;
— Excitement, excitable;

— Exhilaration;

— Frightened easily;

— Sympathetic;

— Offended easily;

— Cowardice, opinion, without courage of own.

This kind of excitability makes the *Graphites* patient quite restless and anxious. There is "Anxiety about future", "Anxiety of conscience" and "Consciousness about trifles". The idea is that each of these emotions creates a kind of restlessness and excitement which can be easily seen. They are the kind of people who get very easily worked up over small things. This also accounts for the "Fastidiousness".

It is called for in a situation where calmness is not going to help, and one has to be excited for survival. One such situation could be where the other members of the family are taking it cool; they do not bother about anything. The house is in a mess, nothing works in order, everybody's work is pending and the husband and children are enjoying themselves. They do not care about the house. So, the wife becomes disappointed and excitable. A *Graphites* lady will probably have a *Calcarea carbonica* or *Sulphur* husband.

These are timid people who lack self-confidence. They are "Cowardly", "Irresolute", and always doubting themselves, which creates "Anxiety". Some features are similar to *Baryta carbonica*. They find concentration difficult and are dull, indolent, absentminded; they can get confused and are unable to plan. There is a strong feeling of inadequacy. It is one of the chief remedies for "Ailments from anticipation". They are always uneasy and fretful with the feeling that misfortune is round the corner or something will happen; a small misfortune can drive them to great "Sadness" and even "Despair".

In their talk they are quite excited and in their actions they are hurried and very restless. They cannot sit long in one place. They know something has to be done but they do not know what: "Fidgety", "Restless while sitting at work". This restlessness while sitting is because they cannot concentrate. Abstracting, theorizing, or analyzing is very difficult for them ("Fatigue from scientific labour" – Phatak's Repertory). When they go to a conference and have to sit and think, it is impossible. They are busy drawing or scribbling and when you ask them later what happened in the conference, word by word will be repeated but they will be no precis, because precis involves thinking, understanding and comprehending. This comes very close to *Baryta carbonica*; both have incapacity to think and abstract. But *Graphites* has much more excitement – "Despair over trifles".

Imagine a woman, whose husband has had a big business loss, whose daughter has eloped and whose son is quarreling with his father. When you ask what is bothering her most, she will say it is that her grandson is not eating properly. The whole house is breaking apart and what bothers her is a trivial thing like this. Big issues are out of her range. When she talks she is so excited, and will give every minute detail.

What *Pulsatilla* is at puberty, *Graphites* is at menopause. *Pulsatilla* is also dependent but she is very protected and does not bother about small things. She sweeps and gets things done. But when she marries and her husband does not treat her like a child, but instead expects her to take care of all these things, she goes into the *Graphites* state but the sense of incapacity remains.

It is mainly a female remedy. A busy executive cannot afford to be *Graphites*. If he is, he has to heavily compensate. So, in a man, *Graphites* is rarely found. What will give them away, even those who are compensated, is the way they describe their complaint, or an incident. This will be in the minutest detail and there will be no thinking behind it. For example, if a man has burning in his chest ameliorated by drinking cold water, *Lycopodium* will say: "I have burning in my chest which is better by cold water." But a *Graphites* will say: "Doctor, when I got up at night, I found there was a burning in my chest, burning like a fire and then when I drank cold water, I felt better, so much better."

When a *Graphites* medical student is asked to talk about a case, he will narrate the whole case in detail in the patient's exact words, he will say each and every thing that the patient said, but there will be no synthesis or comprehension. There will be a lot of sympathy involved in narrating the case, he may even start crying. *Graphites* patients in the clinic will seem quite excited and friendly. They are warm and sympathetic, they laugh easily and loudly, are talkative, expressive and anxious.

The other feature of *Graphites* is "Weeping ameliorates".

The rubrics are:
— Anxiety, weeping ameliorates;
— Sadness, weeping ameliorates;
— Weeping at trifles (Allen's Handbook);
— Apprehension and inclination to weep (Allen's Handbook);
— Weeping ameliorates symptoms;
— Despondency, she must weep (Allen's Handbook).

This feature looks a little like *Pulsatilla* but there is a big difference, which you can see in clinical practice. This weeping is an expression, and the *Graphites* patient is much, much better by expressing her emotions. She becomes totally calm and relaxed, and nothing other than expressing the emotion can give her this relief. Similarly, until she expresses she will be excited, anxious, apprehensive, sad, despairing and despondent. Her mind will be all shaky or vibrating but the moment she expresses, she becomes smooth and calm. She can hardly keep anything to herself; her opinions, doubts, fears, loves and hates, be they good or bad.

These two features blend together to make a unique personality. For example, a housewife whose husband has gone to work and something happens in the house: maybe she received a letter about someone's ill health, or she has had an altercation with the shopkeeper or one of her children has had a slightly raised temperature. She gets all worked up, she frets, and is excited and restless. She cannot do her work, she cannot sit at her work. She is anxiously restless and is waiting for her husband to return. Then, as soon as she opens the door to him, and before he can even come in, she starts describing excitedly and in detail everything that has happened. She goes on and on until she has finished and then she is calm and relaxed.

This quick changeability of moods you can see in the rubrics:
— Moods changeable;
— Anxiety followed by weeping;
— Cheerful followed by melancholy.

The closest thing I can compare this to is a tuning fork. A slight jerk to the fork will cause it to vibrate excitedly and if only it can transmit this vibration to something else, it will become calm immediately.

IGNATIA

The nature of *Ignatia* is like that of a woman who has invested her entire emotional bank balance into an individual. She is very sensitive to the behaviour of that individual; any misbehaviour or rudeness on his parts affects her profoundly and causes grief or sorrow. The only way this mild woman feels she can bring him back to good behaviour (and restore her equipoise) is hysterical manifestation on her part. When she is disturbed, any consolation only aggravates her condition. She is like a young woman in love and her future depends upon her marriage to this man. She has put into this man so much of herself, it is as if she is already married to him. Hence the single symptom: "Delusion, married, she is". She is in love with the man so much that she acts as if she is already married to him.

If she is a housewife, then her survival depends upon her family and she has no other interest. She has sacrificed all her desires and avenues of fulfillment of her "dreams". In short, she has invested all her thoughts, hopes and interests in her family.

Naturally, in these circumstances, when there is a disappointment or loss through death of the person near and dear to her, it produces a feeling of being ruined ("Delusion, ruined, she is"). There is a tremendous grief, anxiety, brooding and shock. It is this element that makes *Ignatia* the acute remedy for most people who are faced with the loss of a dear person, in whom they had invested a great deal of their emotions.

The signs of such emotional investment are twofold:
–   She tries not to hurt anybody; she even suppresses her own feelings, and bears her suffering silently. She is sympathetic, affectionate, caring ("Ailments from cares"), conscientious and duty conscientious ("Delusion, she has neglected her duty"); she is also yielding and cheerful, with undemonstrative grief.
–   The second aspect is attention-seeking behaviour, which is hysterical – convulsions, pain, globus, spasms, choking, sighing, childish behaviour, selfishness, etc. She may also weep, sob or shriek for help. This kind of sadness and weeping are precious to her, because it means that the attention of others is

drawn to her. Therefore, she resists consolation or any attempt to bring down the sadness. She enjoys the sadness ("Sadness, enjoys" – Phatak's Repertory).

Here are some more symptoms:
- Bad news, ailments from;
- Carried, desire to be;
- Confidence, want of self (which shows dependence);
- Industrious;
- Irresolution;
- Laughing;
- Monomania (all thoughts concentrated on one subject);
- Quiet/Secretive;
- Sentimental;
- Involuntary weeping.

The situation of *Ignatia* is of a woman who is dependent upon people who expect her to be the ideal woman. She is going to receive their care and support not by asking for it directly (like *Pulsatilla*) but by behaving in this silent self-sacrificing manner; by being a woman who cares for others at the cost of herself. That is what others expect from her, to be religious, conscientious, warm and caring. Her family casts this role for her. The young woman behaves as if her boyfriend expects this from her (in the actual *Ignatia* situation he does); and she tries to fulfil this role by being the silent sacrificer and taking all the hurts and the pains inside her. In this way, indirectly, she attracts sympathy. If all this fails, she has to become hysterical, which is a back-door entry to his attention.

In the East, these qualities are found in a woman from whom the family expects a lot of sacrifice. In the West, it is the situation of a woman who is dependent on a man who expects her to be the ideal, sacrificing woman.

In the case of a child you will find the following responses to various situations, which call for *Ignatia*:
- Offended easily;
- Sensitive to reprimand;
- Silent (Talk, indisposed to);
- Brooding;
- Sighing;
- Admonition aggravates;
- Weeping from admonition;
- Quiet disposition.

"Conscientious about trifles" has both *Ignatia* and *Silicea*. Both these remedies have to live according to a certain image and both have monomania. They think about particular things to the exclusion of everything else. The difference is that the image which *Silicea* has to live up to has to do with ego. In *Silicea* you have: "Timidity appearing in public" and "Fear of examinations". The image which *Ignatia* has to live up to is to be affectionate and sympathetic, which does not belong to *Silicea*.

But *Aurum metallicum* has a high sense of responsibility which *Ignatia* does not have. Therefore, *Aurum metallicum* is dictatorial whereas *Ignatia* is yielding.

When the young *Ignatia* woman finds again and again that her hopes have been belied, she will no longer enter into a relationship where there is a possibility of disappointment. This is *Natrum muriaticum*. When *Ignatia* gets into a situation where there is no use trying, she needs to become insensitive and apathetic, because now her sensitivity is of no use – even hysteria is of no use – then this insensitive state ("Indifference") is the state of *Phosphoricum acidum*.

Finally, when the *Ignatia* wife is treated very badly and her warm and affectionate nature or quality finds no appreciation, then she develops aversion to her family, the state of *Sepia*.

So, you find the complementary remedies of *Ignatia* in *Aurum metallicum*, *Natrum muriaticum*, *Phosphoricum acidum* and *Sepia*.

KALIUM BROMATUM

Single symptoms:
— Delusion, brother fell overboard in her sight;
— Delusion, about to commit a crime;
— Delusion, thinks she is about to murder her husband and child;
— Delusion, that she he accused of robbery;
— Delusion, thinks he is singled out for divine vengeance;
— Delusion, fancies his mother's house is invaded by lewd women.

These delusions give us a fairly good idea of the situation of *Kalium bromatum*: "Suspicious; looks on all sides; fears people", says Phatak's Materia Medica. One of the fears is that he will do something wrong. The expression of this feeling is:
– Restlessness (fidgety hands –"Hands, restless");
– Suspiciousness (looking to all sides);
– Fear of people.

Morality, crime and guilt are the main features of the *Kalium bromatum* state.

Situation: It is one where he has to be extremely vigilant so as not to do anything wrong. It is as if his survival depends on it; as he will be cast away if something goes wrong. The rubrics are:
— Forsaken feeling;

— Fear of being alone;
— Fear that something will happen;
— Fear of people.

He feels like a thief; answers no questions or "Answers in monosyllables" or "No to all questions". The situation is like one of a child being in a family where the parents are very strict morally. The mother says: "I like you, love you. It's not important that you are perfect, but morally if you move one inch away, I will not accept you." The slightest lie, robbing, dishonesty is a very big crime.

"Thinks he is singled out for divine vengeance": For a child, the mother is God. Vengeance means malice. The child feels that if the slightest wrong is done by him – God (the mother) will never forgive him. He has a tremendous fear and is afraid he might do something wrong. His childish instincts are going to make him do things which are not fully acceptable; and everything is wrong for the mother. So, he always feels like a thief.

"Delusion, brother fell overboard in her sight": This means she was watching and she let it happen! She feels: how could she have been so irresponsible or so negligent in her duty!

"Delusion, fancies mother's house is invaded by lewd women": This delusion means that women who come to his house are lewd and that his mother will find out about this immorality. This gives the idea of sexuality in *Kalium bromatum*. As puberty approaches sexual feelings come up and this is strictly prohibited in his house; so the usual problems of *Kalium bromatum* develop at around puberty.

"Fancies lascivious": There may be masturbation and a tremendous amount of guilt associated with it, and then *Kalium bromatum* starts brooding over these immoral things like *Plumbum*: "Brooding over forbidden things". The more the brooding, the more the guilt and the more he is afraid that people will realize his inner fancies. When he is thinking of such things, he looks around because he thinks people will realize these "dirty" thoughts going on in his mind.

Religion is not such a big issue in *Kalium bromatum* as "Morality". In *Thuja*, religion is very important: "Religious fanaticism". Religion is a kind of group morality, a code of ethics in a group. *Thuja* comes from a situation of religious order in society. Some Arab countries would require this remedy; very fixed ideas about religion. There is also "Fear of strangers" – in *Thuja* anything strange is not acceptable. There is a fear of being exposed and this fixity is combined with brittleness. Fear of ideas, values, of their images getting broken and so you feel delicate and the more delicate you feel, the harder you can get.

LAC CANINUM

The central feeling of *Lac caninum* is: "I am not good enough, I hate myself. I am fat and ugly, and I feel dirty and horrible. Why has it got to be like this? Nobody likes me or can like me. I am not clever enough, everything I say is stupid and foolish." – "Contemptuous of self", "Delusion, she is looked down upon".

"Delusion, she is looked down upon": It is the situation of a child in India, where to be fair is important, and she is a dark child born in a fair-skinned family. She is trying so hard to get fair-skinned, but is sure of failure. She hates herself and suffers in comparison to others. People bring clothes only for her sisters. Nobody listens to her. She is uncared for and neglected because her body looks bad. She washes herself frequently ("Washing always her hands"). People disturb her like snakes and vermin ("Delusion, sees snakes").

She does not trust herself anymore. She is totally "Irresolute" and "Lacking in self-confidence", believes all that she says is a lie. She "Loathes life" and goes into tremendous "Depression". Nothing can be done to make her better. She feels worthless and disgusted with her body ("Delusion, dirty, she is"). She thinks she matters little and it is better for others if she is not there ("Delusion, diminished, short, she is"). She is the untouchable. She is unimportant, not morally but qualitatively. She wants to commit suicide and put an end to her suffering. Sometimes she gets angry with other people for treating her like this. She can get quite rude and quarrelsome. Inside, she knows it is no use, she is dark anyway and nothing can change it. She reacts with "Rage" and "Hatred". She feels suppressed and troubled, and blames other people. She feels she will get an incurable disease and die ("Delusion, incurable disease, has"). She becomes mean. She feels she has been given a raw deal and writes ugly letters to her acquaintances ("Writing meanness to her friends").

It could be in a marital relationship where husband and wife are equal when they are married, but now, after marriage, she is at home bearing children; she becomes obese and develops wrinkles on her face. Her husband remains active and has become famous and popular. Then they go to a social gathering and nobody pays any heed to her. She feels left out and hates herself and also her husband for putting her in this situation. Even her children do not consider her important.

Basically, *Lac caninum* is a feeling within all of us. Dissatisfaction with our natural endowments, and trying our best to bridge the gap between what we are and what we want to be, blaming ourselves and blaming other people and feeling unlovable because of our deficiencies. *Lac caninum* represents the unconditional not-OK. It is a feeling that nothing can be done, because we are not-OK anyway. All of us have this element but in most of us other conditions come up and if we fulfil them, we feel OK.

LACHESIS

Lachesis – a lady who suffers by comparison – imagines she is a daughter-in-law who is being unfavourably compared with the other daughter-in-law: intense sense of competition. She feels also people are out to get her and they are plotting against her: very "Suspicious" of them. The only way she can be worthy is by "Egotism" and "Loquacity", satire, "Mocking", jesting and by feeling "She is under superhuman control". When these fail, she turns to spirituality for salvation. All this competition has to do with interpersonal relationships, so for the time being she has to shut off from work ("Business, aversion to"), and concentrate on sorting out her problem.

It is the spirit of competition and "Jealousy" that differentiates *Lachesis* from *Platinum* and *Palladium*. The remedy that comes close is *Hyoscyamus*. The difference is that *Hyoscyamus* is trying to attract attention by foolish behaviour and by playing antics, and *Hyoscyamus* can get quite threatening with violence and striking, whereas *Lachesis* is more vivacious, more clever and more out to prove that she is better than the other.

Lachesis can be the story of a girl or a woman who has been deserted by her fiance or her husband in favour of somebody who is better than her. This is the situation where she has to be (a bit) cautious about the other person's comparison against her, and at the same time prove her own superiority by her egoistical talk. When this does not work, she has to give up the idea of marriage and take to spiritual things just like a person whose death is near.

Another *Lachesis* situation is of the mother-in-law. After her young daughter-in-law comes in the house, she loses her place to this other woman who is more educated, younger, more attractive, and she tries her best to compete with her. She becomes "Egoistical" and when this does not work, she becomes religious, spiritual and feels her death is near and that she should concentrate on spiritual things. She starts meditating, "Feels she is under a superhuman power". That is why there is a rubric: "Avoids company to indulge in her fancy".

LYCOPODIUM

Some of the prominent components of *Lycopodium* are:
– Lack of self-confidence;
– Egotism;
– Sentimentality;
– Memory poor;
– Irritability;
– Cowardice; fear of people;
– Desires company;
– Contradiction, intolerance of;
– Hurry/Impatience/Restlessness;
– Lascivious;
– Moods changeable;
– Avarice;
– Conscientious.

Every *Lycopodium* patient will have a combination of some of these attributes. Which of them will be prominent will depend upon age, sex and social situation. The ones approved by the society in which he operates will be prominent, while those which are frown upon will appear in a milder or compensated form.

For example, in a society where lasciviousness is considered a sin, you will find the patient has compensated for it by some means. Or where egotism is frowned upon, the patient will try to avoid a display of this quality. Sometimes, he may purposely denigrate himself, so that even by mistake he does not sound egotistical.

Again, in an adult, cowardice my be hidden by an outward show of bravado. This becomes necessary to protect his ego. Occasionally, the *Lycopodium* patient may take recourse to tall talk, boasting with false bravado. This eventually produces a feeling of guilt with a fear of being discovered.

An offshoot of this egotism is the censorious attitude towards others. The *Lycopodium* patient is not unhappy with others, but he nevertheless criticizes them in order to establish his own superiority. At the same time, his "Conscientiousness" will not allow him to overcriticize others. However, he will justify his criticism and say (and feel) that it is his duty to do so in the interest of the person criticized. Thus, *Lycopodium* can be very subtle in his criticism of others.

"Egotism" also makes him "Intolerant of contradiction". His views are supreme and must be accepted. This creates a lot of hurt feelings in those around him, and also for the *Lycopodium* patient himself. In the Repertory, "Egotism" is also to be compared with rubrics like: "Haughty", "Contemptuous", "Presumptuous", etc. This egotism ultimately shapes many symptoms of *Lycopodium*.

The *Lycopodium* child will have: "Fear of new people", "Fear of men", "Fear of strangers", "Cowardice", "Timidity", etc. Hence, he stays away from new situations and new people, sticking always to the familiar and the known. In an adult this quality gets heavily compensated or overcompensated.

Lycopodium's ego does not allow him to accept his "Cowardice", "Lack of self-confidence" and "Fear of men and people". So he creates for himself a world within a world, where he surrounds himself with people whom he does not have to fear, but, in fact, who fear him. He will select a woman who is mild, who will never raise her voice and he will marry her. The *Pulsatilla* woman is the best for him, I suspect. In his work, play and social situation, he will gather around him only such people whom he can dominate and who he needs not fear.

Also such people will praise him and boost his ego. They will never contradict him. In such an environment, *Lycopodium* will dominate, dictate and rule with an iron hand. But outside the safety of his domain, he will still remain anxious and timid. He will never venture out of this domain; yet, at the same time, he will seek to expand it, and will bring more and more people under his power. This situation is found under the rubric "Love of power".

This "Love of power" makes *Lycopodium* very ambitious. He will seek to achieve a position where he can dictate to others and he dare not be contradicted. Whether it is political power, or scientific authority or even an executive post or as the head of an institution, *Lycopodium* seeks power anywhere and everywhere. A frustrated ambition, displacement, even retirement can be a severe blow for *Lycopodium*. He may not give up so easily; nevertheless, there are going to be times when he is deeply upset about the whole incident.

Lycopodium represents the constant struggle of a man between "Cowardice" and "Egotism", between "Lack of confidence" and "Haughtiness", between "Timidity" and "Dictatorial" attitude. The earliest signs of this struggle are seen in childhood. The child is usually lean. He is timid, especially in the presence of new people. For example, it would be difficult for him to approach a shopkeeper for something. He wants to speak on the stage before an audience, but gets a stage-fright. So, he indulges in childish fancies and theories and has to remain content with this for some time. He imagines, or dreams, that he is someone big, a leader of people, a much respected and powerful man – "Delusion, childish fantasies, has".

Lycopodium remains a loner; he cannot make new friends easily and does not like to play. This "Aversion to play in children" arises out of his timidity and also his physical weakness. He is scared also because his brain is more developed than his physique. He is scared of those in authority, of his father and of the head of the college, but not of his mother. So, in his home, he dominates, rules like a tyrant, makes others do what he wishes, commands them; but in the school he is an angel, a pet of his teacher. To those with whom he can be, he is rude and contemptuous – "Contemptuous, hard on subordinates and agreeable to superiors or people he has to fear".

Once, a child of six or seven was brought to the OPD. The parents were describing the child's nature, and I was observing the child. He was mild, reserved, scared, timid and cowardly, whereas his parents were saying that he was very irritable, rude and dictatorial. The contrast between what the child did in a familiar circumstances and what he did in the presence of new people struck me and enabled me to give a prescription of *Lycopodium* with success.

This contrast comes up again when deciding about his profession, his future. His two main considerations in this respect are: security, and a position of power and a challenging job. Therefore, he will have a lot of irresolution while searching for a job that fulfils both these needs. Ultimately security will win, but he will scheme and plan for a better position in the future.

With this basic framework, let us now examine the other aspects of the *Lycopodium* personality.

"Desire for company": Firstly, *Lycopodium* has a fear of being alone in a hostile world, amidst unfamiliar persons. He seeks out known persons, wants someone around him all the time, "even if in the next room", or to accompany him. Thus, he becomes dependent on those few relationships that he develops and he feels anxious if these are threatened by illness or death or if they move away. This makes the *Lycopodium* appears sentimental, desiring company, affectionate, sympathetic and these qualities make

Lycopodium appear like *Phosphorus*, but the big difference is that the *Lycopodium* does not like others to depend on him. He would like to avoid responsibility as far as possible. Hence the rubrics: "Estranged, flies from her own children" and "Escape, attempts to, from her family, children".

"Lasciviousness": Next comes the "Lasciviousness" of *Lycopodium* which, with his desire for company, leads to love affairs. His fear of the new initially makes him shun them, but once he overcomes the fear, he plans the love affair with great care and thought, that is the characteristic approach of *Lycopodium* to all his problems.

He is willing to share and give, but not to commit. So, when an affair reaches a peak, he backs out. Thus, he has a string of love affairs until he eventually decides to settle down. *Lycopodium* usually has late marriage. He now plans the choosing of his spouse seriously – one whom he can depend upon, lean on, who can be his constant companion, one who can be relatively independent but who can reciprocate his warmth and care and allow him to dominate. When he finds such a mate, he marries.

"Strong sense of duty": The third feature of the *Lycopodium* personality is his "Strong sense of duty". Once he commits, he accepts full responsibility, as he is duty bound to do. In short, once he commits himself he is not irresponsible.

"Affectionate": Another feature of the *Lycopodium* personality is that behind his irritable exterior he can be very "Affectionate", "Sentimental" and "Emotional". Hence, the rubric: "Abrupt, rough, yet affectionate". The sentimental and emotional part of *Lycopodium* is rarely seen; it is often hidden. He can weep when seeing sentimental scenes, both of joy and sorrow. Nostalgia, pleasant memories, relationships with his parents, memories of his relatives – these can cause tears. Thus the rubric: "Weeps when thanks". He can be sentimental also from scenes in novels and cinema.

Naturally, with all these contradictions in his nature – his irritability and sympathy, his cowardice and love of power, his lack of confidence and dictatorial tendency – all these are bound to create a split in his personality and give rise to two symptoms: "Irresolution" and "Moods changeable".

Let me now emphasize two more aspects of *Lycopodium*, viz. hurry and impatience, and restlessness.

"Hurry": "Hurry" is a component which usually does not need to be compensated, as it is encouraged and approved by social standards. In this fast paced world, hurry can be an asset. Therefore, this symptom of *Lycopodium* will be found directly in most patients. They do things fast, but not necessarily in an orderly manner. They are impatient and cannot wait for anything (like *Histaminum*). In the clinic during the interview, especially during the follow-ups, they are quite impatient and want to get away quickly. Combined with their poor memory, this impatience accounts for a lot of mistakes. So, there are mistakes in speech, writing, etc. Their mind works too fast, and is always racing ahead (*Natrum muriaticum* lives in the past, while *Lycopodium* lives in the future).

"Weakness of memory": Another aspect of *Lycopodium* is his "Weakness of memory" and "Mistakes in speech and writing". The weakness of memory is especially for proper names; it also extends to dates, events and the things he has to do. This poor memory is a big handicap for *Lycopodium*.

In some aspects, *Lycopodium* resembles *Nux vomica* with the irritability, impatience and dictatorial nature. These two remedies may come close, but the main difference is that *Nux vomica* is not so cowardly inside; he is more rash and audacious. He is more forceful and expressive, more impulsive and explosive. From a young age we can see this difference. *Lycopodium* has a shy and introverted childhood, while *Nux vomica* has a daring and mischievous one.

In adulthood, when given a job, a *Nux vomica* will do it "by hook or crook" and he will break all the obstacles in his way like a "road roller". He can often get violent. The *Lycopodium* is not so ardent and daring; he weighs each step and does not rush into things. If the obstacle is big, he will hesitate and may even withdraw.

Other remedies to be compared are *Aurum metallicum, Staphysagria, Chelidonium, Phosphoricum acidum, Platinum, Medorrhinum, Sulphur* (*Lycopodium* is called vegetable *Sulphur*), *China, Silicea, Argentum nitricum, Bryonia, Calcarea carbonica* (the exact opposite of *Lycopodium* in that *Calcarea carbonica* is slow and indolent while *Lycopodium* is fast paced and emotional).

Lycopodium is a man who was told that he is not loved as he is, but only if he achieves something in his life. So his feelings are connected with achievement. He feels he must achieve in order to be loved. A mother tells her son: "Look on, you must achieve a position of eminence for me to care for you, to feel good about you and value you." He receives the message that in order to get her love he must achieve, reach somewhere which is not easy, but difficult, because the circumstances around him are difficult. When Shivaji's mother told him: "You must reach that fort and conquer it", he had no army and the fort belonged to the Emperor, so he had an uphill task. He had to collect an army around him, to conquer and achieve what his mother wanted to do; and when he said: "Mother, I have done it", she replied: "Conquer another fort." *Lycopodium* is the son of a mother who demands achievement, the son of a father demanding achievement.

In order to conquer and achieve he needs people to whom he can dictate, he needs an army around him, and he is afraid that he will not reach the goal, it is too difficult. So, he has "Anticipatory anxiety" and "Lack of self-confidence". On one side he has "Egotism", "Ambition", "Love of power" and "Dominance" and on the other side he feels uneasy without achievement. It is the feeling of inferiority which requires him to be egoistic. *Lycopodium* is duty conscious because he feels it is his duty to please the person who demands, yet he feels that his slender means reduce his capacity, therefore the rubric: "Fear, unable to reach his destination".

This feature of love of power and achievement never leaves a *Lycopodium* patient even when he tries to look for a wife; he feels that a woman can love him only if he achieves. When he is close to a woman, he wants her to like him not because he is what he is, but because of his achievements. He does not like a woman who likes him for what he is. He feels the need to show her that he is achieving, and he constantly emphasizes that he is a great achiever. The moment he knows that it is not so, the whole relationship breaks down. He always likes to be on a pedestal; if he steps down from the pedestal, he is low/short. He has to be on a pedestal. He has to be an achiever.

When a woman leaves a *Lycopodium* person, he feels she left him because he had not achieved. He will now be more busy in achieving; he has no attachment to his children – rubrics: "Children, flies from his own", "Indifference to her children", "Estranged, flies from her own children", "Escape, attempts to, from her own children".

LYSSINUM

In the chapter "Unsuitable Postures", I have given a case of *Lyssinum*. In this chapter I shall examine in further detail its situational Materia Medica and compare it with the situations of some other remedies.

The main feeling of *Lyssinum* is the "feeling of being tormented":
— Delusion, tormented, that she is (*China*, *Lyssinum*);
— Praying;
— Violence;
— Mortification;
— Impulse to kill;
— Impulse to stab his flesh with the knife he held;
— Forsaken feeling;
— Delusion, fancies he has suffered wrong;
— Anger alternating with quick repentance (*Crocus sativus*);
— Rage followed by repentance (*Crocus sativus*).

With these fundamental rubrics, let us construct the situation of *Lyssinum*.

"Rage followed by repentance" (*Crocus sativus*, *Lyssinum*): What is the meaning of the rubric? Rage is violent anger, almost frenzied violence. It is required in a situation where a person has to lash out against somebody because if he keeps quiet he will be further troubled. But this rage has to be followed by repentance because if it persists too long, it is not good for him. He has to repent and this gives the idea that the rage is directed towards somebody on whom he is dependent but who is troubling him also. This is the situation of both *Lyssinum* and *Crocus sativus*. But this the only common feature of the situations. Otherwise there is difference between the situations. This is because *Crocus sativus* has other components:
– Singing;
– Dancing;

321

- Cheerful;
- Attractive behaviour (*Tarentula*).

Lyssinum does not have this attractive behaviour. So, *Crocus sativus* has the need to attract alternating with the need for rage; so, also, cheerfulness alternating with quarrel-someness. *Crocus sativus* is the situation of a woman who is being neglected by her husband who is dominating her at the same time. There is a threat of his going away because he is no longer attracted by her and, at the same time, he is dominating. In this situation, the combination of attractive behaviour keeps him attracted towards her, and rage prevents him from being too dominating and too troublesome.

The *Lyssinum* situation is one of a woman who is being insulted, tormented and injured by her own husband, the very person on whom she is dependent, and she reacts with rage. The rage is quite violent in *Lyssinum*. It is wild behaviour, with the impulse to cut, bite, stab and kill. This is because *Lyssinum* is not merely being troubled but is actually tormented. There is threat, so she becomes very sensitive and a dog-like behaviour sets in:

— Delusion, he is a dog;
— Growling like a dog.

If you hurt a dog too much and then touch him he will growl, become wild and will bite. So, whenever people trouble him again he becomes violent and gets into a rage. Later on he cools down. He is not always in a rage, but only when he is troubled. He is like a dog dependent on his master for food.

The heightened sensitivity of *Lyssinum* to light and noise is a characteristic feature of his "Alertness". *Lyssinum* will respond to any situation in this manner. For example, if the roof is leaking, he will tolerate it for some time, but then will get so angry that he takes a hammer and breaks off the plaster. In a few minutes his anger subsides and he goes to get cement and fills it up again.

I remember the case of a homoeopath who would tear his Kent's Repertory into bits and stick it up again. When I asked him why he did this, he said that when he does not find the right rubric he just tears up the Repertory. After tearing it up, he repents and then carefully pastes the whole book back again. If he is trying to put a nail into the wall and it will not go in, he will break the wall. Once, there was some flooring work going on in a room upstairs which made a lot of noise. He got so angry that he broke the glass cupboard in his clinic with his fist and got cut. He immediately repented and went to another doctor and got it stitched up.

We too can get similar feelings in some situations. For example, we are going in a car and it is giving us a lot of trouble. It stops once, we push it in the hot sun, get into it and again there is some noise, some smoke and after some time we feel like getting out of the car and kicking it or breaking it. We may even do something like this, yet we have to repent because we are dependent on the car. So, we get into it and tow it to the nearest mechanic. The *Lyssinum* situation is therefore one in which he is tormented by a thing on which he is dependent, and this torment is not merely an insult but actually causes physical and mental pain. It is not merely being treated badly or unjustly. It is much worse than that; it brings about a situation of rage, of insane rage, of wildness, of fury, or biting, or growling like dog, attacking and then withdrawing.

The *Staphysagria* situation is similar but on a much milder level. It is a situation of being unjustly treated by a person on whom he is dependent and so there is:

- Injustice, cannot support;
- Egotism;
- Insulted feeling;
- Mortification;
- Suppressed anger;
- Occasional violent outbursts of anger.

But the anger in *Staphysagria* is not like the rage of *Lyssinum* with its biting and kicking. It is not a situation of being tormented like *Lyssinum* but just being treated unfairly, mortified, insulted. It is not something active, not taking a stick and poking the ribs. Telling you to get out creates *Staphysagria*, whereas taking a stick poking your ribs three times a day creates *Lyssinum*. Both are similar, very much complementary remedies, being in the same situation but in different degrees.

China also feels tormented like *Lyssinum* but it lacks the violence and wild behaviour, the anger with quick repentance and the frenzy of *Lyssinum*. The torment in *China* is constant whereas the torment in *Lyssinum* is episodic, periodical and sudden. *China* as long-standing persecution, hindered at work; something that is going on for a long time, chronically and so, out of all this, he becomes indolent, he does not want to do anything and just sits and daydreams. This is the situation of *China*. He also has an unfortunate feeling, suicidal disposition and sad feeling.

So, one can say that *China* has the same situation in a more dragged out and less intense way. When we talk of persecution, the other remedy which comes in is *Drosera*. Its other components are:

- Anxiety when alone;
- Desire for company.

The *Drosera* persecution is not from people on whom he is dependent. There are people on whom he can depend and he seeks their company. There are outside agencies that are persecuting him and he can turn to nobody for support and security – this is missing in the *Lyssinum* situation.

The remedy that comes closest to *Lyssinum* is *Stramonium*. *Stramonium* also has the wild behaviour, the insanity, the dog-like behaviour and the doglike attacking rage. But the delusion that he has suffered wrong is not present in *Stramonium*; the situation of *Stramonium* is one of threat. He is being threatened by somebody outside and he runs and seeks light and people. He likes to escape from the position of threat, whereas *Lyssinum*

323

has no escape, therefore *Lyssinum* is not present in "Escape, desire to", in which *Stramonium* is prominently seen. *Stramonium* is threatened and afraid, he reacts with violence, trying to get out of this, trying to cling to somebody for support and looking for a secure and safe place. *Stramonium* has fear of strangers; therefore, he seeks the familiar. He is terrorized by the unfamiliar, whereas *Lyssinum* is tormented by someone familiar and so there is no question of clinging in *Lyssinum*.

Hyoscyamus also has the feeling of being wronged and injured, but he does not have the tormented feeling like *Lyssinum*. There is a desire to escape like *Stramonium*. He also has a fear of being poisoned, unlike *Lyssinum*. *Lyssinum* is therefore not a suspicious person whereas *Hyoscyamus* is one of the most suspicious people in our Materia Medica. In *Hyoscyamus* there is also attractive behaviour:

- Lascivious;
- Singing;
- Jesting;
- Shameless;
- Amativeness.

All this is not seen in *Lyssinum*.

Jealousy and suspiciousness of one's partner are the strong features of *Hyoscyamus*, whereas sudden anger with quick repentance is the main feature in *Lyssinum*. The *Hyoscyamus* situation is one where he has an unfaithful partner whom he loves, but who can even kill him. So, it is a situation of threat, a feeling that he has been wronged. *Hyoscyamus* on one hand is trying to keep the relationship going, but is also cautious and suspicious on the other hand. He has the need to be attractive. So, this is not a situation of being tormented but of being injured and wronged.

Lyssinum is a situation of being tormented by a person on whom she is dependent. The torment is episodic or periodical and the person needs to react to it with rage which is followed by quick repentance. This is the situation of *Lyssinum* but it can take various forms in a child, in a man or in a woman. Not only can it exist in the relationship between people but also in the relationship between a man and his house or his machine, etc. Whenever dependence and torment are seen together, and the torment is episodic or periodic in its course, one is reminded of *Lyssinum*. Also if a person reacts to any situation as if it is this one, then he requires *Lyssinum*.

NATRUM CARBONICUM

Natrum carbonicum is the outcast. She is the one who does not fit into the majority's idea of the norm and, therefore, is always at the receiving end of abuse ("Offended easily"). Most of the society have "ganged up" in order to pursue her, making her feel that she is abnormal and not a part of the group. They isolate her, creating a division between herself and others, which include her own family and intimate friends. She develops a "Fear of people" and a "Sensitivity to certain people", especially those who are against her. At the same time she develops a "Sympathetic" and sensitive attitude towards those who are similarly cast out by society. She reacts to this kind of criticism with "Quarrelsomeness", anxiety and courage. She becomes "Suspicious", "Violent", indignant, heedless of behaviour, imagining herself to be sick and seeing no hope in this "no win" (therefore inconsolable) situation. She experiences sadness, weeping, "Suicidal feeling", and "Indifference". Certain situations aggravate her problem, namely company and crowds.

A thunderstorm signifies the coming together of dark clouds in preparation for a storm and downpour. It symbolizes the way people get together to shower her with abuse. To this very strong weather she reacts with anxiety and fear. This is so every time there is a sudden change in the temperature, signifying the coming of a thunderstorm.

Music, for a *Natrum carbonicum* patient, signifies several individual notes coming together to form a meaningful sound of harmony. The piano is the instrument through which such a coming together of individual notes is most obvious. It reminds her of the situation when totally different individuals come together for the sole purpose of harming her. It is this music that she has to face and she gets anxious and sad, even suicidal from doing so. In this "no win" situation there is anxiety and fear about the future. She is confused and such confusion is only made worse by dwelling on the problem. This is not something that thinking can solve and so she has to stop; there is "Dullness", "Prostration in mind", "Indifference", "Discouragement" and "Despair". It is at such times that she will avoid the sight of even her intimate friends. However, she will turn to a sympathizer for support in the form of being "Magnetized" (suggestions). As things get taken away from her, she becomes "Avaricious", developing a "Fear of robbers". All this naturally keeps her in a "Discontented", uncomfortable and "Sad" state which will sometimes end up with cheerfulness, singing and loquacity. Such a sad person is unable to indulge in, and therefore, reacts to excessive joy. The main rubric of *Natrum carbonicum* is: "Delusion, division between himself and others". Other notable rubrics are:

— Fear, society, of;
— Estranged, family, from her;
— Estranged, friends, from;
— Ailments from anger;
  – with anxiety;
  – with fright;
  – with silent grief.

It is interesting that *Natrum carbonicum* does not have any fear or delusions of animals. It is only fear of man and people. The quality that he is afraid of is not the animal quality of attack but the human quality of forming a group and casting out people if they do not fit into the expected norms of the group. The creation of such norms, the judgement, criticism and the "ganging up" against a few individuals is a speciality of the human race, and is probably unique to man.

In this sense, *Natrum carbonicum* has a problem with qualities which are human. Therefore, it is one of the prominent remedies for "Fear of men and people".

OPIUM

Morphine is a derivative of opium. This is used in medical treatment for a particular state, i.e. a state of too much pain, one of extreme physical or mental suffering.

The components of *Opium* are:
–   Indifference to pain and suffering;
–   Rash;
–   Bold, courageous;
–   Does not complain;
–   Delusion, says he is well when sick.

The situation of *Opium* is given under the rubrics:
—   Delusion, of frightful animals, i.e. people around him appear to be frightening like animals;
—   Delusion, sees hideous faces;
—   Delusion, that he is away from home;
—   Delusion, that he would be murdered;
—   Fright, complaints from;
—   Frightened easily;
—   Fear, of being murdered;
—   Fear, of being approached;
—   Fear, of death;
—   Delusion, sees soldiers;
—   Delusion, that people are fighting.

"Delusion, that people are fighting": It is a situation of war. Before a soldier goes to war, he may need *Opium* because he needs to be bold, courageous and indifferent to suffering and pain. He should not complain even though he is going to see persons who will attack him like animals to kill him, or he may see hideous faces. His own people are going to die and there will be bloodshed and much pain. If the person is sensitive to all this, he is going to collapse.

This has been well portrayed in the Bhagavad Gita, where there is a situation of war. The warrior asks the Lord what he should do in such a situation where there is pain and suffering all around. The Lord replies:

"When man gives up all desires of mind and delights in himself, then he is said to be a man of steady wisdom. He who is imperturbable in misery and free from desires amidst pleasures, who has denied all attachment, fear and anger – that state is said to be one of steady wisdom. He who is free from affection everywhere and who, when faced with good or evil, neither welcomes or hates them, has steady wisdom and when he completely withdraws his senses from the sense objects as a tortoise does to his limbs, then he is wise. From the abstemious embodied being sense of objects fall off but not the relish, but even this relish of man of steady wisdom ceases when, that supreme being is realized."

Indifference, getting rid of fear and anger and being calm amidst suffering are the features required by a warrior. "Delusion, people want to execute him": it is a painful situation that calls for such indifference.

The *Opium* state eases the anxiety and makes a person more courageous. A timid person becomes bold under its influence. Complementary to *Opium* is *Baryta carbonica*, which is one of the most timid, dependent and anxious individuals in the Materia Medica. *Opium* produces an anaesthetic effect – a numbness and painless and a pleasant feeling. It also makes the person sluggish, dreamy, dull and wanting nothing.

Opium comes from a state of suffering, a great threat and fright, so much that the person becomes numb, insensitive and indifferent in order to survive because the situation is too much for him to bear. In contrast is another hallucinogen, *Cannabis indica.*

Opium:
— It has hallucinations which are out of context to reality.
— Person is dull and lost in his own world.
— Insensible to what is going on.
— *Laughs involuntary.*

Cannabis indica.
— Sees things as more beautiful, out of proportion to reality.
— Persons are more active, laugh a lot.
— Sees things more clearly, colours are brighter and music sounds louder.
— *Laughs immoderately.*

Cannabis indica: The person becomes more sensitive to what is outside, which is the opposite of *Opium*. What is outside is boring, dull, unexciting and without interest, so he seeks excitement. "Delusion, he is leading a vegetable existence": These individuals take thrill and pleasure in everything. They laugh and they talk a lot.

Opium: They are people who are lost in their own world, who are gentle and mild and those without anxiety and fear. Nothing seems to affect them.

Anhalonium: These people have withdrawn totally from reality and are lost in their own world of delusions of fancy, in which they see colours, shapes, forms and sounds which are completely distorted and unconcerned with reality. They live in a world of light, colour, sound and bliss. Here there is splitting of the self:

– One real;
– One that exists in hallucination. "Splitting" of mind occurs in some cases of schizophrenia and this remedy has a schizophrenia-like state.

This remedy is for people who seek ultimate spiritual experience, who are searching for an out-of-the-world experience.

Situation: Those who have everything and want nothing, i.e. are materially wealthy, such that material things are no challenge for them. They have seen the best of reality as it exists and more of the same thing would only be a repetition, so they seek the thrill of an "out-of-the-world" experience.

Though matching in some symptoms, vast differences exist in the original situation from which the state of *Opium, Cannabis indica* and *Anhalonium* arise.

PSORINUM

Psorinum is a man who has tried to climb a mountain but somewhere along the way is stuck and can neither go up nor down, both being too risky. He is scared to move. Here, an element of tremendous fear is involved: fear with despair. It is not only that he doubts his capacity but he is scared of the mountain itself. It is rather the feeling of danger from outside than a sense of incapacity inside. This fear comes out of a situation in which he finds himself when he has not really assessed the risks involved.

For example, while *Sulphur* is very optimistic and thinks he is great, he can do anything, and *Tuberculinum* has a strong desire for travel and adventure, *Psorinum* will get into adventures where he reaches a particular point from which it is difficult to move forward. *Sulphur* and *Tuberculinum* are complementary to *Psorinum*.

I remember an occasion where I had gone to the Himalayas with a friend. We saw a mountain almost unclimbed and we were thirsty for an adventure. So we started climbing. It was a steep mountain without a path. We reached a particular point about half way up where it became almost impossible to climb further. When we looked back there was no way, not even traces of our footsteps to go down. That was a near death experience. I was almost hanging, holding on to the branch of a tree, with the support of only one foot. At that particular time in my life, I felt totally hopeless, I had a strong fear that this was the last moment of my life and if that was so, why prolong it? So, on one side there was total despair, a feeling that it was better to leave the branch and let go of life – a totally pessimistic approach – and on the other hand, there was great irresolution, anticipation and foreboding. Although I had a friend with me, I felt totally abandoned. It started raining and my rest-lessness increased. Finally, I found a way out by trying very hard and moving inch by inch. I think I was in a *Psorinum* state at that time. The rubrics are:

— Despair;

— Fear of disaster;

— Fear of misfortune;

— Irresolution;

— Ailments from anticipation;

— Anxiety, foreboding;

— Pessimistic;

— Forsaken feeling;

— Estranged from her family;

— Restlessness aggravated during storm;

— Anxiety riding downhill.

The idea of *Psorinum* is that he has reached a very risky point in life, in health, in business, etc. There is nervous foreboding, despair and the fear of disaster.

The rubric "Despair of recovery during convalescence" means that there is danger right up to the last step. He has suffered from such a dangerous illness that he cannot afford to have even the slightest hope. So he has despair until he recovers totally.

Phosphoricum acidum is the situation of a man who has made the effort to climb the mountain and has become so tired that he doubts his capacity to climb further. He is the person who tries but the mountain seems a tough task for him. He feels like taking rest, by lying down. He is totally exhausted and has no energy left. So he sits, sad and broods about his unattainable goal:

— Apathetic from his struggle with unequal circumstances (Phatak's Materia Medica);

— Brooding over one's condition;

— Desires to lie down.

RHUS TOXICODENDRON

The components of *Rhus toxicodendron* are:

— Anxious restlessness;

— Fear of misfortune;

— Fear of evil;

— Forsaken feeling;

— Fear of being murdered;

— Anxiety worse in the house and better walking in the open air;

— Anxiety about her children;

— Anxiety from sitting bent;

— Restless feet;

— Superstitious fear.

The above components indicate that *Rhus toxicodendron* has a tremendous fear that something is going to happen. Restless feet indicate an uncertain fear, an inner restlessness which cannot be explained.

Zincum metallicum	:	has fear as if he had committed a crime, but he does not know what.
Medorrhinum	:	has fear of misfortune as if something will happen, and is clairvoyant.
Rhus toxicodendron	:	has nervous apprehension, a dread, but does not know exactly why.

These three remedies with restless feet have to be cautious and on guard. These remedies are also superstitious – it is a kind of inexplicable fear.

Rhus toxicodendron has:

- Fear of people;
- Fear of being poisoned;
- Fear of being murdered;
- Superstitious fear.

There is always a fear that something bad is going to happen, that someone is going to kill him – a threat inside the house. They are better walking in the open air. The threat is from something inside the house, so he always has to be on guard. If this threat is from outside, he can turn to someone for support, but this is not found in *Rhus toxicodendron*; there is no clinging and no desire for company. So in *Rhus toxicodendron* the threat is from his own people. He cannot turn to anyone for help and he has to keep quiet.

"Talk, indisposed to", "Dwells on past disagreeable occurrences after midnight": As night passes, the anxiety grows. Somebody in the house is going to murder him after midnight when he cannot shout, cannot tell anyone else, and there is no support:

- Weeping involuntarily;
- Weeping causeless, without knowing why;
- Nervous, sad person;
- Cautious , especially after midnight;
- Cannot tell anyone;
- Forsaken feeling.

It is the situation of a woman who has young children and is alone in the house with her husband who is capable of killing her. He is probably drunk and there is no saying what he is going to do; so she has to be on her guard, she is vigilant, nervous, tense, and sad, etc. She is brooding, crying and unable to express her fears. She is dependent on her husband and worried about her children.

I have found that the wife of an alcoholic usually requires *Rhus toxicodendron*, and their children usually develop *Rhus toxicodendron* characteristics. The *Rhus toxicodendron* position is one of threat to a woman from her own husband, due to his drinking or violent habits whereby he may lose control.

Rhus toxicodendron is complementary to *Calcarea carbonica*. A woman who is tense and nervous and feels the threat of being killed, out of proportion to her situation, would be a *Calcarea carbonica* who comes from a world of security and cannot bear horrible things or any cruelty. If such a woman is brought up in a secure environment and then marries a violent individual or a drunkard, she can develop *Rhus toxicodendron* state very easily, even if her husband is not violent – a little anger on his part will make her react with tremendous nervousness, fidgetiness and "Restlessness". Just as *Calcarea carbonica* with a threat from outside can go into a *Stramonium* state, a *Calcarea carbonica* with a threat from her own husband can go into a *Rhus toxicodendron* state.

It has been observed that women who need *Rhus toxicodendron* will need *Calcarea carbonica* some time. Similarly, children with tremendous "Restlessness", fidgetiness, "Desire for cold milk", and for hot baths, and such other characteristics, after being given this remedy, usually go into a *Calcarea carbonica* state.

The actual situation may not be found in the life of the patient or in the life of his parents. If, previously, he was in the situation of the opposite or complementary remedy, then the slightest trigger is enough to move the person into the new state.

SILICEA

The word "Fidgety" is mentioned in Phatak's Repertory about *Silicea*. *Silicea* is tense, especially in the presence of others. The most important about *Silicea* is the feeling: "What do others think about me?"

It is not important that people think of him as a good or a nice person, but that he is thought of in a particular way, a fixed manner. It is not a good opinion that he wants, but a fixed, definite opinion. For example, he does not want others to say: "This man is a very helpful, sympathetic person." But, if he has the idea that he must be a great scientist, then he cares that others should think of him as such. So, one gets the idea that the *Silicea* person as an OK feeling which is conditional to having a very specific image.

The state of *Silicea* therefore arises from a situation where a person's acceptance by people as fulfilling a specific image is a necessary condition. For example, a child is told that he will be accepted and loved if he achieves in a specific way. This could be his doing exceedingly well in sports, becoming a great cricketer. So it is very important for this child that other people think of him as a good cricketer, even better than he is. This creates tension and the timidity in the presence of others:

- Timidity in public;
- Monomania;
- Fixed ideas;
- Fixed actions;
- Counts pins;
- Rigid thinking;

- Egotism;
- Ailments from egotism;
- Fidgety.

Contrast with *Palladium*: *Palladium*'s feeling of well-being (OKness) is subject to having the good opinion of others but not a specific opinion. There is "Longing for the good opinion of others". That means you have to say: "What a nice person this is", or "What a good person he is." You may not say that about *Silicea*.

Palladium comes from the situation where the child needs to get the good opinion of others; otherwise he will be neglected and unappreciated. The *Carcinosinum* situation is similar: the child must be perfect in all ways — his work, his dress, etc., and this "good feeling" is subject to his being perfect and controlled. So, you will see rubrics like:

— Fastidious;

— Sensitive to reprimands;

— Offended easily;

— Desire to travel (*Tuberculinum*).

The *Tuberculinum* situation is where the parent is forcing the child to adopt his standards and so the child tries to revolt – "Audacity" – and to go away – "Desire to travel". That is the connection between *Carcinosinum* and *Tuberculinum*. This illustrates how the situational Materia Medica links remedies together. We went to *Palladium* from *Silicea*, to *Tuberculinum* from *Carcinosinum* – all having similar situations; but note the shades of difference in the situation of each remedy. The difference is in the expression and the state of being. We said that *Silicea* comes from a situation where he must earn a specific image because only then will he be accepted; therefore the need to be accepted is a part of the situation:

— Yielding;

— Mildness.

So, *Silicea* is actually fulfilling an image made for him by somebody else. In that sense he yields to that image, but he also becomes fixed to it and so he is "Obstinate". This combination of "Obstinate" and "Yielding" is found in *Silicea* in a peculiar way. On one hand there is "Desire to be magnetized", i.e. he wants to be completely under the suggestion of somebody else, and on the other hand he is so fixed in his opinions that if he is contradicted he can become violent: "Contradiction, intolerance of, has to restrain from violence" (*Aloe socotrina*, *Silicea*). *Silicea* does not openly revolt but sticks to her opinion. Samuel Butler used to say: "Convinced against her will, but of the same opinion still." So, she will say "Yes" finally and not make an issue, but inside the feeling is: "No, this is wrong." *Silicea* is "Dependent". She is unable to revolt but if she yields completely and gives up her goals and images, then whoever she is dependent on will start disliking her. This is a peculiar contradiction.

Situation: A man has married a woman who is not well-educated and soon she discovers that her husband only wants an educated wife, a woman of a particular learning.

If she does not fulfil this, her husband will start disliking her. So, she becomes a student of literature, starts studying very hard and tries to become perfect. Therefore, the rubrics are:

— Ailments from anticipation;
— Anticipation, examination, before;
— Fear of failure;
— Delusion, fail, he will.

So, she concentrates completely on literature and tries to build up her image in this way – she is very nervous when people come to visit because her ignorance may be exposed. She is dependent on and yields to the man. At the same time if the man says: "Forget about literature, let's go out", she will become stubborn because if she gives that up, he will lose respect for her. The man wants her to be yielding and at the same time he wants her to have an individuality so he is pushing both messages at her and she responds in this way. She cannot yield too much, yet she cannot be too stubborn; this is her situation. Her survival depends on constantly proving to others that she is very good in a specific way.

Lycopodium is similar to *Silicea*. *Lycopodium*'s survival depends upon reaching a particular goal rather than fulfilling a particular image. Therefore, *Lycopodium* is not present in rubrics such as:

— Timidity appearing in public;
— Monomania.

The fixity of *Silicea* is not present in *Lycopodium*. Once *Lycopodium* reaches one goal, he sets another for himself, but in *Silicea* it is a very specific image which she never reaches.

One of the situations of *Silicea* is that of being the eldest child in the family. The eldest child is the torchbearer, the one who keeps up the family name, the crown-prince. The crown-prince has a tremendous image to keep up. People may pressurize the second and third child, but the focus of everyone's attention is the crown-prince. This is how *Silicea* comes close to *Aurum metallicum* since *Aurum metallicum* is also the eldest son. The difference is that *Silicea* is image-bound whilst *Aurum metallicum* is duty-bound. *Silicea* does not have responsibility whereas *Aurum metallicum* has the responsibility of the whole family.

Aurum metallicum: The situational Materia Medica is one where his survival is dependent on his fulfilling his duty. *Aurum metallicum* is the eldest child of the family and the father is dead. Society will blame *Aurum metallicum* if he does not take charge of his siblings. So *Aurum metallicum*'s survival depends on his being moral. He sacrifices his interests for those of the family. He raises the family. He is the duty-bound son who is rigid in his views, very moral and conscientious. The feeling of duty of *Aurum metallicum* is totally missing in *Silicea*. *Aurum metallicum* is more concerned about how he appears to himself. He always checks whether he has done it rightly, since his survival depends on this, and not how he appears to other people. Consequently there is no timidity when appearing in public. As long as he is straight and he has done his job, he is safe. So, feelings of guilt, morality feeling, religious feeling are all strong in *Aurum metallicum*. "If I do my job, nobody can say anything about me." This is the state of *Aurum metallicum*. *Aurum metallicum* is also much adamant about principles. His value systems are very strict and he imposes the same values on others, described by the rubric: "Dictatorial".

Baryta carbonica: This is another remedy which comes close to *Silicea*; it is the exact opposite of *Silicea*. This is because *Baryta carbonica* is someone who does not care about his image. He is a fool, and he knows it and he knows others know it too. However, this does not bother him. *Baryta carbonica* is the dependent child of the family. He is the child everybody takes care of and nobody is really concerned whether he does well or not. It is accepted that he is a fool, that he will do badly and that he will have to be supported. This is *Baryta carbonica*, the exact opposite of *Silicea*, and therefore they are complementary. *Baryta carbonica* feels he is inferior:

— Delusion, legs are cut off;

— Delusion, he walks on his knees;

— Taking the support of others.

Silicea has: "Contradiction, intolerant of", "Haughty" and "Egotism".

Sulphur: Here is another remedy that comes close to *Silicea*. *Sulphur* already has a good opinion of himself. Therefore, *Sulphur* appears in the opposite rubric: "Indifference to personal appearance". The difference between *Silicea* and *Sulphur* are as follows:

Silicea	**Sulphur**
Cold moist palms and soles	Burning palms and soles
Chilly	Hot
Clean	Dirty
Very particular about his image	Careless about his personal appearance

This kind of fixity is not present in *Lycopodium*. Once he reaches the goal, another one is taken up, but in *Silicea* it is a very specific image which she never reaches. This idea of an image also gives the rubrics:

— Conscientious about trifles;

— Remorse about trifles (where *Silicea* is the main remedy).

She has to be very particular about every little thing so that she does not reveal her real self which is opposed to the image. She is very careful about perfection in a particular way.

Silicea is the princess. A princess is of royal descent and her survival depends upon fulfilling a particular image. She has to talk, walk, sit, stand, etc., in a particular way in public. If she goes to a discotheque, no one will care for her anymore, nobody will love her.

So, whenever there is a demand from others to fulfill an image in order to be accepted, *Silicea* will be present. It is hardly surprising that childhood, the time when these images are not yet established, is the time that *Silicea* enjoys most. Even in the dreams you see "Dreams of youth time". This is the most prominent dream of *Silicea*.

I saw a Swiss doctor who, when asked: "Tell me about your father", replied: "My father was the chief doctor" of a particular place. Again he saw the need for an image. Why did he have to emphasize that his father was the chief doctor? What happens is that his anxiety to maintain an image (a fixed image which is threatened all the time), *Silicea* concentrates on himself. If there were such a rubric as: "Anxiety only about himself", this would have been a good rubric for *Silicea*. *Silicea* people lack emotions. Their emotions are blunted. This includes their ability to communicate, their affection and their warmth. These are lacking unless this too is a part of the image. I have seen *Silicea* people who are social workers, working in the slums, but this is part of their image.

Silicea does not require company, it is not a prerequisite for their situation. *Silicea* does not react well to consolation either, so they will not display much gratitude or affection and therefore can be quite difficult to get along with. A *Silicea* may break but will not bend. Slowly another phenomena results — you find that they cannot take or accept affection just as they cannot give it. They can only accept praise, someone's acknowledgment that they are excellent in their field. But if you say: "I like you as you are", they will run away from you because they cannot accept themselves as they are. They are not OK as they are and if you like them as they are, then they assume that something must be wrong with you.

Silicea people can be: "Late to develop relationships and to marry". They will occupy themselves with books. One can call them "eternal" students. So at the age of sixty, *Silicea* is still attending university, trying to add more degrees to her name.

Some expressions of *Silicea*

If a *Silicea* girl likes you, she may not tell you so because it is below her dignity; this does not form part of her image. The princess cannot go and tell anybody: "I like you." So, she will come to you with some work that concerns her image.

For example, if she is a student/colleague, she will come with an essay and ask your opinion about it. In this way she meets you three times, once to give the essay, another time to take it back and again to discuss it. It also gives her an opportunity to show you how good she is.

The fixity of thinking, the difficulty in accepting things from outside and the violence against everything that goes against her fixed ideas, all find their expression at the physical level in the form of asthma, intolerance of vaccination and foreign bodies and also a strong chronic defence against them.

When *Silicea* works, she does so with great precision, great calculation and great exactitude, but with little feeling. There will be much analysis but no synthesis. There will be facts and figures but no philosophy. Most of the work will only have theoretical value.

The *Silicea* homoeopath uses a computer because this represents exactness. A large number of symptoms can be taken, much detailed analysis can be made (which remedy carries how many marks and in that way it is more than the other remedies, etc.), but there will be very little feeling. The way the homoeopath analyzes his patients is very similar. I have seen my *Silicea* students argue very stubbornly over why I chose a particular remedy when other remedies carried the same number of marks (and sometimes more)! When I try to explain that the central feeling of the remedy I have chosen is given exactly in the book, they say: "So what, what about the rest of the symptoms?"

You can read a letterhead and say this is a *Silicea* person as there will be so many letters following his name, from various universities around the world, and below that will be written the important posts he has held. Three quarters of the letterhead will be taken up with the credentials and there will be little space below for writing the letter!

How he appears is very important. When a doctor is called to give a lecture – for instance he is asked to talk on *Silicea* – he will say: "My dear colleagues, I remember the time when I was dining with the Queen of England and she turned around and said: 'Doctor so and so, you are one of the greatest homoeopaths in the world and I would like to know which is your favourite remedy.' I answered '*Silicea*' ", and the rest of the lecture follows only after his credentials have been thoroughly established.

The lecture will be prepared word for word. It will be typed, printed and distributed to all the participants. It will be exact with quotations from books and a large bibliography and references at the end. Everything will be neatly marked, but the article will convey nothing that is not known, no new revelations, no imagination. It will be an absolute dry copy of what everybody else has said before, but put forth very beautifully, perfectly and impressively.

STRAMONIUM

— Chases imaginary objects.

Meaning : Chases: drives away. Imaginary: not real, or what exists only in imagination. Object: material thing or something one directs attention to.

Interpretation : To drive away imaginary things to which his attention is directed.

Expression : Patient: "I keep getting these colds. I am determined to find the root cause and to eliminate it."

This has other elements too:
– The colds are troubling ("Delusion, injured, he is being");
– Wants to find out ("Desire for light", "Fear of dark");

- Determined to chase/hunt;
- Root cause (imaginary object);
- Eliminate ("Kill").

Rubrics:
— Hide, desire to;
— Fear, of bright objects;
— Sadness in sunshine;
— Aversion to light;
— Delusion, objects, fright from bright;
— Fear, of looking at glass;
— Fear, of being approached;
— Fear, of mirrors.

These rubrics indicate that whenever there is a fear of being exposed, there is a desire for darkness. They feel very vulnerable to attack. On the other hand, when they have to find something or they want to expose something, bring it into the open, then they want light. This is fear of the unknown. For example: Europe is cut into two, one part buried, the other alive. Parents separate: the child is cut into two, remaining with one parent. One side alive, the other buried, not to be mentioned.

"Chasing imaginary objects" : philosophical, psychological devils. Pretends that all is well and happy. Each person chooses his own Bible, the old Bible has crumbled and new Bibles (cults) come up; each group speaks a foreign language.

Vulnerable to being exposed, to injury, to hurt, to even look at themselves; they compensate with psychotherapy. The feeling is of being "Alone in the wilderness". Manic reaction, wild dancing, loud music, split personality, sensation of being double.
— Familiar things seem strange;
— Feels forsaken;
— Violence when approached and provoked;
— Compensation: meditation, relaxation, yoga, spirituality.

There is a subculture in Europe, where several hundred people cling together in broken down houses, wearing black, reacting violently to any attempt to remove them. They react well to loud music, sit in dark rooms with flashes of rhythmic light giving a scary, strange effect. They cling to the drugs of their culture.

People who feel split up (alive on one side, buried on the other), they are split off from society which they claim to be buried and the other side of them is more than alive. The part which they have buried is their connection with society, the orthodox traditional side. The part which is alive, or even more than alive is the one which is unorthodox, new, different (rubric: "Delusion, everything is new").

— Familiar things seem strange

They cannot form the balance and just split up in the alive and buried side. The most extreme form of this is probably a terrorist, where one side is totally buried and the other terribly alive. Each person can chase what in his imaginary are the symbols of the society he is fighting against. So, when they break the windows of a bank, they are merely attacking an image and not reality.

Jumping out of bed: suddenly jumping out of one's resting place. This occurs due to a feeling of impending threat in the place of rest.

In *Stramonium* the feeling is that the familiar bed and house become too oppressive and almost threaten to suffocate ("Fear of suffocation"). There is a claustrophobic feeling ("Fear of narrow places"), "Forsaken feeling", a feeling that he does not belong there ("Lost", "Familiar things seem strange"). He suddenly jumps out of his home, society, family, relationship, etc. He escapes only to find some other company, family or society.

TARENTULA HISPANICA

Tarentula hispanica is a fascinating study of the situational Materia Medica. It has the following elements:
- Desire for music;
- Desire for dancing;
- Desire for painting;
- Very active;
- Very industrious;
- Very deceitful;
- Very cunning;
- Mischievous.

When does a person need to sing and dance? Which situation demands that a person should dance and wear colourful clothes in order to survive? A person who dances and wears colourful clothes does so in order to be seen and noticed, in order to attract attention. So, when does a person need to attract attention?

A person needs to attract attention in a situation where he wants to be noticed and is not. Such a situation arises when a person tries to attract the attention of the opposite sex. For example, person A is interested in person B but person B is not looking at person A. It is not a situation where person A has gone up to person B and has been rejected, but where the person A, being very much interested in person B will try any tactic to win over that person.

Such a situation is not one of disappointed love; it is a situation of unrequited love. Phatak gives in his Materia Medica the causation of *Tarentula hispanica* as: "Ill effects of unrequited love".

THUJA

Thuja comes from a situation which demands rigidity of thinking. This occurs when religion becomes very strict. Social security lies in adhering or at least appearing to adhere strictly to religious norms. Inside however, the person feels as if his real self will be exposed; he therefore feels brittle or fragile. In his manner, he looks straight and fixed, and his ideas and views do not allow for any freedom of thinking. Yet from inside, there is always a fear of being exposed and his whole cover breaking down; this makes him stiff and cautious in the presence of strangers. The fall from grace is symbolized in: "Dreams of falling", from which he wakes up with a fright. The theme of religion is represented by the rubrics: "Religious fanaticism" and "Fanaticism" in general. The fixed idea is shown by the rubric: "Monomania". The guilt is expressed by the rubrics: "Anxiety of conscience, as if guilty of a crime", "Delusion, sees strangers in the room" and "Presence of strangers aggravates". The brittle feeling in the mind is represented in the body too, and can be seen in: "Delusion, body is made of glass".

VERATRUM ALBUM

The most beautiful symptom of *Veratrum album* given in the Synthetic Repertory is: "Despair, social position of". If we understand this symptom correctly, it will be very easy to understand the picture of *Veratrum album.*

The state of a remedy can be understood as a set of components, as a characteristic combination of components. The important components of *Veratrum album* are as follows (rubrics from Synthetic Repertory):
— Liar;
— Deceitful;
— Courageous;
— Squanders money;
— Extravagance;
— Praying;
— Religious;
— Shameless;
— Smiling;
— Laughing
— High-spirited;
— Haughty.

Now, we will try to understand how these components are connected to each other. We can make a connection between them if we understand that this man behaves as if he is reacting to a loss of social position. It is like a king who has suddenly become a pauper. If this man is to survive, he has to tell lies and make a show of wealth. He has to squander money and speak highly of himself. He needs to create an aura of grandeur. So, all these components of *Veratrum album* can be connected together if we imagine that this is state which has arisen as a survival mechanism in this particular situation.

42

COMPARISON OF REMEDIES
USING SITUATIONAL MATERIA MEDICA

APIS, LACHESIS, HYOSCYAMUS

We are going to compare the jealousy of *Apis* with the jealousy of *Hyoscyamus* and *Lachesis*. *Apis, Hyoscyamus, Lachesis* and *Nux vomica* are among the most jealous remedies, along with *Calcarea sulphurica, Medorrhinum, Pulsatilla, Staphysagria* and *Stramonium*. How do we differentiate between these remedies in this rubric? It is the other components of each remedy which will differentiate them from each other.

This is a very simple way to explain it. *Apis* will be busy and restless, *Lachesis* will be sarcastic, *Hyoscyamus* will be shameless and foolish, *Nux vomica* will be quarrelsome, along with being jealous.

This is a practical way in which we usually explain the difference. But there is another way and that is to try and understand why and how the jealousy of *Apis* comes and why and how the jealousy of *Hyoscyamus* comes. If we understand the context in which the jealousy arises in each of these remedies, then we shall also be able to understand the other components. First it is necessary to look at all the components.

One of the components of *Apis* is violence: there is shrieking and violent activities. Violence is called for as an adjustment when there is a situation of threat. When a person feels threatened, he becomes violent. Therefore, the *Apis* situation is one in which is required some kind of threat. The kind of threat has something to do with death, because there is a presentiment of death and a fear of being poisoned. Death and this fear have something to do with being alone because there is fear of being alone and desire for company.

This is therefore a situation where there is a threat from outside. There is also a lot of crying. Crying is usually the reaction to grief. So, along with this threatening situation, there is grief involved. This is a situation which involves both fright and grief. Now, there is also jealousy and busy industriousness. So there is fright as well as grief; she has to be busy and she has to be jealous. Also she has to be lascivious. When you combine all these, the situation which you come to is of a young widow, or any person who has lost his

341

partner. Left to herself, this widow feels threatened, feels grief, feels frightened and needs to find the company of a person of the opposite sex, therefore she has to become more lascivious. She also has to compare herself with the position of other people. She has to feel jealous of the people who are secure. Unless she feels jealous of their position, she is not going to try for security. *Apis* is a known remedy for widow. All these components come together to form the situation which is *Apis*. Once you understand the situation of a threatened widow, that is *Apis*, you know how all the components come in this state.

What we have to remember is that the states we are talking about are very common. We must not imagine that they are to be found in a very special and rare situation. Then you will not see any *Apis* people around. You will see a remedy indicated as frequently as that situation is found in human life. If the stress situation which causes the state of the remedy is frequently found, then that remedy will be found often in practice. The rarer the stress situation required to cause the state of that remedy, the rarer that remedy is found in practice. That is why *Sulphur* is found frequently indicated. What most of us require in today's world is hope, a good self-image and philosophy in order to survive the stress. *Sulphur* provides these three qualities. It is a much needed state and so it is a most frequently indicated remedy.

If we look at the components of *Hyoscyamus*, we will find violence like *Apis*, which again means a threatened situation. There is also jealousy, like *Apis*, which means the need to compete. Thirdly, we will see "Cheerful", "Laughing", "Joking", "Smiling", etc.; "Lasciviousness" is also present, as in *Apis*, as well as "Suspicion".

When we put these components together, we can see that the situation is similar to *Apis*, but there is no grief. This is not a person who has lost something. Cheerfulness, laughing and singing are usually to attract attention. That means somebody is not giving him proper attention or somebody is going away. At the same time, he is very suspicious because this is also a threatening situation. So, he is threatened and he needs to attract attention. This is a typical situation of a man who is in love with his wife, but she is having some kind of extramarital affair. Here, the man is suspicious and jealous. He feels afraid and threatened that his wife may do something to him, and he can get violent. At the same time, he loves her and so needs to attract her attention by laughing, shamelessness and by sexual behaviour. The jealousy of *Hyoscyamus* is what he actually needs, to be jealous of the other person, in order to do something to get his wife back.

The *Lachesis* situation will have different components from both *Apis* and *Hyoscyamus* because *Lachesis* is deceitful and egoistical. *Lachesis* is always talking about himself and slandering other people. The *Apis* jealousy is not going to be helped by slandering others or being egoistical or deceitful, nor will *Hyoscyamus* be helped by this kind of behaviour, but this state will help a person who is in a very strong competition. There is only one place and that place has got to be filled by the most able person. This person has to prove he is better than others to get that one place. You can say *Lachesis* is a person in a competition.

43

REMEDY RELATIONSHIP

In this chapter we shall examine the basis of complementarity and inimical relationships between remedies.

Complementary remedies

Complementary remedies are those that are frequently found to be indicated after each other; and we shall attempt to find out why this is so. For example, a *Staphysagria* state is one in which a person feels humiliated and insulted. Naturally, this state will arise more easily in one who originally had pride and egotism than in a one who did not. We know that *Staphysagria* is often followed by *Sulphur*. In other words, a *Sulphur* state of egotism predisposes to a *Staphysagria* state of humiliation. Therefore, when we see *Staphysagria* in a person, it would be worthwhile examining whether there is a *Sulphur* state behind it, which therefore may follow it. Of course, a particular state can exist independently, but there is a good chance that it exists because of the predisposition caused by another state in the background, and this background state is usually the opposite.

To take another example, *Stramonium* has a state of tremendous terror and violence coming from feelings of being lost and forsaken in a dangerous place. The predisposition required to develop this state may well be one of great security, like living in a shell. Such a need for security is found in the *Calcarea carbonica* state and it is this kind of person who, with only a slight exciting cause of fear, will easily develop a *Stramonium* state. So, we have to understand that the *Stramonium* state may come about easily in a *Calcarea carbonica* person. Therefore, you can suspect a background of *Calcarea carbonica* when you see a *Stramonium* state.

We have also talked, in the chapter "Unsuitable postures" about the transmission of roots from one generation to another. It is possible that when a *Stramonium* root is transmitted (which means probably the father or the mother had a strong *Stramonium* state), the root of *Calcarea carbonica* is also transmitted, being the background state. Thus, you find these remedies forming a pair, just like *Staphysagria* and *Sulphur*.

Another relationship I have seen in practice is the one between *Hyoscyamus* and *Staphysagria*. *Staphysagria* is a state of suppressed hostility and suppressed sexuality. When he breaks down, the *Staphysagria* patient may develop a state like manic depressive psychosis, and in the manic state there will be overt sexuality and expressed hostility. This is the *Hyoscyamus* state. Some years ago I saw a patient who presented with a mania requiring *Hyoscyamus*, which gave immediate relief. There was a *Staphysagria* state in the background which became apparent after the *Hyoscyamus* state had subsided, and after *Staphysagria* was given, the patient did not suffer a relapse (case given in chapter "Acute processes").

So we see one state predisposing to another. The two states form a pair and are usually in some way opposite to each other.

Another well-known pair is *Natrum muriaticum* and *Ignatia*. We find that when *Ignatia* comes up as an acute remedy, it is usually followed by *Natrum muriaticum*. Again, they seem to be in opposite state with *Ignatia* having constant and active grief, while in *Natrum muriaticum*, it is passive, chronic and underlying. Similarly, if you take anxiety which is subconscious, reserved and unexpressed, you have *Thuja* and its complement is *Arsenicum album* with overt anxiety, tremendous restlessness, and expressed fear. Another good example is the relationship between *Aconitum* and *Sulphur*. The contrast is quite striking. *Sulphur* is indifferent, philosophical, careless, cheerful and imaginative. He is not really bothered about anything. But when this person has a sudden fright or fever, his state changes to one of tremendous anxiety and excitement with heat and restlessness. So, when the indifference of *Sulphur* is suddenly jolted, he will develop the *Aconitum* state.

If a person is already very anxious, like one who is in an *Arsenicum album* state, then a sudden stress would not make him go into an *Aconitum* state.

Let us take an example on the physical level. A person is indolent, fat, fair and flabby and not used to exercise. If this *Calcarea* patient lifts a heavy object suddenly, he will get a sprain. So, his indolence predisposes him to a *Rhus toxicodendron* state. These two remedies are complementary, the one with tremendous restlessness and the other with indolence.

If we examine complementary relationships in this way, we find a lot of pairs with opposite states to each other: *Nux vomica* and *Sulphur* for example. *Nux vomica* is so clean and *Sulphur* so dirty, *Nux vomica* so chilly and *Sulphur* so hot; *Nux vomica* is ardent and vehement while *Sulphur* is careless and lazy. So, *Sulphur* predisposes to *Nux vomica* and *Nux vomica* to *Sulphur*. *Lachesis* and *Lycopodium* is another set of complementary remedies. Here again the contrast is obvious. *Lachesis* is always competing with others, he wants to do better than others, and *Lycopodium* is always competing with himself and doubting his own capacity. A person who keeps doubting his own capacity is predisposed to developing lack of self-confidence. *Lachesis* predisposes to *Lycopodium* and *Lycopodium* predisposes to *Lachesis*. They are such opposite states that *Lachesis* is left-sided and *Lycopodium* right-sided; *Lachesis* does not like hot drinks and *Lycopodium* craves them; *Lachesis* is worse in the morning after sleep and *Lycopodium* in the evening before sleep.

We can look at another famous relationship: the one between *Pulsatilla* and *Silicea*. *Silicea* is so obstinate and *Pulsatilla* so mild; *Silicea* is rigid in his views, while *Pulsatilla* is irresolute; *Silicea* is averse to consolation, and *Pulsatilla* craves it; *Silicea* is so egoistical and *Pulsatilla* so humble; *Silicea* is hard, *Pulsatilla* is soft; *Silicea* is chilly and *Pulsatilla* hot; *Silicea* cannot tolerate a draft of air, and *Pulsatilla* cannot live without it. These two opposite states complement each other. Hardness predisposes to softness, and softness predisposes to hardness, just like a philosophical attitude predisposes to anxiety and anxiety predisposes to a philosophical attitude.

We can give many more examples, but this much is sufficient to convey the point that when we see a remedy in a patient we have to examine whether it exists independently or whether it exists because of a predisposition caused by some other remedy state. When doing so, it is necessary to consider those remedies which are some way opposite in nature to the present one. We may find that after giving the first remedy we have symptoms of the complementary remedy appearing.

Change of remedy or change within a remedy

Same remedy but different facets:

When we see a change of symptoms in the life span of a patient, especially a change in the mental state, we should not always jump to the conclusion that his remedy has changed. It is equally possible that he is exhibiting a different form of the same remedy. Each remedy does not present a fixed picture at all times, but takes many forms. A person can change from one form to another of the same remedy depending on the situation and also the strength of the internal dynamic disease. For example, we could meet a *Staphysagria* man who is so sweet and pleasant, but in another situation he may become angry and violent. These are merely different facets of the same state, since both come from the same source.

Get down to basic components:

Therefore, each time we have to get down to the basic components of the person and examine which remedy is indicated. The expressions of facets may vary, but we have to trace the source of the expression to come to the basic feeling which caused it. Only a change in such basic feeling justifies a change of remedy.

Also, such a change will invariably be accompanied by definite changes in the physical generals of the patient, his cravings and aversions, his modalities and also the characteristic particulars and concomitants.

Only such confirmation would entitle us to conclude that there is indeed a change of state and another remedy is needed to complete the action of the earlier one. For example, a *Lycopodium* patient may present with a particular state of great anxiety about how he is going to accomplish a certain task. But once that task is done, the situation becomes less challenging, the anxiety lessens, he becomes cheerful, and his talk even becomes egoistical. This does not make him a *Sulphur* as yet. If he has changed to *Sulphur*, then we must see signs of total change. He would exude a definite sense of confidence and real egotism, a feeling that he is great, not merely showing or proving that he is great. The *Lycopodium* often needs to prove to himself and others that he is someone who is capable. The wish to prove himself shows that the *Lycopodium* state – of lack of self-confidence – still exists even though it may not now be so apparent.

When can we say that a *Staphysagria* person has changed and is now in a *Causticum* state? The change has to be in the basic mental parameters. *Staphysagria* is concerned about his honour, which is wounded easily ("Honour, effects of, wounded"). The *Causticum* state does not have this basic parameter. So, as long as wounded honour and the sensitivity to being insulted are the main parameters, *Staphysagria* remains his remedy, no matter what changes are shown in the expression. But, the point at which this changes and the person starts thinking of others rather than of himself, when he is concerned about the injustice done to others rather than to him, and when sympathy and anxiety for others become the dominant parameters, *Staphysagria* is no longer the remedy and *Causticum* is now indicated ("Anxiety for others", "Sympathetic").

How states change

"Doctor", says the patient, "I have recurrent congestion in my chest, I am taking allopathic drugs but I am losing my weight and strength due to them."

Interpretation into rubrics:
— Theorizing... (his theory regarding the action of the drugs);
— Delusion, injured, is being... (by the drugs);
— Delusion, she is getting thin... (losing weight and strength);
— Egotism... ("I know everything, I have no doubt that this is so!").
The remedy that emerges is *Sulphur*.

On taking his history we see that when he was young, he was fat and was being insulted by schoolmates and he used to go home weeping.

Rubrics (as that time):
— Mortification;
— Ailments from suppressed anger;
— Weeps from vexation;
— Timidity.
The remedy of that time: *Staphysagria*.

His mother says that sometime in his youth he underwent a big change and after this change he has developed the following characteristics:
– Feeling, he is superior;
– The need for others to know this fact;
– Great achiever;
– Anger followed by quick repentance;
– Dipsomania.
The remedy after this change: *Sulphur*.

How, and why, did this change of state (from *Staphysagria* to *Sulphur*) occur? It occurred because, at some point, the situation became so intense and the *Staphysagria* state proved insufficient to cope with it. Then, change to the opposite (*Sulphur*) state was called for.

Consider the case of a man running in front of a lion which catches up with him; so, his state has to change to one complementing the earlier state.

First state (when the man is running):
– Timidity;
– Fear;
– Desire to run away;
– Feels inferior to lion.

Second state (when lion catches up), opposite of the first state:
– Courage;
– Thinks he is superior to the lion;
– Desire to fight (rather than escape).

In this way, when one state reaches an extreme on account of the situation, and yet the person is not able to cope with the situation, then the state changes into another one which is complementary to the first one, and in some ways opposite. Take one more example, namely of *Gelsemium* and *Argentum nitricum*. The *Gelsemium* state is like that of a man sitting in a plane which is about to crash; he clings to his seat, immobilized, unable to do anything, the slightest jerk deeply upsets him, he anticipates disaster.

When this plane somehow lands on the runway, he has to get out of the plane as soon as possible. His state now changes to the *Argentum nitricum* one, with its desire to escape, trapped feeling, impulse to run, desire for open air. There is no clinging now, no immobility; rather there is the opposite: forsaken feeling and desire to run.

We have already studied the situational Materia Medica. Now, we can readily understand that the complementary remedies will come from situations which are complementary, i.e. the situations of two complementary remedies will be such as to be found very close to each other or one following the other.

Inimical remedies

So far we have examined remedies which are complementary to one another and see that in some way they are opposite. Because of this difference one seems to predispose to the other. We can get confirmation of this idea if we examine the other relationship between remedies, namely the relationship of incompatibility.

Some remedies are known to be incompatible to one another, which means that they do not follow each other well. This probably signifies that when one state exists, the other cannot exist behind it. This means that these two states are in some way very close to each other, very similar, so that one cannot predispose to the other. It is the same idea we saw above but applied in the reverse direction. If remedies that are in some way opposite to each other are naturally predisposed to one another, then remedies that are similar will naturally repeal each other.

The best known example of incompatibility between remedies is that of *Causticum* and *Phosphorus*. These two remedies are very close to one another, both of them being sympathetic and anxious for others. They are both chilly, both desire cold drinks and are averse to sweets. Both may have paralysis of the right side of the face. They seem so close to each other that if a *Causticum* state exists, it is very seldom that a situation can arise which creates in this person a *Phosphorus* state. Therefore, *Causticum* and *Phosphorus* states will rarely be found in the same person. It is interesting to note that *Causticum* is listed as a collateral (similar) remedy to *Phosphorus*, and yet they are incompatible and are unlikely to be needed in the same person.

It is a similar story with *Bryonia* and *Calcarea*. Here again, the remedies are so similar in nature, both having aversion to movement and need for security, both having fear of poverty, and therefore desiring stability. *Bryonia* and *Calcarea* can hardly exist together in the same person and they are known to be incompatible.

I will give one more example of incompatibility between remedies, viz. *Chamomilla* and *Nux vomica*. Both are such highly irritable remedies, so sensitive, violent, and intolerant of pain, that we could easily mistake between the two. When we examine the incompatibility between remedies, we find that those which are similar in one way will have similar exciting factors and similar effects.

Marital relationships

In marital relationship (or where two persons live together in harmony), you will usually find that each will belong to a different remedy state and that their states are complementary, i.e. they are opposite in some way.

This happens because each one of us has within himself roots of several remedies. When the need arises from an exciting cause, which may be the behaviour of one partner, a particular root in the other partner is stimulated into a state. For example, if the husband is careless and indifferent to details of household problems (*Sulphur*), then the *Graphites* root ("Carefulness about trifles") in the wife will be stimulated. If the husband is spending extravagantly, then the wife must become avaricious. Where one of the partners is dominating (*Lycopodium*), the other has to be yielding (*Pulsatilla*) if the relationship is to survive. People do it voluntarily in the beginning but over a course of time, it becomes an involuntary state, especially if the person already has such a root.

This is also the reason why a child is often born with roots of two complementary remedies, for instance roots of *Arsenicum album* and *Sulphur*, *Lycopodium* and *Pulsatilla*, etc. These remedies can occur in pairs in the child because if he gets one root from one parent, the complementary root is derived from the other parent. If both roots are pretty strong and excitable, then the states may alternate in the child.

This teaches us to study the nature of both the spouses (or parents of the patient). A proper understanding of this approach can be useful in prescribing.

If you see a typical *Graphites* lady, just look into the nature of her husband, and if you see a very strong *Sulphur* in him, your remedy is doubly confirmed.

If you see a strong *Lycopodium* man, then you can almost predict that the partner is going to be a *Pulsatilla*, especially if they have adjusted themselves to each other, and are living harmoniously!

44

LESSER USED REMEDIES

Introduction

The purpose of this chapter is to focus the reader's attention on the need to be unprejudiced when taking a case. Most of the time we are tempted to match the patient with one of the remedies we know well. We convince ourselves that the patient must have this or that feeling, and therefore requires this or that remedy. We are even clever enough to somehow confirm this idea. The main pitfall of a homoeopath is to fall into the rut of prescribing a specific range of remedies, fitting all his patients into that group. The idea of this chapter, therefore, is to show the necessity of keeping an open mind to all peculiarities, whether mental or physical, and to allow ourselves to see the patient as he is, without fitting him into a particular idea. In doing so, we shall not only expand our Materia Medica, but it is also a unique opportunity to discover new remedies and to see them work.

I am not advocating prescribing on one or two symptoms even if they may be peculiar. However, when you do come across something peculiar you should open your reference books and try to find that exact symptom, instead of brushing it aside because it does not fit in with your preconceived idea about the patient's remedy.

I hope that the cases given here will convince you about the usefulness of opening your books more often, especially you Repertories. I must add that probably I shall be one of the biggest beneficiaries of reading this chapter because I see myself falling into the same routine; the mind refuses to move into anything new since it is so easy to stick to the old and familiar. In the cases presented here, I am only giving the main characteristics, not the whole case. You can assume that there was nothing very prominent in the case.

Case n. 1

This is the case of a child aged nine months. He had been brought for constipation and recurrent coughs and colds. I observed that he was very restless and could not remain in one position even for a short time. Among the peculiar things about him was that he was very stubborn. If he wanted a particular thing, he insisted on having it without delay, and would not be satisfied with anything else. He never asked for it softly, but would always scream and demand impatiently.

Another peculiarity of the child was that he seemed to require very little sleep. Even though he might have had just two hours of sleep, he was refreshed. He never demanded food. Despite the fact that he had not been fed for a long time, he would not cry or show hunger in any other way. His sweat stained yellow and was profuse, especially on the head. In the history of the parents I could not elicit much, except that both the parents were working and in the initial months the child was left alone. From these symptoms I gathered the following rubrics:

— Craving for particular things (Phatak's Repertory);
— Need for sleep, little (Phatak's Repertory);
— Need for food, little (Phatak's Materia Medica);
— Desires impatiently many things dislikes its favourite playthings (Synthetic Repertory);
— Demands things with great impatience and shrieking (Clarke's Dictionary);
— Perspiration staining yellow (Kent's Repertory).

From these symptoms I came to the remedy *Rheum*, which worked beautifully. Incidentally, I learned many things about *Rheum* from this case, the most important of which is that *Rheum* is placed in the Materia Medica between *Magnesium carbonicum* and *Chamomilla*. *Magnesium carbonicum* is the orphan child who demands nothing, who needs little sleep and little food. On the other hand, the *Chamomilla* child is not being given any attention even though his parents are in the house. *Rheum* is the child who is orphaned sometimes and at other times needs to demand attention. It is like the child whose parents are away for work but are also sometimes present in the house; when they are at home the child demands their attention. This was more or less the situation of the child. This case taught me something about the situational Materia Medica of *Rheum*, and its relationship to the other two remedies.

Case n. 2

A colleague from Switzerland, Dr. Hansjorg Hee, narrated a case to me while he was in India. This was the case of a child aged eight to nine years, who suffered from two major problems. One was an eczema which affected her face, and the other was that she was completely withdrawn, taciturn and psychologically disturbed. One peculiarity about her eczema was there was no itching despite it being a wet eczema with oozing and crust formation. Her psychological problem started a few years earlier when her father told her a story of a girl, an angel, who was put into a coffin by her father (or some other man) when she was still alive. The coffin was buried and the girl woke up and found all kinds of creeping creatures around her. After hearing this story, the girl was completely shocked, and from this time her whole attitude and mood changed. I suggested that she should be given *Cicuta*:

— Horrible things, sad stories affect her profoundly;
— Sadness from sad stories;
— Talk, indisposed to, desire to be silent, taciturn;
— Men, shuns the foolishness of;
— Sensitive to sad stories;

— Company, aversion to; avoids the sight of people;

— Quiet disposition;

— Dullness, sluggishness.

Combined with this, Phatak's Repertory gives only two remedies for eruptions without itching, of which *Cicuta* is one. Reading the skin symptoms of *Cicuta* I found a close similarity with the patient. I heard from Dr. Hee later that she did very well on *Cicuta*, both mentally and physically.

Case n. 3

A businessman gave me a symptom, resembling a mental problem. He said he just could not continue talking to me for long since it produced in him the need to stop and to go away. Similar feelings were produced when he was calculating, reading or in conversation. He just felt the need to go away from the place. I did not know how to interpret this symptom and I tried to question him in various ways to elicit exactly how he felt. I asked him whether he felt that if he continued something would happen, or some thing would break, or what. He denied all this but kept repeating that if he did any of the above actions he felt the need to leave the place immediately. After thinking for sometime I opened the Repertory to the rubric "Restless, mental labour, during and after", and one of the most important remedies there is *Kalium phosphoricum*. On studying his other symptoms I was able to confirm this remedy, and it helped him a lot.

Case n. 4

A Swiss violinist came to me with the problem of severe anticipatory anxiety and nervousness before a concert. He had been given various medicines, including *Argentum nitricum*, *Gelsemium* and others for the problem, but without any result. On studying his symptoms what came out prominently was that he seemed to have absolutely no emotions. He never got angry, was never sad and never too happy. When I asked why, he said he did not see the need to have emotions since everything happens the way it is supposed to; for example: "Why should I get angry with a man who is behaving badly with me? It is in his nature. Why should I let this affect me? So, I don't get angry." He had a very strict upbringing. In his house pop music and other modern music was anathema, since it was not considered suitable for intellectual people. He never did anything adventurous even in his teen years, and he sorely missed this. I chose the rubric from the synthetic Repertory "Emotions predominated by the intellect" and found the remedy *Viola odorata*. Incidentally, *Viola odorata* is the only remedy mentioned under the rubric "Sensitive, music of violin, to". I gave him *Viola odorata* and heard that he had benefited.

Case n. 5

In the case of a woman aged fifty, I could not differentiate between two remedies as far as her mental symptoms were concerned. There was a lot of anxiety in her about her family, which looked like *Kalium carbonicum*, yet she was extremely mild and yielding, which looked like *Pulsatilla*. While I was debating between these two remedies, I looked into her physical symptoms. She had come with pains which affected most of her joints, and for these pains she had been prescribed Aspirin. She had been taking fifteen to sixteen Aspirin tablets everyday, for the past twelve years! Aspirin was the only thing that gave her relief. Not only did it relieve her pains, but it made her feel better on the whole and emotionally calmed her down. I was curious. I looked up the remedy *Salicylicum acidum* in Clark's Dictionary, and to my surprise the first symptoms I found in the mind were "Anxiety; worry, restless, yet mild".

On examining her physical symptoms I found the confirmation that they were much worse by movement like *Bryonia* and better by dry heat like *Rhus toxicodendron*. With *Salicylicum acidum* in potency, not only was she able to come off Aspirin very quickly, but she found great relief in her complaints.

Case n. 6

Several years ago, I was called to see a young, recently married woman. She had covered herself with layers and layers of quilts. There must have been twelve or thirteen layers, and she was there under all of them shivering. She had no temperature. She said that she felt frozen despite all these quilts, and that this coldness came in waves which were ascending all around to her head. I prescribed the remedy *Heloderma horridus* (the Gila monster) and with this she improved rapidly from a condition which could not even be diagnosed by her physicians. The description of this remedy is to be found in Boericke's Materia Medica and I came to it from the Repertories.

Case n. 7

My teacher, Dr. Sarabhai Kapadia, has described several cases of a little known remedy called *Taxus baccata*. He found this remedy by accident. We routinely ask the patient what happens if he remains hungry and how long he can bear the hunger. One of the patients said that he cannot bear hunger for more than two hours, and if he remains hungry, he gets all kinds of noises in his stomach. One would easily overlook such as symptom; however, Sarabhai's attention to detail made him open the Repertory to the rubrics: "Abdomen, rumbling, fasting while" and "Stomach, appetite, ravenous, eating, two hours after". In both rubrics there is only one remedy listed: *Taxus baccata*. On these two symptoms alone Dr. Sarabhai has prescribed *Taxus baccata* in several different types of cases with good results.

Case n. 8

A patient was admitted to the homoeopathic hospital with very severe pains in her abdomen. The surgeon who was consulted diagnosed an ulcer and advised surgical procedure. When I saw the patient she was lying on her abdomen and said this was the only comfortable position for her. When I asked her the effect of hot and cold drinks, she said cold drinks suited a lot and she continued saying that when she drank something cold she could feel the coldness going down through the oesophagus and then into the stomach which felt very cold. The whole process of drinking cold gave her some relief. I was struck by this description and opened the Repertory to the rubrics:

— Stomach, coldness ice-like, after cold drinks;

— Stomach, coldness internal, as if ice water were rising and descending through a cylindrical tube;

— Stomach pain, lying on abdomen ameliorates.

The remedy which emerged prominently was *Elaps*. There was a very dramatic relief of her pains with this remedy.

Case n. 9

A young man aged twenty used to come to me for various problems which were mainly functional. He would experience some dizziness and rush to me asking that his blood pressure be checked. Or he would suffer from pain in the chest and rush to me asking that the electrocardiogram be taken immediately. He had several electrocardiograms and even an echocardiogram. What surprised me was that a man of his age was spending many hours over several days of the week in my clinic, when he could have been out enjoying himself. Another feature was that he was a very miserly person and would save the pocket money given to him by his parents. This is also the age where a person may steal in order to spend, and this boy was saving money. In fact, he would even prevent his parents from spending lavishly. The two symptoms that come out of his case were:

– Anxiety about health;
– Anxiety about money matters.

The only remedy that emerges from these rubrics in the Synthetic Repertory is *Calcarea silicata*. In Kent's "Lectures and Lesser Writings" I found a very close similarity and, with *Calcarea silicata*, this young man did well, regaining much more confidence. I utilized this case to make some observations about *Calcarea silicata*:

– Lean, chilled person;
– Coldness, especially in the tips of the fingers;
– Sweaty palms;
– Desire for sour and milk;
– Blue or dark line on the margin of the gums, like *Plumbum*;
– Dream of talking with his dead relatives.

I have been able to confirm this group of symptoms again and again, especially in young people who come with very anxious expressions on their faces for relatively minor complaints.

In the chapter on "Situational Materia Medica", I have described this remedy more extensively. The idea of mentioning it here is to show the need to make observations about these lesser known remedies, and to confirm these observations, so that we can add to the storehouse of information.

Case n. 10

A man aged thirty-five, came to me with the complaint of pain in the knee joint. I tried one or two remedies based upon my understanding of his case but with no result. Eventually he told me that he had one more problem which he wanted to be treated. This had to do with his beard. There were some bald spots in the beard and from these bald spots appeared a little fluffy white hair. I decide to look up this symptom, and in Kent's Repertory I found it as follows: "Head, hair, falling, spots, in, and comes in white". The only remedy there is *Vinca minor*. With great caution I prescribed *Vinca minor* and to my surprise not only did the bald spots go but he found relief from the joint pains.

Case n. 11

I was treating a businessman from a large family. He was living with his elderly father, mother, his brothers and sisters. The expression on his face was very bitter. From his history I could see that he felt he had been treated badly by the whole family and subjected to a lot of injustice. He felt nobody really appreciated him or his efforts. He was particularly angry with his parents and this had been going on for a long time. The only relief he found was from listening very sad music. He would somehow feel in tune with this kind of music and feel very much better from it. I took the rubrics:

— Embittered;

— Sadness, sad music ameliorates.

From these rubrics the remedy that emerged was *Manganum* and this remedy benefitted him.

Case n. 12

This case is of a medical doctor who was treated by my colleague, Dr. Praful Barvalia. The main complaint was psychological. He was sleepless for several nights, despite the strongest tranquilizers and sedatives. When Praful saw him, the doctor refused to talk and he had been pacing up and down the room restlessly the whole day and night. The only thing that Praful observed was that there was a photograph of the doctor's father in the room, towards which the doctor would glance frequently with a sorry look. The history was that the doctor has been married twice, and both marriages had failed. He had married against the wishes of his father. The doctor was also a very resourceful man and was planning to build a large hospital in Bombay using funds from abroad. He was a very hardworking man and all this stress had resulted in an acute peptic ulcer; consequently immediate surgery had been advised.

Praful took the rubrics:

— Remorse;

— Plans, making many;

— Sleepless from thoughts and activity of the mind, the same thought is repeated;

— Industrious.

From these rubrics he came to the remedy *Coffea* which helped the doctor to sleep immediately and also get rid of the ulcer. In mentioning these cases I wish to emphasize the need to look at the case exactly as it is without bringing remedies into our mind. The second point that needs emphasis is the necessity for attention to the smallest detail of the case. You may get a clue to the remedy from anywhere and you need to be open to it. The third point that needs emphasis is that our Repertories and Materia Medica are reliable, and our provings symptoms have been recorded accurately. Therefore, we should never hesitate to prescribe a new remedy if its important and peculiar symptoms match the patient's. You can place as much faith in these small remedies as you can in the more well-known remedies of the Materia Medica.

In the other chapters of this book I have described several remedies which are less known and also described aspects of well-known remedies which are not so well known. For example, *Calcarea sulphurica*, *Chelidonium*, the mental states of *China*, *Graphites*, *Magnesium muriaticum* and *Kalium iodatum*. I would never have come to these remedies if I had persisted in using the few remedies I know well.

The last point is that the peculiar physical symptoms must be very carefully considered when selecting the remedy. You must not become too focused on the body, but try to understand the state behind the mind and body through the peculiar expressions in both spheres. It is very useful to understand these lesser used remedies through cases, and slowly they will be ranked among your most important remedies. Through case work, I have understood more about remedies like *Graphites* and *Calcarea sulphurica* and I find I am now using them more frequently.

It is also useful to share knowledge about these lesser used remedies through journals, seminars and case conferences.

GLOSSARY

I have given here some terms that have appeared in the text and their meanings.

Basic delusion

The most basic feeling of the person, his false view of the situation which explains all his other feelings and expressions.

Basic parameter

A feature of a person that is basic to him, not explainable by any other feature.

Central disturbance

The functional disturbance of the central controlling systems of the body, namely the psyche, the nervous system, the endocrine system and immunologic system, which is together called the P-N-E-I system.

Compensation

A voluntary act of will which is against one's basic feeling or impulses.

Components

Basic features of a person that make up his state.

Concomitant

Something that exists along with one symptom, without any obvious connection with it.

Delusion

False perception of reality, the way things seem to be rather than how they are.

Disease

A disturbance in the organism's general state of health, a state of being which is maladapted to the present situation.

Dominating state

The state of the body which is at present producing all the effects.

Epidemic cause

A cause that produces a similar effect in the large majority of people.

Pathology

Organic changes in organ systems.

Peripheral disturbance

The disturbance of the organ systems resulting from the central disturbance.

P-N-E-I

Refer Central disturbance.

Root of disease

An impression from a past state which creates the tendency of the organism to go into the same state from an exciting cause.

Silent state

A state which exists without being the dominating one, rather like a silent partner in a partnership, or a minority party in parliament.

Single symptoms

Symptoms for which only one remedy is known, as given in the Repertory.

Situational Materia Medica

A description of a remedy in terms of the original situation from which a state of a remedy is likely to have come as a survival mechanism.

To the reader

After reading this book you may have several ideas and may have some new experiences. You may relate what I have said to what you are already familiar with. I would be grateful to receive a communication from you on the following:

- The concurrence or divergence of your views and experiences from what is stated in the book.

- Examples from your practice of life regarding case taking techniques, use of the Repertory, imaginative use of rubrics, Homoeo-psychotherapy, etc.

- Your ideas on the "situational Materia Medica" of various remedies, even those not mentioned in this book.

- Similarity or difference from the views (expressed in the book) observed by you in any literature, even if not on Homoeopathy.

- Any cases in your experience where delusions, dreams, perceptions, etc., have helped.

In case I include your contribution in any future edition of the book, I will acknowledge the source. I am sure I will benefit personally from your communication. Many thanks.

Rajan Sankaran

"Dinar"
20, Station Road
Santa Cruz (West),
Mumbai – 400 054
INDIA

INDEX